Diabetes
SOURCEBOOK

Seventh Edition

Health Reference Series

Seventh Edition

Diabetes
SOURCEBOOK

*Basic Consumer Health Information about Type 1 and
Type 2 Diabetes, Gestational Diabetes, and Other Types of
Diabetes and Prediabetes, with Details about Medical, Dietary,
and Lifestyle Disease Management Issues, Including Blood
Glucose Monitoring, Meal Planning, Weight Control,
Oral Diabetes Medications, and Insulin*

*Along with Facts about the Most Common Complications
of Diabetes and Their Prevention, Current Research in
Diabetes Care, Tips for People following a Diabetic Diet,
a Glossary of Related Terms, and a Directory of
Resources for Further Help and Information*

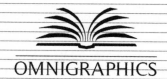

OMNIGRAPHICS

615 Griswold, Ste. 901, Detroit, MI 48226

Bibliographic Note

Because this page cannot legibly accommodate all the copyright notices, the Bibliographic Note portion of the Preface constitutes an extension of the copyright notice.

* * *

OMNIGRAPHICS

Angela L. Williams, *Managing Editor*

***

Copyright © 2018 Omnigraphics

ISBN 978-0-7808-1648-0
E-ISBN 978-0-7808-1649-7

Library of Congress Cataloging-in-Publication Data

Names: Omnigraphics, Inc., issuing body.

Title: Diabetes sourcebook: basic consumer health information about type 1 and type 2 diabetes, gestational diabetes, and other types of diabetes and prediabetes, with details about medical, dietary, and lifestyle disease management issues, including blood glucose monitoring, meal planning, weight control, oral diabetes medications, and insulin; along with facts about the most common complications of diabetes and their prevention, current research in diabetes care, tips for people following a diabetic diet, a glossary of related terms, and a directory of resources for further help and information.

Description: Seventh edition. | Detroit, MI: Omnigraphics, Inc., [2018] | Series: Health reference series | Includes bibliographical references and index.

Identifiers: LCCN 2018034651 (print) | LCCN 2018034961 (ebook) | ISBN 9780780816497 (ebook) | ISBN 9780780816480 (hard cover: alk. paper) | ISBN 9780780816497 (ebook)

Subjects: LCSH: Diabetes--Popular works.

Classification: LCC RC660.4 (ebook) | LCC RC660.4.D56 2018 (print) | DDC 616.4/62--dc23

LC record available at https://lccn.loc.gov/2018034651

This book is printed on acid-free paper meeting the ANSI Z39.48 Standard. The infinity symbol that appears above indicates that the paper in this book meets that standard.

Printed in the United States

Table of Contents

Part III: Medications and Diabetes Care

Part V: Complications of Diabetes and Co-Occurring Disorders

Part VIII: Additional Help and Information

Preface

About This Book

Diabetes is a chronic disorder characterized by high levels of blood sugar. It can lead to a host of complications, including heart disease, stroke, high blood pressure, blindness, kidney disease, nervous system disease, and limb amputation. Although many of the complications of diabetes occur over long periods of time, poorly controlled blood glucose levels can also result in acute medical emergencies, such as seizures or coma or even death.

The number of people with diabetes in the United States is growing. According to the Centers for Disease Control and Prevention (CDC), more than 100 million U.S. adults are now living with diabetes or prediabetes. Over 30.3 million Americans—9.4 percent of the U.S. population—have diabetes. Another 84.1 million have prediabetes, a condition that if not treated often leads to type 2 diabetes within five years. Despite its prevalence, many Americans are unaware of the basic facts about diabetes and the progress being made in the fight against it. For example, new forms of treatment such as pancreatic islet transplantation and artificial pancreas offer hope for an eventual cure.

Diabetes Sourcebook, Seventh Edition provides basic consumer information about the different types of diabetes and how they are diagnosed. It discusses strategies for controlling diabetes and managing daily life challenges. It includes information about the complications of diabetes and their prevention and offers guidelines for recognizing and treating diabetic emergencies. The book concludes with updated information regarding the most recent research in diabetes care, a glossary of related terms, and a list of resources for additional help and information.

How to Use This Book

This book is divided into parts and chapters. Parts focus on broad areas of interest. Chapters are devoted to single topics within a part.

Part I: Understanding Diabetes explains how the body processes glucose and what can go wrong. It describes different types of diabetes and provides statistics on the prevalence of diabetes and diabetes-related complications.

Part II: Identifying and Managing Diabetes describes metabolic syndrome and other risk factors for developing diabetes. It gives details about the tests most commonly used to diagnose diabetes and monitor blood glucose levels. It also explains the importance of achieving good diabetes control. The part concludes with a description of the tests, check-ups, and vaccinations doctors recommend for people with diabetes.

Part III: Medications and Diabetes Care discusses the medications used to manage diabetes. It describes different types of insulin and the methods used to administer insulin, including injections, external insulin pumps, and other new and emerging insulin delivery systems. It also describes oral and noninsulin injectable medications, new diabetes medications, and alternative and complementary diabetes treatments.

Part IV: Dietary and Other Lifestyle Issues Important for Diabetes Control describes the components of the diabetic diet and the types of meal planning that can be used to control blood glucose levels. It explains the importance of physical activity and weight management and offers tips for handling the challenges diabetics face in daily life. The part concludes with information about identifying and dealing with emergency situations.

Part V: Complications of Diabetes and Co-Occurring Disorders provides facts about the impact diabetes can have on the eyes, feet, skin, cardiovascular system, kidneys, mouth, and elsewhere in the body. It describes the symptoms of these complications and discusses ways to prevent their occurrence. It also describes disorders that often accompany diabetes and offers suggestions for their prevention and treatment.

Part VI: Diabetes in Specific Populations discusses the particular challenges of managing diabetes among pregnant women, the elderly, and children. It offers suggestions for overcoming such challenges as managing diabetes at school, coping with sick days, and celebrating special occasions.

Part VII: Research in Diabetes Care describes the most current research into the management and prevention of diabetes. It explains the results of recent research studies and details the most current advances in stem cell research, pancreatic islet transplantation, and efforts toward developing an artificial pancreas. It concludes with a discussion of clinical trials currently being conducted.

Part VIII: Additional Help and Information includes a glossary of terms related to diabetes, recipes for diabetics and their families, information about sources of financial assistance, and a directory of other resources for additional help and support.

Bibliographic Note

This volume contains documents and excerpts from publications issued by the following government agencies: Centers for Disease Control and Prevention (CDC); National Center for Complementary and Integrative Health (NCCIH); National Heart, Lung, and Blood Institute (NHLBI); National Highway Traffic Safety Administration (NHTSA); National Institute of Diabetes and Digestive and Kidney Diseases (NIDDK); National Institute on Aging (NIA); National Institutes of Health (NIH); *NIH News in Health*; NIH Osteoporosis and Related Bone Diseases~National Resource Center (NIH ORBD~NRC); Office on Women's Health (OWH); U.S. Department of Veterans Affairs (VA); U.S. Equal Employment Opportunity Commission (EEOC); and the U.S. Food and Drug Administration (FDA).

It may also contain original material produced by Omnigraphics and reviewed by medical consultants.

About the Health Reference Series

The *Health Reference Series* is designed to provide basic medical information for patients, families, caregivers, and the general public. Each volume takes a particular topic and provides comprehensive coverage. This is especially important for people who may be dealing with a newly diagnosed disease or a chronic disorder in themselves or in a family member. People looking for preventive guidance, information about disease warning signs, medical statistics, and risk factors for health problems will also find answers to their questions in the *Health Reference Series*. The *Series*, however, is not intended to serve as a tool for diagnosing illness, in prescribing treatments, or as a substitute for the physician/patient relationship. All people concerned about medical symptoms or the possibility of disease are encouraged to seek professional care from an appropriate healthcare provider.

A Note about Spelling and Style

Health Reference Series editors use *Stedman's Medical Dictionary* as an authority for questions related to the spelling of medical terms and the *Chicago Manual of Style* for questions related to grammatical structures, punctuation, and other editorial concerns. Consistent adherence is not always possible, however, because the individual volumes within the *Series* include many documents from a wide variety of different producers, and the editor's primary goal is to present material from each source as accurately as is possible. This sometimes means that information in different chapters or sections may follow other guidelines and alternate spelling authorities. For example, occasionally a copyright holder may require that eponymous terms be shown in possessive forms (Crohn's disease vs. Crohn disease) or that British spelling norms be retained (leukaemia vs. leukemia).

Medical Review

Omnigraphics contracts with a team of qualified, senior medical professionals who serve as medical consultants for the *Health Reference Series*. As necessary, medical consultants review reprinted and originally written material for currency and accuracy. Citations including the phrase, "Reviewed (month, year)" indicate material reviewed by this team. Medical consultation services are provided to the *Health Reference Series* editors by:

Dr. Vijayalakshmi, MBBS, DGO, MD
Dr. Senthil Selvan, MBBS, DCH, MD
Dr. K. Sivanandham, MBBS, DCH, MS (Research), PhD

Our Advisory Board

We would like to thank the following board members for providing initial guidance on the development of this series:

- Dr. Lynda Baker, Associate Professor of Library and Information Science, Wayne State University, Detroit, MI

- Nancy Bulgarelli, William Beaumont Hospital Library, Royal Oak, MI

- Karen Imarisio, Bloomfield Township Public Library, Bloomfield Township, MI

- Karen Morgan, Mardigian Library, University of Michigan-Dearborn, Dearborn, MI

- Rosemary Orlando, St. Clair Shores Public Library, St. Clair Shores, MI

Health Reference Series *Update Policy*

The inaugural book in the *Health Reference Series* was the first edition of *Cancer Sourcebook* published in 1989. Since then, the *Series* has been enthusiastically received by librarians and in the medical community. In order to maintain the standard of providing high-quality health information for the layperson the editorial staff at Omnigraphics felt it was necessary to implement a policy of updating volumes when warranted.

Medical researchers have been making tremendous strides, and it is the purpose of the *Health Reference Series* to stay current with the most recent advances. Each decision to update a volume is made on an individual basis. Some of the considerations include how much new information is available and the feedback we receive from people who use the books. If there is a topic you would like to see added to the update list, or an area of medical concern you feel has not been adequately addressed, please write to:

Managing Editor
Health Reference Series
Omnigraphics
615 Griswold, Ste. 901
Detroit, MI 48226

Part One

Understanding Diabetes

Chapter 1

Introduction to Diabetes

What Is Diabetes?

Diabetes is a disease that occurs when your blood glucose, also called blood sugar, is too high. Blood glucose is your main source of energy and comes from the food you eat. Insulin, a hormone made by the pancreas, helps glucose from food get into your cells to be used for energy. Sometimes your body doesn't make enough—or any—insulin or doesn't use insulin well. Glucose then stays in your blood and doesn't reach your cells.

Over time, having too much glucose in your blood can cause health problems. Although diabetes has no cure, you can take steps to manage your diabetes and stay healthy.

Sometimes people call diabetes "a touch of sugar" or "borderline diabetes." These terms suggest that someone doesn't really have diabetes or has a less serious case, but every case of diabetes is serious.

What Are the Different Types of Diabetes?

The most common types of diabetes are type 1, type 2, and gestational diabetes.

This chapter includes text excerpted from "What Is Diabetes?" National Institute of Diabetes and Digestive and Kidney Diseases (NIDDK), November 2016.

Type 1 Diabetes

If you have type 1 diabetes, your body does not make insulin. Your immune system attacks and destroys the cells in your pancreas that make insulin. Type 1 diabetes is usually diagnosed in children and young adults, although it can appear at any age. People with type 1 diabetes need to take insulin every day to stay alive.

Type 2 Diabetes

If you have type 2 diabetes, your body does not make or use insulin well. You can develop type 2 diabetes at any age, even during childhood. However, this type of diabetes occurs most often in middle-aged and older people. Type 2 is the most common type of diabetes.

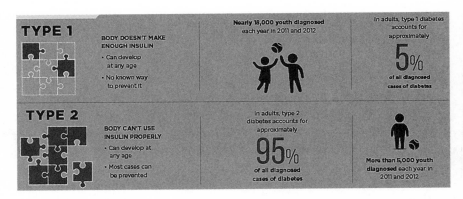

Figure 1.1. *Type 1 and Type 2 Diabetes* (Source: "A Snapshot of Diabetes in the United States," Centers for Disease Control and Prevention (CDC).)

Gestational Diabetes

Gestational diabetes develops in some women when they are pregnant. Most of the time, this type of diabetes goes away after the baby is born. However, if you've had gestational diabetes, you have a greater chance of developing type 2 diabetes later in life. Sometimes diabetes diagnosed during pregnancy is actually type 2 diabetes.

Other Types of Diabetes

Less common types include monogenic diabetes, which is an inherited form of diabetes, and cystic fibrosis-related diabetes (CFRD).

4

How Common Is Diabetes?

As of 2015, 30.3 million people in the United States, or 9.4 percent of the population, had diabetes. More than 1 in 4 of them didn't know they had the disease. Diabetes affects 1 in 4 people over the age of 65. About 90–95 percent of cases in adults are type 2 diabetes.

Who Is More Likely to Develop Type 2 Diabetes?

You are more likely to develop type 2 diabetes if you are age 45 or older, have a family history of diabetes, or are overweight. Physical inactivity, race, and certain health problems such as high blood pressure also affect your chance of developing type 2 diabetes. You are also more likely to develop type 2 diabetes if you have prediabetes or had gestational diabetes when you were pregnant.

What Health Problems Can People with Diabetes Develop?

Over time, high blood glucose leads to problems such as:

- heart disease
- stroke
- kidney disease
- eye problems
- dental disease
- nerve damage
- foot problems

You can take steps to lower your chances of developing these diabetes-related health problems.

Chapter 2

Symptoms and Causes of Diabetes

What Are the Symptoms of Diabetes?

Symptoms of diabetes include:

- increased thirst and urination

- increased hunger

- fatigue

- blurred vision

- numbness or tingling in the feet or hands

- sores that do not heal

- unexplained weight loss

Symptoms of type 1 diabetes can start quickly, in a matter of weeks. Symptoms of type 2 diabetes often develop slowly—over the course of several years—and can be so mild that you might not even notice them. Many people with type 2 diabetes have no symptoms. Some people do not find out they have the disease until they have diabetes-related health problems, such as blurred vision or heart trouble.

This chapter includes text excerpted from "Symptoms and Causes of Diabetes," National Institute of Diabetes and Digestive and Kidney Diseases (NIDDK), November 2016.

What Causes Type 1 Diabetes?

Type 1 diabetes occurs when your immune system, the body's system for fighting infection, attacks and destroys the insulin-producing beta cells of the pancreas. Scientists think type 1 diabetes is caused by genes and environmental factors, such as viruses, that might trigger the disease. Studies are working to pinpoint causes of type 1 diabetes and possible ways to prevent or slow the disease.

What Causes Type 2 Diabetes?

Type 2 diabetes—the most common form of diabetes—is caused by several factors, including lifestyle factors and genes.

Overweight, Obesity, and Physical Inactivity

You are more likely to develop type 2 diabetes if you are not physically active and are overweight or obese. Extra weight sometimes causes insulin resistance and is common in people with type 2 diabetes. The location of body fat also makes a difference. Extra belly fat is linked to insulin resistance, type 2 diabetes, and heart and blood vessel disease. To see if your weight puts you at risk for type 2 diabetes, check out the Body Mass Index (BMI) charts (www.niddk.nih.gov/health-information/diabetes/overview/risk-factors-type-2-diabetes#BMI).

Insulin Resistance

Type 2 diabetes usually begins with insulin resistance, a condition in which muscle, liver, and fat cells do not use insulin well. As a result, your body needs more insulin to help glucose enter cells. At first, the pancreas makes more insulin to keep up with the added demand. Over time, the pancreas can't make enough insulin, and blood glucose levels rise.

Genes and Family History

As in type 1 diabetes, certain genes may make you more likely to develop type 2 diabetes. The disease tends to run in families and occurs more often in these racial/ethnic groups:

- African Americans
- Alaska Natives
- American Indians

- Asian Americans
- Hispanics/Latinos
- Native Hawaiians
- Pacific Islanders

Genes also can increase the risk of type 2 diabetes by increasing a person's tendency to become overweight or obese.

What Causes Gestational Diabetes?

Scientists believe gestational diabetes, a type of diabetes that develops during pregnancy, is caused by the hormonal changes of pregnancy along with genetic and lifestyle factors.

Insulin Resistance

Hormones produced by the placenta contribute to insulin resistance, which occurs in all women during late pregnancy. Most pregnant women can produce enough insulin to overcome insulin resistance, but some cannot. Gestational diabetes occurs when the pancreas can't make enough insulin.

As with type 2 diabetes, extra weight is linked to gestational diabetes. Women who are overweight or obese may already have insulin resistance when they become pregnant. Gaining too much weight during pregnancy may also be a factor.

Genes and Family History

Having a family history of diabetes makes it more likely that a woman will develop gestational diabetes, which suggests that genes play a role. Genes may also explain why the disorder occurs more often in African Americans, American Indians, Asians, and Hispanics/Latinas.

What Else Can Cause Diabetes?

Genetic mutations, other diseases, damage to the pancreas, and certain medicines may also cause diabetes.

Genetic Mutations

- Monogenic diabetes is caused by mutations, or changes, in a single gene. These changes are usually passed through families, but sometimes the gene mutation happens on its own. Most of these gene mutations cause diabetes by making the pancreas less able to make insulin. The most common types of monogenic diabetes are neonatal diabetes and maturity-onset diabetes of the young (MODY). Neonatal diabetes occurs in the first six months of life. Doctors usually diagnose MODY during adolescence or early adulthood, but sometimes the disease is not diagnosed until later in life.

- Cystic fibrosis (CF) produces thick mucus that causes scarring in the pancreas. This scarring can prevent the pancreas from making enough insulin.

- Hemochromatosis causes the body to store too much iron. If the disease is not treated, iron can build up in and damage the pancreas and other organs.

Hormonal Diseases

Some hormonal diseases cause the body to produce too much of certain hormones, which sometimes cause insulin resistance and diabetes.

- Cushing syndrome occurs when the body produces too much cortisol—often called the "stress hormone."

- Acromegaly occurs when the body produces too much growth hormone.

- Hyperthyroidism occurs when the thyroid gland produces too much thyroid hormone.

Damage to or Removal of the Pancreas

Pancreatitis, pancreatic cancer, and trauma can all harm the beta cells or make them less able to produce insulin, resulting in diabetes. If the damaged pancreas is removed, diabetes will occur due to the loss of the beta cells.

Medicines

Sometimes certain medicines can harm beta cells or disrupt the way insulin works. These include:

- niacin, a type of vitamin B_3

- certain types of diuretics, also called water pills

- antiseizure drugs

- psychiatric drugs

- drugs to treat human immunodeficiency virus (HIV)

- pentamidine, a drug used to treat a type of pneumonia

- glucocorticoids—medicines used to treat inflammatory illnesses such as rheumatoid arthritis (RA), asthma, lupus, and ulcerative colitis (UC)

- antirejection medicines, used to help stop the body from rejecting a transplanted organ

Statins, which are medicines to reduce low-density lipoproteins (LDL) ("bad") cholesterol levels, can slightly increase the chance that you'll develop diabetes. However, statins help protect you from heart disease and stroke. For this reason, the strong benefits of taking statins outweigh the small chance that you could develop diabetes.

If you take any of these medicines and are concerned about their side effects, talk with your doctor.

Chapter 3

Diabetes Prevalence in America

More than 100 million U.S. adults are now living with diabetes or prediabetes, according to a report released by the Centers for Disease Control and Prevention (CDC). The report finds that as of 2015, 30.3 million Americans—9.4 percent of the U.S. population—have diabetes. Another 84.1 million have prediabetes, a condition that if not treated often leads to type 2 diabetes within five years.

The report confirms that the rate of new diabetes diagnosis remains steady. However, the disease continues to represent a growing health problem. Diabetes was the seventh leading cause of death in the United States in 2015. The report also includes county-level data for the first time, and shows that some areas of the country bear a heavier diabetes burden than others.

"Although these findings reveal some progress in diabetes management and prevention, there are still too many Americans with diabetes and prediabetes," said CDC Director Brenda Fitzgerald, M.D. "More than a third of U.S. adults have prediabetes, and the majority don't know it. Now, more than ever, we must step up our efforts to reduce the burden of this serious disease."

Diabetes is a serious disease that can often be managed through physical activity, diet, and the appropriate use of insulin and other

---

This chapter includes text excerpted from "New CDC Report: More than 100 Million Americans Have Diabetes or Prediabetes," Centers for Disease Control and Prevention (CDC), July 18, 2017.

medications to control blood sugar levels. People with diabetes are at increased risk of serious health complications including premature death, vision loss, heart disease, stroke, kidney failure, and amputation of toes, feet, or legs.

The National Diabetes Statistics Report (NDSR), released approximately every two years, provides information on diabetes prevalence and incidence, prediabetes, risk factors for complications, acute and long-term complications, mortality, and costs in the United States.

Key Findings from the National Diabetes Statistics Report

The report finds that:

- In 2015, an estimated 1.5 million new cases of diabetes were diagnosed among people ages 18 and older.

- Nearly one in four adults living with diabetes—7.2 million Americans—didn't know they had the condition. Only 11.6 percent of adults with prediabetes knew they had it.

- Rates of diagnosed diabetes increased with age. Among adults ages 18–44, four percent had diabetes. Among those ages 45–64 years, 17 percent had diabetes. And among those ages 65 years and older, 25 percent had diabetes.

Rates of diagnosed diabetes were higher among American Indians/ Alaska Natives (15.1%), non-Hispanic blacks (12.7%), and Hispanics (12.1%), compared to Asians (8.0%) and non-Hispanic whites (7.4%). Other differences include:

- Diabetes prevalence varied significantly by education. Among U.S. adults with less than a high school education, 12.6 percent had diabetes. Among those with a high school education, 9.5 percent had diabetes; and among those with more than a high school education, 7.2 percent had diabetes.

- More men (36.6%) had prediabetes than women (29.3%). Rates were similar among women and men across racial/ethnic groups or educational levels.

- The southern and Appalachian areas of the United States had the highest rates of diagnosed diabetes and of new diabetes cases.

"Consistent with previous trends, our research shows that diabetes cases are still increasing, although not as quickly as in previous years," said Ann Albright, Ph.D., R.D., director of the CDC's Division of Diabetes Translation (DDT). "Diabetes is a contributing factor to so many other serious health conditions. By addressing diabetes, we limit other health problems such as heart disease, stroke, nerve and kidney diseases, and vision loss."

Chapter 4

Diabetes among Children and Women

Diabetes among Children and Youth

The common type of diabetes in children and teens was type 1. It was called juvenile diabetes. With type 1 diabetes, the pancreas does not make insulin. Insulin is a hormone that helps glucose, or sugar, get into your cells to give them energy. Without insulin, too much sugar stays in the blood.

Now younger people are also getting type 2 diabetes. Type 2 diabetes used to be called adult-onset diabetes. But now it is becoming more common in children and teens, due to more obesity. With Type 2 diabetes, the body does not make or use insulin well.

Children have a higher risk of type 2 diabetes if they are overweight or have obesity, have a family history of diabetes, or are not active. Children who are African American, Hispanic, Native American/Alaska Native, Asian American, or Pacific Islander also have a higher risk. To lower the risk of type 2 diabetes in children:

• have them maintain a healthy weight

This chapter contains text excerpted from the following sources: Text under the heading "Diabetes among Children and Youth" is excerpted from "Diabetes in Children and Teens," MedlinePlus, National Institutes of Health (NIH), June 30, 2016; Text beginning with the heading "Diabetes among Women" is excerpted from "Diabetes," National Women's Health Information Center (NWHIC), Office on Women's Health (OWH), August 7, 2018.

17

- be sure they are physically active

- have them eat smaller portions of healthy foods

- limit time with the TV, computer, and video

Children and teens with type 1 diabetes may need to take insulin. Type 2 diabetes may be controlled with diet and exercise. If not, patients will need to take oral diabetes medicines or insulin. A blood test called the A1C can check on how you are managing your diabetes.

Diabetes among Women

Diabetes is a disease in which blood sugar (glucose) levels in your body are too high. Diabetes can cause serious health problems, including heart attack or stroke, blindness, problems during pregnancy, and kidney failure. More than 13 million women have diabetes, or about one in 10 women ages 20 and older.

Are You at Risk for Diabetes?

A risk factor is something that puts you at a higher risk for a disease compared with an average person.

Risk factors for type 1 diabetes in women and girls include:

- **Age.** It often develops in childhood.

- **Family health history.** Having a parent or brother or sister with type 1 diabetes.

- Certain **viral infections or illnesses**, such as coxsackievirus B (a common cause of hand, foot, and mouth disease), rotavirus (also called stomach flu), and mumps

- **Where you live.** It is more common in people who live in colder climates.

Risk factors for type 2 diabetes in women and girls include:

- **Overweight or obesity.** Body mass index (BMI) of 25 or higher for adults. Find out your BMI (www.cdc.gov/healthyweight/ assessing/bmi/adult_bmi/english_bmi_calculator/bmi_calculator. html). Children and teens weighing above the 85th percentile based on their BMI are at risk for type 2 diabetes.

- **Older age.** 45 or older. After menopause, women are at higher risk for weight gain, especially more weight around the waist, which raises the risk for type 2 diabetes.

- **Family health history.** Having a mother, father, brother, or sister with diabetes.

- **Race/ethnicity.** Family background of African-American, American Indian/Alaska Native, Hispanic, Asian-American, and Native Hawaiian/Pacific Islander

- Having a baby that weighed 9 pounds or more at birth

- Having diabetes during pregnancy (gestational diabetes)

- **High blood pressure.** Taking medicine for high blood pressure or having a blood pressure of 140/90 mmHg or higher. (Both numbers are important. If one or both numbers are usually high, you have high blood pressure.)

- **High cholesterol.** High-density lipoproteins (HDL) cholesterol of 35 mg/dL or lower and triglycerides of 250 mg/dL or higher

- **Lack of physical activity.** Women who are active less than three times a week

- Having polycystic ovary syndrome (PCOS)

- Personal history of heart disease or stroke

If you have any of these risk factors, talk to your doctor about ways to lower your risk for diabetes.

Do Women of Color Need to Worry about Diabetes?

Yes. Certain racial and ethnic groups have a higher risk for type 2 diabetes. These groups include:

- **African-Americans.** African-American women are twice as likely to develop diabetes as white women. African-Americans are also more likely to have health problems caused by diabetes and excess weight.

- **Hispanics.** Hispanic women are twice as likely to develop diabetes as white women. Diabetes affects more than one in 10 Hispanics. Among Hispanic women, diabetes affects Mexican-Americans and Puerto Ricans most often.

- **American Indian/Alaskan Native.** Diabetes affects nearly 16 percent of American Indian/Alaskan Native adults

- **Native Hawaiian/Pacific Islander.** Native Hawaiians/Pacific Islanders are about twice as likely to develop diabetes as whites

- **Asian-Americans.** Diabetes is the fifth-leading cause of death for Asian-Americans. Asian-American women are also more likely to develop gestational diabetes than white women and usually develop gestational diabetes at a lower body weight.

How Does Diabetes Affect Women Differently than Men?

Diabetes affects women and men in almost equal numbers. However, diabetes affects women differently than men.

Compared with men with diabetes, women with diabetes have:

- A higher risk for heart disease. Heart disease is the most common complication of diabetes.

- Lower survival rates and a poorer quality of life (QOL) after heart attack

- A higher risk for blindness

- A higher risk for depression. Depression, which affects twice as many women as men, also raises the risk for diabetes in women.

Does Diabetes Raise Your Risk for Other Health Problems?

Yes. The longer you have type 2 diabetes, the higher your risk for developing serious medical problems from diabetes. Also, if you smoke and have diabetes, you are even more likely to develop serious medical problems from diabetes, compared with people who have diabetes and do not smoke.

The extra glucose in the blood that leads to diabetes can damage your nerves and blood vessels. Nerve damage from diabetes can lead to pain or a permanent loss of feeling in your hands, feet, and other parts of your body.

Blood vessel damage from diabetes can also lead to:

- heart disease

- stroke

- blindness

- kidney failure

- leg or foot amputation

- hearing loss

Women with diabetes are also at higher risk for:

- problems getting pregnant

- problems during pregnancy, including possible health problems for you and your baby

- repeated urinary and vaginal infections

Is It Safe for Women with Diabetes to Get Pregnant?

Yes. If you have type 1 or type 2 diabetes, you can have a healthy pregnancy. If you have diabetes and you want to have a baby, you need to plan ahead, before you get pregnant.

Talk to your doctor before you get pregnant. He or she can talk to you about steps you can take to keep your baby healthy. This may include a diabetes education program to help you better understand your diabetes and how to control it during pregnancy.

Chapter 5

Type 1 Diabetes

Type 1 diabetes (previously called insulin-dependent or juvenile diabetes) is usually diagnosed in children, teens, and young adults, but it can develop at any age.

If you have type 1 diabetes, your pancreas isn't making insulin or is making very little. Insulin is a hormone that enables blood sugar to enter the cells in your body where it can be used for energy. Without insulin, blood sugar can't get into cells and builds up in the bloodstream. High blood sugar is damaging to the body and causes many of the symptoms and complications of diabetes.

Type 1 diabetes is less common than type 2—about five percent of people with diabetes have type 1. Currently, no one knows how to prevent type 1 diabetes, but it can be managed by following your doctor's recommendations for living a healthy lifestyle, controlling your blood sugar, getting regular health checkups, and getting diabetes self-management education.

For Parents

If your child has type 1 diabetes, you'll be involved in diabetes care on a day-to-day basis, from serving healthy foods to giving insulin injections to watching for and treating hypoglycemia (low blood sugar;

This chapter includes text excerpted from "Type 1 Diabetes," Centers for Disease Control and Prevention (CDC), August 15, 2018.

see below). You'll also need to stay in close contact with your child's healthcare team; they will help you understand the treatment plan and how to help your child stay healthy.

Causes

Type 1 diabetes is caused by an autoimmune reaction (the body attacks itself by mistake) that destroys the cells in the pancreas that make insulin, called beta cells. This process can go on for months or years before any symptoms appear.

Some people have certain genes (traits passed on from parent to child) that make them more likely to develop type 1 diabetes, though many won't go on to have type 1 diabetes even if they have the genes. Being exposed to a trigger in the environment, such as a virus, is also thought to play a part in developing type 1 diabetes. Diet and lifestyle habits don't cause type 1 diabetes.

Symptoms and Risk Factors

It can take months or years for enough beta cells to be destroyed before symptoms of type 1 diabetes are noticed. Type 1 diabetes symptoms can develop in just a few weeks or months. Once symptoms appear, they can be severe.

Some type 1 diabetes symptoms are similar to symptoms of other health conditions. Don't guess—if you think you could have type 1 diabetes, see your doctor right away to get your blood sugar tested. Untreated diabetes can lead to very serious—even fatal—health problems.

Risk factors for type 1 diabetes are not as clear as for prediabetes and type 2 diabetes, though family history is known to play a part.

Getting Tested

A simple blood test will let you know if you have diabetes. If you've gotten your blood sugar tested at a health fair or pharmacy, follow up at a clinic or doctor's office to make sure the results are accurate.

If your doctor thinks you have type 1 diabetes, your blood may also tested for autoantibodies (substances that indicate your body is attacking itself) that are often present with type 1 diabetes but not with type 2. You may have your urine tested for ketones (produced when your body burns fat for energy), which also indicate type 1 diabetes instead of type 2.

Management

Unlike many health conditions, diabetes is managed mostly by you, with support from your healthcare team (including your primary care doctor, foot doctor, dentist, eye doctor, registered dietitian nutritionist, diabetes educator, and pharmacist), family, teachers, and other important people in your life. Managing diabetes can be challenging, but everything you do to improve your health is worth it!

If you have type 1 diabetes, you'll need to take insulin shots (or wear an insulin pump) every day to manage your blood sugar levels and get the energy your body needs. Insulin can't be taken as a pill because the acid in your stomach would destroy it before it could get into your bloodstream. Your doctor will work with you to figure out the most effective type and dosage of insulin for you.

You'll also need to check your blood sugar regularly. Ask your doctor how often you should check it and what your target blood sugar levels should be. Keeping your blood sugar levels as close to target as possible will help you prevent or delay diabetes-related complications.

Stress is a part of life, but it can make managing diabetes harder, including controlling your blood sugar levels and dealing with daily diabetes care. Regular physical activity, getting enough sleep, and relaxation exercises can help. Talk to your doctor and diabetes educator about these and other ways you can manage stress.

Healthy lifestyle habits are really important, too:

- Making healthy food choices

- Being physically active

- Controlling your blood pressure

- Controlling your cholesterol

Make regular appointments with your healthcare team to be sure you're on track with your treatment plan and to get help with new ideas and strategies if needed.

Whether you just got diagnosed with type 1 diabetes or have had it for some time, meeting with a diabetes educator is a great way to get support and guidance, including how to:

- Develop and stick to a healthy eating and activity plan.

- Test your blood sugar and keep a record of the results.

- Recognize the signs of high or low blood sugar and what to do about it.

- Give yourself insulin by syringe, pen, or pump.

- Monitor your feet, skin, and eyes to catch problems early.

- Buy diabetes supplies and store them properly.

- Manage stress and deal with daily diabetes care.

Ask your doctor about diabetes self-management education and to recommend a diabetes educator. You can also search the American Association of Diabetes Educators' (AADE) nationwide directory (www. diabeteseducator.org/living-with-diabetes/find-an-education-program) for a list of educators in your community.

Hypoglycemia

Hypoglycemia (low blood sugar) can happen quickly and needs to be treated immediately. It's most often caused by too much insulin, waiting too long for a meal or snack, not eating enough, or getting extra physical activity. Hypoglycemia symptoms are different from person to person; make sure you know your specific symptoms, which could include:

- Shakiness

- Nervousness or anxiety

- Sweating, chills, or clamminess

- Irritability or impatience

- Dizziness and difficulty concentrating

- Hunger or nausea

- Blurred vision

- Weakness or fatigue

- Anger, stubbornness, or sadness

If you have hypoglycemia several times a week, talk to your doctor to see if your treatment needs to be adjusted.

Connect with Others

Tap into online diabetes communities for encouragement, insights, and support. The American Diabetes Association's (ADA) Community page (community.diabetes.org/home) and the American Association of Diabetes Educators' (AADE) Peer Support Resources (www.dia-beteseducator.org/living-with-diabetes/tip-sheets-and-handouts/peer-support) are great ways to connect with others who share your experience.

Chapter 6

Insulin Resistance and Prediabetes

Insulin resistance and prediabetes occur when your body doesn't use insulin well.

What Is Insulin?

Insulin is a hormone made by the pancreas that helps glucose in your blood enter cells in your muscle, fat, and liver, where it's used for energy. Glucose comes from the food you eat. The liver also makes glucose in times of need, such as when you're fasting. When blood glucose, also called blood sugar, levels rise after you eat, your pancreas releases insulin into the blood. Insulin then lowers blood glucose to keep it in the normal range.

What Is Insulin Resistance?

Insulin resistance is when cells in your muscles, fat, and liver don't respond well to insulin and can't easily take up glucose from your blood. As a result, your pancreas makes more insulin to help glucose enter your cells. As long as your pancreas can make enough insulin

---

This chapter includes text excerpted from "Insulin Resistance and Prediabetes," National Institute of Diabetes and Digestive and Kidney Diseases (NIDDK), May 2018.

to overcome your cells' weak response to insulin, your blood glucose levels will stay in the healthy range.

What Is Prediabetes?

Prediabetes means your blood glucose levels are higher than normal but not high enough to be diagnosed as diabetes. Prediabetes usually occurs in people who already have some insulin resistance or whose beta cells in the pancreas aren't making enough insulin to keep blood glucose in the normal range. Without enough insulin, extra glucose stays in your bloodstream rather than entering your cells. Over time, you could develop type 2 diabetes.

How Common Is Prediabetes?

More than 84 million people ages 18 and older have prediabetes in the United States. That's about 1 out of every 3 adults.

Who Is More Likely to Develop Insulin Resistance or Prediabetes?

People who have genetic or lifestyle risk factors are more likely to develop insulin resistance or prediabetes. Risk factors include

- overweight or obesity
- age 45 or older
- a parent, brother, or sister with diabetes
- African American, Alaska Native, American Indian, Asian American, Hispanic/Latino, Native Hawaiian, or Pacific Islander American ethnicity
- physical inactivity
- health conditions such as high blood pressure and abnormal cholesterol levels
- a history of gestational diabetes
- a history of heart disease or stroke
- polycystic ovary syndrome, also called PCOS

People who have metabolic syndrome—a combination of high blood pressure, abnormal cholesterol levels, and large waist size—are more likely to have prediabetes.

Along with these risk factors, other things that may contribute to insulin resistance include

- certain medicines, such as glucocorticoids, some antipsychotics, and some medicines for human immunodeficiency virus (HIV)

- hormonal disorders, such as Cushing syndrome and acromegaly

- sleep problems, especially sleep apnea

Although you can't change risk factors such as family history, age, or ethnicity, you can change lifestyle risk factors around eating, physical activity, and weight. These lifestyle changes can lower your chances of developing insulin resistance or prediabetes.

What Causes Insulin Resistance and Prediabetes?

Researchers don't fully understand what causes insulin resistance and prediabetes, but they think excess weight and lack of physical activity are major factors.

Excess Weight

Experts believe obesity, especially too much fat in the abdomen and around the organs, called visceral fat, is a main cause of insulin resistance. A waist measurement of 40 inches or more for men and 35 inches or more for women is linked to insulin resistance. This is true even if your body mass index (BMI) falls within the normal range. However, research has shown that Asian Americans may have an increased risk for insulin resistance even without a high BMI.

Researchers used to think that fat tissue was only for energy storage. However, studies have shown that belly fat makes hormones and other substances that can contribute to chronic, or long-lasting, inflammation in the body. Inflammation may play a role in insulin resistance, type 2 diabetes, and cardiovascular disease (CVD).

Excess weight may lead to insulin resistance, which in turn may play a part in the development of fatty liver disease.

Physical Inactivity

Not getting enough physical activity is linked to insulin resistance and prediabetes. Regular physical activity causes changes in your body that make it better able to keep your blood glucose levels in balance.

What Are the Symptoms of Insulin Resistance and Prediabetes?

Insulin resistance and prediabetes usually have no symptoms. Some people with prediabetes may have darkened skin in the armpit or on the back and sides of the neck, a condition called acanthosis nigricans. Many small skin growths called skin tags often appear in these same areas.

Even though blood glucose levels are not high enough to cause symptoms for most people, a few research studies have shown that some people with prediabetes may already have early changes in their eyes that can lead to retinopathy. This problem more often occurs in people with diabetes.

How Do Doctors Diagnose Insulin Resistance and Prediabetes?

Doctors use blood tests to find out if someone has prediabetes, but they don't usually test for insulin resistance. The most accurate test for insulin resistance is complicated and used mostly for research.

Doctors most often use the fasting plasma glucose (FPG) test or the A1C test to diagnose prediabetes. Less often, doctors use the oral glucose tolerance test (OGTT), which is more expensive and not as easy to give.

The A1C test reflects your average blood glucose over the past 3 months. The FPG and OGTT show your blood glucose level at the time of the test. The A1C test is not as sensitive as the other tests. In some people, it may miss prediabetes that the OGTT could catch. The OGTT can identify how your body handles glucose after a meal—often before your fasting blood glucose level becomes abnormal. Often doctors use the OGTT to check for gestational diabetes, a type of diabetes that develops during pregnancy.

People with prediabetes have up to a 50 percent chance of developing diabetes over the next 5–10 years. You can take steps to manage your prediabetes and prevent type 2 diabetes.

The following test results show prediabetes

- A1C—5.7 to 6.4 percent

- FPG—100 to 125 mg/dL (milligrams per deciliter)

- OGTT—140 to 199 mg/dL

You should be tested for prediabetes if you are overweight or have obesity and have one or more other risk factors for diabetes, or if your parents, siblings, or children have type 2 diabetes. Even if you don't have risk factors, you should start getting tested once you reach age 45.

If the results are normal but you have other risk factors for diabetes, you should be retested at least every 3 years.

How Can I Prevent or Reverse Insulin Resistance and Prediabetes?

Physical activity and losing weight if you need to may help your body respond better to insulin. Taking small steps, such as eating healthier foods and moving more to lose weight, can help reverse insulin resistance and prevent or delay type 2 diabetes in people with prediabetes.

The National Institutes of Health (NIH)-funded research study, the Diabetes Prevention Program (DPP), showed that for people at high risk of developing diabetes, losing 5 to 7 percent of their starting weight helped reduce their chance of developing the disease. That's 10–14 pounds for someone who weighs 200 pounds. People in the study lost weight by changing their diet and being more physically active.

The DPP also showed that taking metformin, a medicine used to treat diabetes, could delay diabetes. Metformin worked best for women with a history of gestational diabetes, younger adults, and people with obesity. Ask your doctor if metformin might be right for you.

Making a plan, tracking your progress, and getting support from your healthcare professional, family, and friends can help you make lifestyle changes that may prevent or reverse insulin resistance and prediabetes. You may be able to take part in a lifestyle change program as part of the National Diabetes Prevention Program.

Chapter 7

Type 2 Diabetes

What Is Type 2 Diabetes?

Type 2 diabetes, the most common type of diabetes, is a disease that occurs when your blood glucose, also called blood sugar, is too high. Blood glucose is your main source of energy and comes mainly from the food you eat. Insulin, a hormone made by the pancreas, helps glucose get into your cells to be used for energy. In type 2 diabetes, your body doesn't make enough insulin or doesn't use insulin well. Too much glucose then stays in your blood, and not enough reaches your cells.

The good news is that you can take steps to prevent or delay the development of type 2 diabetes.

Who Is More Likely to Develop Type 2 Diabetes?

You can develop type 2 diabetes at any age, even during childhood. However, type 2 diabetes occurs most often in middle-aged and older people. You are more likely to develop type 2 diabetes if you are age 45 or older, have a family history of diabetes, or are overweight or obese. Diabetes is more common in people who are African American, Hispanic/Latino, American Indian, Asian American, or Pacific Islander.

Physical inactivity and certain health problems such as high blood pressure affect your chances of developing type 2 diabetes. You are

---

This chapter includes text excerpted from "Type 2 Diabetes," National Institute of Diabetes and Digestive and Kidney Diseases (NIDDK), May 2017.

also more likely to develop type 2 diabetes if you have prediabetes or had gestational diabetes when you were pregnant.

What Are the Symptoms of Diabetes?

Symptoms of diabetes include

- increased thirst and urination
- increased hunger
- feeling tired
- blurred vision
- numbness or tingling in the feet or hands
- sores that do not heal
- unexplained weight loss

Symptoms of type 2 diabetes often develop slowly—over the course of several years—and can be so mild that you might not even notice them. Many people have no symptoms. Some people do not find out they have the disease until they have diabetes-related health problems, such as blurred vision or heart disease.

What Causes Type 2 Diabetes?

Type 2 diabetes is caused by several factors, including

- overweight and obesity
- not being physically active
- insulin resistance
- genes

How Do Healthcare Professionals Diagnose Type 2 Diabetes?

Your healthcare professional can diagnose type 2 diabetes based on blood tests.

How Can I Manage My Type 2 Diabetes?

Managing your blood glucose, blood pressure, and cholesterol, and quitting smoking if you smoke, are important ways to manage your type 2 diabetes. Lifestyle changes that include planning healthy meals, limiting calories if you are overweight, and being physically active are also part of managing your diabetes. So is taking any prescribed medicines. Work with your healthcare team to create a diabetes care plan that works for you.

What Medicines Do I Need to Treat My Type 2 Diabetes?

Along with following your diabetes care plan, you may need diabetes medicines, which may include pills or medicines you inject under your skin, such as insulin. Over time, you may need more than one diabetes medicine to manage your blood glucose. Even if you don't take insulin, you may need it at special times, such as during pregnancy or if you are in the hospital. You also may need medicines for high blood pressure, high cholesterol, or other conditions.

What Health Problems Can People with Diabetes Develop?

Following a good diabetes care plan can help protect against many diabetes-related health problems. However, if not managed, diabetes can lead to problems such as

- heart disease and stroke
- nerve damage
- kidney disease
- foot problems
- eye disease
- gum disease and other dental problems
- sexual and bladder problems

Many people with type 2 diabetes also have nonalcoholic fatty liver disease (NAFLD). Losing weight if you are overweight or obese can improve NAFLD. Diabetes is also linked to other health problems such as sleep apnea, depression, some types of cancer, and dementia.

How Can I Lower My Chances of Developing Type 2 Diabetes?

Research such as the Diabetes Prevention Program (DPP), sponsored by the National Institutes of Health (NIH), has shown that you can take steps to reduce your chances of developing type 2 diabetes if you have risk factors for the disease. Here are some things you can do to lower your risk:

- **Lose weight if you are overweight, and keep it off.** You may be able to prevent or delay diabetes by losing 5–7 percent of your current weight. For instance, if you weigh 200 pounds, your goal would be to lose about 10–14 pounds.

- **Move more.** Get at least 30 minutes of physical activity, such as walking, at least 5 days a week. If you have not been active, talk with your healthcare professional about which activities are best. Start slowly and build up to your goal.

- **Eat healthy foods.** Eat smaller portions to reduce the amount of calories you eat each day and help you lose weight. Choosing foods with less fat is another way to reduce calories. Drink water instead of sweetened beverages.

Ask your healthcare team what other changes you can make to prevent or delay type 2 diabetes.

Most often, your best chance for preventing type 2 diabetes is to make lifestyle changes that work for you long term.

Chapter 8

Gestational Diabetes

Facts about Gestational Diabetes

What Is Gestational Diabetes?

Gestational diabetes is a type of diabetes that develops during pregnancy. Diabetes means your blood glucose, also called blood sugar, is too high. Too much glucose in your blood is not good for you or your baby.

Gestational diabetes is usually diagnosed in the 24th to 28th week of pregnancy. Managing your gestational diabetes can help you and your baby stay healthy. You can protect your own and your baby's health by taking action right away to manage your blood glucose levels.

How Can Gestational Diabetes Affect My Baby?

High blood glucose levels during pregnancy can cause problems for your baby, such as

- being born too early
- weighing too much, which can make delivery difficult and injure your baby
- having low blood glucose, also called hypoglycemia, right after birth
- having breathing problems

This chapter includes text excerpted from "Gestational Diabetes," National Institute of Diabetes and Digestive and Kidney Diseases (NIDDK), May 2017.

High blood glucose also can increase the chance that you will have a miscarriage or a stillborn baby. Stillborn means the baby dies in the womb during the second half of pregnancy.

Your baby also will be more likely to become overweight and develop type 2 diabetes as he or she gets older.

How Can Gestational Diabetes Affect Me?

If you have gestational diabetes, you are more likely to develop preeclampsia, which is when you develop high blood pressure and too much protein in your urine during the second half of pregnancy.

Preeclampsia can cause serious or life-threatening problems for you and your baby. The only cure for preeclampsia is to give birth. If you have preeclampsia and have reached 37 weeks of pregnancy, your doctor may want to deliver your baby early. Before 37 weeks, you and your doctor may consider other options to help your baby develop as much as possible before he or she is born.

Gestational diabetes may increase your chance of having a cesarean section, also called a C-section, because your baby may be large. A C-section is major surgery.

If you have gestational diabetes, you are more likely to develop type 2 diabetes later in life. Over time, having too much glucose in your blood can cause health problems such as diabetic retinopathy, heart disease, kidney disease, and nerve damage. You can take steps to help prevent or delay type 2 diabetes.

Symptoms and Causes

What Are the Symptoms of Gestational Diabetes?

Usually, gestational diabetes has no symptoms. If you do have symptoms, they may be mild, such as being thirstier than normal or having to urinate more often.

What Causes Gestational Diabetes?

Gestational diabetes occurs when your body can't make the extra insulin needed during pregnancy. Insulin, a hormone made in your pancreas, helps your body use glucose for energy and helps control your blood glucose levels.

During pregnancy, your body makes special hormones and goes through other changes, such as weight gain. Because of these changes, your body's cells don't use insulin well, a condition called insulin resistance. All pregnant women have some insulin resistance during late pregnancy. Most pregnant women can produce enough insulin to overcome insulin resistance, but some cannot. These women develop gestational diabetes.

Being overweight or obese is linked to gestational diabetes. Women who are overweight or obese may already have insulin resistance when they become pregnant. Gaining too much weight during pregnancy may also be a factor.

Having a family history of diabetes makes it more likely that a woman will develop gestational diabetes, which suggests that genes play a role.

Tests and Diagnosis

When Will I Be Tested for Gestational Diabetes?

Testing for gestational diabetes usually occurs between 24 and 28 weeks of pregnancy.

If you have an increased chance of developing gestational diabetes, your doctor may test for diabetes during the first visit after you become pregnant.

How Do Doctors Diagnose Gestational Diabetes?

Doctors use blood tests to diagnose gestational diabetes. You may have the glucose challenge test (GCT), the oral glucose tolerance test (OGTT), or both. These tests show how well your body uses glucose.

Glucose Challenge Test (GCT)

You may have the GCT first. Another name for this blood test is the glucose screening test. In this test, a healthcare professional will draw your blood 1 hour after you drink a sweet liquid containing glucose. You do not need to fast for this test. Fasting means having nothing to eat or drink except water. If your blood glucose is too high—140 or more—you may need to return for an OGTT while fasting. If your blood glucose is 200 or more, you may have type 2 diabetes.

Oral Glucose Tolerance Test (OGTT)

The OGTT measures blood glucose after you fast for at least eight hours. First, a healthcare professional will draw your blood. Then you will drink the liquid containing glucose. You will need your blood drawn every hour for two to three hours for a doctor to diagnose gestational diabetes.

High blood glucose levels at any two or more blood test times—fasting, one hour, two hours, or three hours—mean you have gestational diabetes. Your healthcare team will explain what your OGTT results mean.

Your healthcare professional may recommend an OGTT without first having the GCT.

Management and Treatment

How Can I Manage My Gestational Diabetes?

Many women with gestational diabetes can manage their blood glucose levels by following a healthy eating plan and being physically active. Some women also may need diabetes medicine.

Follow a Healthy Eating Plan

Your healthcare team will help you make a healthy eating plan with food choices that are good for you and your baby. The plan will help you know which foods to eat, how much to eat, and when to eat. Food choices, amounts, and timing are all important in keeping your blood glucose levels in your target range.

If you're not eating enough or your blood glucose is too high, your body might make ketones. Ketones in your urine or blood mean your body is using fat for energy instead of glucose. Burning large amounts of fat instead of glucose can be harmful to your health and your baby's health.

Your doctor might recommend you test your urine or blood daily for ketones or when your blood glucose is above a certain level, such as 200. If your ketone levels are high, your doctor may suggest that you change the type or amount of food you eat. Or, you may need to change your meal or snack times.

Be Physically Active

Physical activity can help you reach your target blood glucose levels. If your blood pressure or cholesterol levels are too high, being physically active can help you reach healthy levels. Physical activity can also relieve stress, strengthen your heart and bones, improve muscle strength, and keep your joints flexible. Being physically active will also help lower your chances of having type 2 diabetes in the future.

Talk with your healthcare team about what activities are best for you during your pregnancy. Aim for 30 minutes of activity 5 days of the week, even if you weren't active before your pregnancy. If you are already active, tell your doctor what you do. Ask your doctor if you may continue some higher intensity activities, such as lifting weights or jogging.

How Will I Know Whether My Blood Glucose Levels Are on Target?

Your healthcare team may ask you to use a blood glucose meter to check your blood glucose levels. This device uses a small drop of blood from your finger to measure your blood glucose level. Your healthcare team can show you how to use your meter.

Recommended daily target blood glucose levels for most women with gestational diabetes are

- Before meals, at bedtime, and overnight: 95 or less

- 1 hour after eating: 140 or less

- 2 hours after eating: 120 or less

Ask your doctor what targets are right for you.

You can keep track of your blood glucose levels using My Daily Blood Glucose Record (www.niddk.nih.gov/-/media/Files/Diabetes/BloodGlucose_508.pdf). You can also use an electronic blood glucose tracking system on your computer or mobile device. Record the results every time you check your blood glucose. Your blood glucose records can help you and your healthcare team decide whether your diabetes care plan is working. Take your tracker with you when you visit your healthcare team.

How Is Gestational Diabetes Treated If Diet and Physical Activity Aren't Enough?

If following your eating plan and being physically active aren't enough to keep your blood glucose levels in your target range, you may need insulin.

If you need to use insulin, your healthcare team will show you how to give yourself insulin shots. Insulin will not harm your baby and is usually the first choice of diabetes medicine for gestational diabetes. Researchers are studying the safety of the diabetes pills metformin and glyburide during pregnancy, but more long-term studies are needed.

Talk with your healthcare professional about what treatment is right for you.

Prevention

What Increases My Chance of Developing Gestational Diabetes?

Your chance of developing gestational diabetes are higher if you

- are overweight
- had gestational diabetes
- have a parent, brother, or sister with type 2 diabetes
- have prediabetes, meaning your blood glucose levels are higher than normal yet not high enough for a diagnosis of diabetes
- are African American, American Indian, Asian American, Hispanic/Latina, or Pacific Islander American
- have a hormonal disorder called polycystic ovary syndrome, also known as PCOS

How Can I Lower My Chance of Developing Gestational Diabetes?

If you are thinking about becoming pregnant and are overweight, you can lower your chance of developing gestational diabetes by losing extra weight and increasing physical activity before you become pregnant. Taking these steps can improve how your body uses insulin and help your blood glucose levels stay normal.

Once you are pregnant, don't try to lose weight. You need to gain some weight for your baby to be healthy. However, gaining too much weight too quickly may increase your chance of developing gestational diabetes. Ask your doctor how much weight gain and physical activity during pregnancy are right for you.

After Your Baby Is Born

After I Have My Baby, How Can I Find out Whether I Have Diabetes?

You should get tested for diabetes no later than 12 weeks after your baby is born. If your blood glucose is still high, you may have type 2 diabetes. Even if your blood glucose is normal, you still have a greater chance of developing type 2 diabetes in the future. Therefore, you should be tested for diabetes every 3 years.

How Can I Prevent or Delay Type 2 Diabetes Later in Life?

You can do a lot to prevent or delay type 2 diabetes. Here are steps you should take if you had gestational diabetes:

- Be more active and make healthy food choices to get back to a healthy weight.
- Breastfeed your baby. Breastfeeding gives your baby the right balance of nutrients and helps you burn calories.
- If your test results show that you could get diabetes and you are overweight, ask your doctor about what changes you can make to lose weight and for help in making them. Your doctor may recommend that you take medicine such as metformin to help prevent type 2 diabetes.

How Can I Help My Child Be Healthy?

You can help your child be healthy by showing him or her how to make healthy lifestyle choices, including

- being physically active
- limiting time watching TV, playing video games, or using a mobile device or computer
- making healthy food choices
- staying at a healthy weight

Making healthy choices helps the whole family and may protect your child from becoming obese or developing diabetes later in life.

Chapter 9

Diabetes Insipidus

What Is Diabetes Insipidus?

Diabetes insipidus (DI) is a rare disorder that occurs when a person's kidneys pass an abnormally large volume of urine that is insipid—dilute and odorless. In most people, the kidneys pass about 1–2 quarts of urine a day. In people with diabetes insipidus, the kidneys can pass 3–20 quarts of urine a day. As a result, a person with diabetes insipidus may feel the need to drink large amounts of liquids.

Diabetes insipidus (DI) and diabetes mellitus (DM)—which includes both type 1 and type 2 diabetes—are unrelated, although both conditions cause frequent urination and constant thirst. Diabetes mellitus causes high blood glucose, or blood sugar, resulting from the body's inability to use blood glucose for energy. People with diabetes insipidus have normal blood glucose levels; however, their kidneys cannot balance fluid in the body.

What Are the Kidneys and What Do They Do?

The kidneys are two bean-shaped organs, each about the size of a fist. They are located just below the rib cage, one on each side of the spine. Every day, the kidneys normally filter about 120–150 quarts of blood to produce about 1–2 quarts of urine, composed of wastes and

This chapter includes text excerpted from "Diabetes Insipidus," National Institute of Diabetes and Digestive and Kidney Diseases (NIDDK), October 2015.

extra fluid. The urine flows from the kidneys to the bladder through tubes called ureters. The bladder stores urine. When the bladder empties, urine flows out of the body through a tube called the urethra, located at the bottom of the bladder.

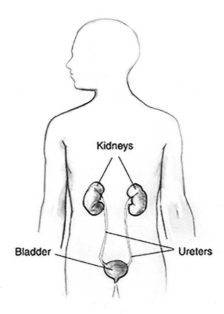

Figure 9.1. *Human Urinary System*

How Is Fluid Regulated in the Body?

A person's body regulates fluid by balancing liquid intake and removing extra fluid. Thirst usually controls a person's rate of liquid intake, while urination removes most fluid, although people also lose fluid through sweating, breathing, or diarrhea. The hormone vasopressin, also called antidiuretic hormone (ADH), controls the fluid removal rate through urination. The hypothalamus, a small gland located at the base of the brain, produces vasopressin. The nearby pituitary gland stores the vasopressin and releases it into the bloodstream when the body has a low fluid level. Vasopressin signals the kidneys to absorb less fluid from the bloodstream, resulting in less urine. When the body has extra fluid, the pituitary gland releases smaller amounts of vasopressin, and sometimes none, so the kidneys remove more fluid from the bloodstream and produce more urine.

What Are the Types of Diabetes Insipidus?

The types of diabetes insipidus include

- central
- nephrogenic
- dipsogenic
- gestational

Each type of diabetes insipidus has a different cause.

Central Diabetes Insipidus (CDI)

Central diabetes insipidus (CDI) happens when damage to a person's hypothalamus or pituitary gland causes disruptions in the normal production, storage, and release of vasopressin. The disruption of vasopressin causes the kidneys to remove too much fluid from the body, leading to an increase in urination. Damage to the hypothalamus or pituitary gland can result from the following:

- surgery
- infection
- inflammation
- a tumor
- head injury

CDI can also result from an inherited defect in the gene that produces vasopressin, although this cause is rare. In some cases, the cause is unknown.

Nephrogenic Diabetes Insipidus (NDI)

Nephrogenic diabetes insipidus (NDI) occurs when the kidneys do not respond normally to vasopressin and continue to remove too much fluid from a person's bloodstream. NDI can result from inherited gene changes, or mutations, that prevent the kidneys from responding to vasopressin.

Other causes of NDI include:

- chronic kidney disease
- certain medications, particularly lithium

- low potassium levels in the blood

- high calcium levels in the blood

- blockage of the urinary tract

The causes of NDI can also be unknown.

Dipsogenic Diabetes Insipidus

A defect in the thirst mechanism, located in a person's hypothalamus, causes dipsogenic diabetes insipidus. This defect results in an abnormal increase in thirst and liquid intake that suppresses vasopressin secretion and increases urine output. The same events and conditions that damage the hypothalamus or pituitary—surgery, infection, inflammation, a tumor, head injury—can also damage the thirst mechanism. Certain medications or mental health problems may predispose a person to dipsogenic diabetes insipidus.

Gestational Diabetes Insipidus (GDI)

Gestational diabetes insipidus (GDI) occurs only during pregnancy. In some cases, an enzyme made by the placenta—a temporary organ joining mother and baby—breaks down the mother's vasopressin. In other cases, pregnant women produce more prostaglandin, a hormone-like chemical that reduces kidney sensitivity to vasopressin. Most pregnant women who develop GDI have a mild case that does not cause noticeable symptoms. GDI usually goes away after the mother delivers the baby; however, it may return if the mother becomes pregnant again.

What Are the Complications of Diabetes Insipidus?

The main complication of diabetes insipidus is dehydration if fluid loss is greater than liquid intake. Signs of dehydration include

- thirst

- dry skin

- fatigue

- sluggishness

- dizziness

- confusion

- nausea

Severe dehydration can lead to seizures, permanent brain damage, and even death.

How Is Diabetes Insipidus Diagnosed?

A healthcare provider can diagnose a person with diabetes insipidus based on the following:

- medical and family history
- physical exam
- urinalysis
- blood tests
- fluid deprivation test
- magnetic resonance imaging (MRI)

Medical and Family History

Taking a medical and family history can help a healthcare provider diagnose diabetes insipidus. A healthcare provider will ask the patient to review his or her symptoms and ask whether the patient's family has a history of diabetes insipidus or its symptoms.

Physical Exam

A physical exam can help diagnose diabetes insipidus. During a physical exam, a healthcare provider usually examines the patient's skin and appearance, checking for signs of dehydration.

Urinalysis

Urinalysis tests a urine sample. A patient collects the urine sample in a special container at home, in a healthcare provider's office, or at a commercial facility. A healthcare provider tests the sample in the same location or sends it to a lab for analysis. The test can show whether the urine is dilute or concentrated. The test can also show the presence of glucose, which can distinguish between diabetes insipidus and diabetes mellitus. The healthcare provider may also have the patient collect urine in a special container over a 24-hour period to measure the total amount of urine produced by the kidneys.

Blood Tests

A blood test involves drawing a patient's blood at a healthcare provider's office or a commercial facility and sending the sample to a lab for analysis. The blood test measures sodium levels, which can help diagnose diabetes insipidus and in some cases determine the type.

Fluid Deprivation Test

A fluid deprivation test measures changes in a patient's body weight and urine concentration after restricting liquid intake. A healthcare provider can perform two types of fluid deprivation tests:

- **A short form of the deprivation test.** A healthcare provider instructs the patient to stop drinking all liquids for a specific period of time, usually during dinner. The next morning, the patient will collect a urine sample at home. The patient then returns the urine sample to his or her healthcare provider or takes it to a lab where a technician measures the concentration of the urine sample.

- **A formal fluid deprivation test.** A healthcare provider performs this test in a hospital to continuously monitor the patient for signs of dehydration. Patients do not need anesthesia. A healthcare provider weighs the patient and analyzes a urine sample. The healthcare provider repeats the tests and measures the patient's blood pressure every one to two hours until one of the following happens:

  - The patient's blood pressure drops too low or the patient has a rapid heartbeat when standing.

  - The patient loses 5 percent or more of his or her initial body weight.

  - Urine concentration increases only slightly in two to three consecutive measurements.

At the end of the test, a healthcare provider will compare the patient's blood sodium, vasopressin levels, and urine concentration to determine whether the patient has diabetes insipidus. Sometimes, the healthcare provider may administer medications during the test to see if they increase a patient's urine concentration. In other cases, the healthcare provider may give the patient a concentrated sodium solution intravenously at the end of the test to increase the patient's blood sodium level and determine if he or she has diabetes insipidus.

Magnetic Resonance Imaging (MRI)

Magnetic resonance imaging (MRI) is a test that takes pictures of the body's internal organs and soft tissues without using X-rays*. A specially trained technician performs the procedure in an outpatient center or a hospital, and a radiologist—a doctor who specializes in medical imaging—interprets the images. A patient does not need anesthesia, although people with a fear of confined spaces may receive light sedation. An MRI may include an injection of a special dye, called contrast medium. With most MRI machines, the person lies on a table that slides into a tunnel-shaped device that may be open ended or closed at one end. Some MRI machines allow the patient to lie in a more open space. MRIs cannot diagnose diabetes insipidus. Instead, an MRI can show if the patient has problems with his or her hypothalamus or pituitary gland or help the healthcare provider determine if diabetes insipidus is the possible cause of the patient's symptoms.

* *A type of high-energy radiation. In low doses, X-rays are used to diagnose diseases by making pictures of the inside of the body.*

How Is Diabetes Insipidus Treated?

The primary treatment for diabetes insipidus involves drinking enough liquid to prevent dehydration. A healthcare provider may refer a person with diabetes insipidus to a nephrologist—a doctor who specializes in treating kidney problems—or to an endocrinologist—a doctor who specializes in treating disorders of the hormone-producing glands. Treatment for frequent urination or constant thirst depends on the patient's type of diabetes insipidus:

- **Central diabetes insipidus (CDI).** A synthetic, or human-made, hormone called desmopressin treats CDI. The medication comes as an injection, a nasal spray, or a pill. The medication works by replacing the vasopressin that a patient's body normally produces. This treatment helps a patient manage symptoms of CDI; however, it does not cure the disease.

- **Nephrogenic diabetes insipidus (NDI).** In some cases, NDI goes away after treatment of the cause. For example, switching medications or taking steps to balance the amount of calcium or potassium in the patient's body may resolve the problem. Medications for NDI include diuretics, either alone or combined with aspirin or ibuprofen. Healthcare providers commonly prescribe diuretics to help patients' kidneys remove fluid from the body. Paradoxically, in people with NDI, a class of diuretics called thiazides reduces urine production and helps patients' kidneys concentrate urine. Aspirin or ibuprofen also helps reduce urine volume.

- **Dipsogenic diabetes insipidus.** Researchers have not yet found an effective treatment for dipsogenic diabetes insipidus. People can try sucking on ice chips or sour candies to moisten their mouths and increase saliva flow, which may reduce the desire to drink. For a person who wakes multiple times at night to urinate because of dipsogenic diabetes insipidus, taking a small dose of desmopressin at bedtime may help. Initially, the healthcare provider will monitor the patient's blood sodium levels to prevent hyponatremia, or low sodium levels in the blood.

- **Gestational diabetes insipidus (GDI).** A healthcare provider can prescribe desmopressin for women with GDI. An expecting mother's placenta does not destroy desmopressin as it does vasopressin. Most women will not need treatment after delivery.

Most people with diabetes insipidus can prevent serious problems and live a normal life if they follow the healthcare provider's recommendations and keep their symptoms under control.

Eating, Diet, and Nutrition

Researchers have not found that eating, diet, and nutrition play a role in causing or preventing diabetes insipidus.

Chapter 10

Monogenic Diabetes

The most common forms of diabetes, type 1 and type 2, are polygenic, meaning they are related to a change, or defect, in multiple genes. Environmental factors, such as obesity in the case of type 2 diabetes, also play a part in the development of polygenic forms of diabetes. Polygenic forms of diabetes often run in families. Doctors diagnose polygenic forms of diabetes by testing blood glucose, also known as blood sugar, in individuals with risk factors or symptoms of diabetes.

Genes provide the instructions for making proteins within the cell. If a gene has a change or mutation, the protein may not function properly. Genetic mutations that cause diabetes affect proteins that play a role in the ability of the body to produce insulin or in the ability of insulin to lower blood glucose. People typically have two copies of most genes, with one gene inherited from each parent.

What Are Monogenic Forms of Diabetes?

Some rare forms of diabetes result from mutations or changes in a single gene and are called monogenic. In the United States, monogenic forms of diabetes account for about 1–4 percent of all cases of diabetes. In most cases of monogenic diabetes, the gene mutation is inherited from one or both parents. Sometimes the gene mutation develops spontaneously, meaning that the mutation is not carried by

This chapter includes text excerpted from "Monogenic Diabetes (Neonatal Diabetes Mellitus and MODY)," National Institute of Diabetes and Digestive and Kidney Diseases (NIDDK), November 2017.

either of the parents. Most mutations that cause monogenic diabetes reduce the body's ability to produce insulin, a protein produced in the pancreas that helps the body use glucose for energy.

Neonatal diabetes mellitus (NDM) and maturity-onset diabetes of the young (MODY) are the two main forms of monogenic diabetes. NDM occurs in newborns and young infants. MODY is much more common than NDM and usually first occurs in adolescence or early adulthood.

Most cases of monogenic diabetes are incorrectly diagnosed. For example, when high blood glucose is first detected in adulthood, type 2 diabetes is often diagnosed instead of monogenic diabetes. If your healthcare provider thinks you might have monogenic diabetes, genetic testing may be needed to diagnose it and to identify which type. Testing of other family members may also be indicated to determine whether they are at risk for or already have a monogenic form of diabetes that is passed down from generation to generation. Some monogenic forms of diabetes can be treated with oral diabetes medicines (pills), while other forms require insulin injections. A correct diagnosis allows for proper treatment and can lead to better glucose control and improved health in the long term.

What Is Neonatal Diabetes Mellitus?

NDM is a monogenic form of diabetes that occurs in the first 6–12 months of life. NDM is a rare condition accounting for up to 1 in 400,000 infants in the United States. Infants with NDM do not produce enough insulin, leading to an increase in blood glucose. NDM is often mistaken for type 1 diabetes, but type 1 diabetes is very rarely seen before six months of age. Diabetes that occurs in the first six months of life almost always has a genetic cause. Researchers have identified a number of specific genes and mutations that can cause NDM. In about half of those with NDM, the condition is life-long and is called permanent neonatal diabetes mellitus (PNDM). In the rest of those with NDM, the condition is transient, or temporary, and disappears during infancy but can reappear later in life. This type of NDM is called transient neonatal diabetes mellitus (TNDM).

Clinical features of NDM depend on the gene mutations a person has. Signs of NDM include frequent urination, rapid breathing, and dehydration. NDM can be diagnosed by finding elevated levels of glucose in blood or urine. The lack of insulin may cause the body to produce chemicals called ketones, resulting in a potentially life-threatening condition called diabetic ketoacidosis. Most fetuses with NDM do not grow well in the womb, and newborns with NDM are much smaller than those of the same gestational age, a condition called intrauterine growth restriction. After birth, some infants fail to gain weight and grow as rapidly as other infants of the same age and sex. Appropriate therapy may improve and normalize growth and development.

What Is Maturity Onset Diabetes of the Young?

MODY is a monogenic form of diabetes that usually first occurs during adolescence or early adulthood. MODY accounts for up to two percent of all cases of diabetes in the United States in people ages 20 and younger.

A number of different gene mutations have been shown to cause MODY, all of which limit the ability of the pancreas to produce insulin. This leads to high blood glucose levels and, in time, may damage body tissues, particularly the eyes, kidneys, nerves, and blood vessels.

Clinical features of MODY depend on the gene mutations a person has. People with certain types of mutations may have slightly high blood sugar levels that remain stable throughout life, have mild or no symptoms of diabetes, and do not develop any long-term complications. Their high blood glucose levels may only be discovered during routine blood tests. However, other mutations require specific treatment with either insulin or a type of oral diabetes medication called sulfonylureas.

MODY may be confused with type 1 or type 2 diabetes. In the past, people with MODY have generally not been overweight or obese, or have other risk factors for type 2 diabetes, such as high blood pressure or abnormal blood fat levels. However, as more people in the United States become overweight or obese, people with MODY may also be overweight or obese.

Although both type 2 diabetes and MODY can run in families, people with MODY typically have a family history of diabetes in multiple successive generations, meaning MODY is present in a grandparent, a parent, and a child.

How Is Monogenic Diabetes Diagnosed?

Genetic testing can diagnose most forms of monogenic diabetes. A correct diagnosis with proper treatment should lead to better glucose control and improved health in the long term.

Genetic testing is recommended if:

- diabetes is diagnosed within the first six months of age
- diabetes is diagnosed in children and young adults, particularly those with a strong family history of diabetes, who do not have

typical features of type 1 or type 2 diabetes, such as the presence of diabetes-related autoantibodies, obesity, and other metabolic features

- a person has stable, mild fasting hyperglycemia, especially if obesity is not present

What Do You Need to Know about Genetic Testing and Counseling?

Genetic testing for monogenic diabetes involves providing a blood or saliva sample from which deoxyribonucleic acid (DNA) is isolated. The DNA is analyzed for changes in the genes that cause monogenic diabetes. Genetic testing is done by specialized labs.

Abnormal results can determine the gene responsible for diabetes in a particular individual or show whether someone is likely to develop a monogenic form of diabetes in the future. Genetic testing can be helpful in selecting the most appropriate treatment for individuals with monogenic diabetes. Testing is also important in planning for pregnancy and to understand the risk of having a child with monogenic diabetes if you, your partner, or your family members have monogenic diabetes.

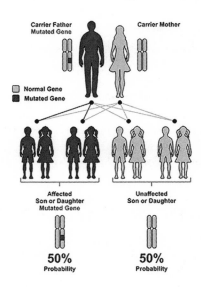

Figure 10.1. *Autosomal Dominant*

Most forms of NDM and MODY are caused by autosomal dominant mutations, meaning that the condition can be passed on to children when only one parent carries or has the disease gene. With dominant mutations, a parent who carries the gene has a 50 percent chance of having an affected child with monogenic diabetes.

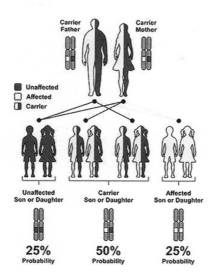

Figure 10.2. *Autosomal Recessive*

In contrast, with autosomal recessive disease, a mutation must be inherited from both parents. In this instance, a child has a 25 percent chance of having monogenic diabetes.

For recessive forms of monogenic diabetes, testing can indicate whether parents or siblings without disease are carriers for recessive genetic conditions that could be inherited by their children.

While not as common, it is possible to inherit mutations from the mother only (X-linked mutations). Also not as common are mutations that occur spontaneously.

If you suspect that you or a member of your family may have a monogenic form of diabetes, you should seek help from healthcare professionals—physicians and genetic counselors—who have specialized knowledge and experience in this area. They can determine whether genetic testing is appropriate; select the genetic tests that should be performed; and provide information about the basic principles of genetics, genetic testing options, and confidentiality issues. They also can review the test results with the patient or parent after testing, make recommendations about how to proceed, and discuss testing options for other family members.

How Is Monogenic Diabetes Treated and Managed?

Treatment varies depending on the specific genetic mutation that has caused a person's monogenic diabetes. People with certain forms of MODY and NDM can be treated with a sulfonylurea, an oral diabetes medicine that helps the body release more insulin into the blood. Other people may need insulin injections. Some people with MODY may not need medications and are able to manage their diabetes with lifestyle changes alone, which include physical activity and healthy food choices. Your physician and diabetes care team will work with you to develop a plan to treat and manage your diabetes based on the results of genetic testing.

Chapter 11

Diabetes Myths

Diabetes is a complex disease. You may have heard conflicting theories on what causes it, how it is diagnosed, and how it is managed. If you are affected by diabetes, you will want the truth about the disease.

Myths about Diabetes

Here are some common myths that you may have heard:

There Is No Diabetes in Your Family, So You Don't Have to Worry

Diabetes does run in families, but many people diagnosed with the disease have no close family members who have it. Lifestyle, heredity, and possibly other factors, such as certain viruses, may increase the risk for the disease.

It's Called Sugar Diabetes, So It Must Come from the Sugar You Eat

When you eat food, the body turns it into a form of energy called glucose, also known as "blood sugar." Glucose is not the refined sugar that you buy in stores. Insulin helps move the blood sugar into the body's cells for energy. When the body's own insulin does not work

---

This chapter includes text excerpted from "Diabetes Myths," Centers for Disease Control and Prevention (CDC), June 2017.

well or when not enough is made, the blood sugar level rises. Then the person has diabetes.

You'll Know That You Have Diabetes by Your Symptoms

A person with type 1 diabetes, usually seen in children and young adults, will have obvious symptoms, because they have little or no insulin, the hormone that controls the blood sugar level. However, people with type 2 diabetes, which usually occurs later in life, or women who have gestational diabetes, the diabetes that only appears during pregnancy, may have few or no symptoms. Their symptoms are milder since they still produce some insulin. Unfortunately, they don't make enough insulin, or it is not being used properly. Only a blood test can tell for sure if someone has diabetes.

You Don't Have to Worry for You Have Only "Borderline Diabetes" or "Touch of Sugar"

There is no such thing as borderline diabetes. To many people, "borderline" means they don't really have the disease, so they don't have to make any changes to control it. This is wrong. If you have diabetes, you have diabetes. Diabetes must be treated and taken seriously.

By Drinking Water, You Can Wash Away the Extra Sugar in Your Blood and Cure Your Diabetes

Although you can wash away sugar spilled on a table, you cannot wash away a high blood sugar level by drinking water. However, you can control diabetes by eating healthy food, being physically active, controlling your weight, seeing your medical team regularly, taking prescribed medications, and monitoring your blood sugar often.

Insulin Is a Cure for Diabetes

Insulin is not a cure for diabetes. At this point, there is no cure; there are only medicine and behaviors that can control diabetes. Insulin helps to control diabetes by keeping the blood sugar from rising.

Your Friend Takes Insulin Pills to Control Her Diabetes

Insulin is a protein; it cannot be taken by mouth because the stomach would not digest it. Insulin must be given by injection or insulin pump through the skin. Diabetes pills help by making the body produce more insulin, use its own insulin better, produce less blood sugar from the liver, or limit carbohydrate absorption after a meal.

If You Don't Take Diabetes Medicine, Your Diabetes Must Not Be Serious

Not everyone who has diabetes takes diabetes medicine. If the body produces some insulin, weight loss, healthy eating habits, and regular physical activity can help insulin work more effectively. However, diabetes does change over time, and diabetes medicine may be needed later.

If You Get Diabetes, You Will Never Be Able to Eat Any Sugar

To control one's blood sugar, all sources of carbohydrates must be controlled. Carbohydrates include starchy foods like pasta and bread as well as sugary foods like candy. Even juice, milk, and fruit all contain carbohydrates, so they must be eaten in moderate amounts. With careful planning, small amounts of sugar can replace other carbohydrates usually eaten at a meal. Too much sugar is bad for everyone. It provides only empty calories.

If You Have Diabetes, You Can Not Do Anything about It

Remember that diabetes is serious, common, costly, and CONTROLLABLE. There are many things people with diabetes can do to live a full life, while preventing or delaying complications. You can control your diabetes by eating healthy foods, staying active, losing weight if needed, taking medicine as prescribed, testing your blood sugar, and seeing your healthcare team.

Part Two

Identifying and
Managing Diabetes

Chapter 12

Diabetes: Assessing Your Risk

Who's at Risk?

Prediabetes

You're at risk for developing prediabetes if you:

- are overweight

- are 45 years or older

- have a parent, brother, or sister with type 2 diabetes

- are physically active less than three times a week

- have ever had gestational diabetes (diabetes during pregnancy) or given birth to a baby who weighed more than nine pounds

- are African American, Hispanic/Latino American, American Indian, or Alaska Native (some Pacific Islanders and Asian Americans are also at higher risk)

You can prevent or reverse prediabetes with simple, proven lifestyle changes such as losing weight if you're overweight, eating healthier, and getting regular physical activity. The Centers for Disease Control

---

This chapter includes text excerpted from "Diabetes Home—Who's at Risk?" Centers for Disease Control and Prevention (CDC), July 25, 2017.

and Prevention (CDC)-led National Diabetes Prevention Program (NDPP) can help you make healthy changes that have lasting results.

Type 2 Diabetes

You're at risk for developing type 2 diabetes if you:

- have prediabetes
- are overweight
- are 45 years or older
- have a parent, brother, or sister with type 2 diabetes
- are physically active less than three times a week
- have ever had gestational diabetes (diabetes during pregnancy) or given birth to a baby who weighed more than nine pounds
- are African American, Hispanic/Latino American, American Indian, or Alaska Native (some Pacific Islanders and Asian Americans are also at higher risk)

You can prevent or delay type 2 diabetes with simple, proven lifestyle changes such as losing weight if you're overweight, eating healthier, and getting regular physical activity.

Type 1 Diabetes

Type 1 diabetes is thought to be caused by an immune reaction (the body attacks itself by mistake). Risk factors for type 1 diabetes are not as clear as for prediabetes and type 2 diabetes. Known risk factors include:

- **Family history.** Having a parent, brother, or sister with type 1 diabetes.
- **Age.** You can get type 1 diabetes at any age, but it's more likely to develop when you're a child, teen, or young adult.

In the United States, whites are more likely to develop type 1 diabetes than African Americans and Hispanic/Latino Americans.

As of now, no one knows how to prevent type 1 diabetes.

Gestational Diabetes

You're at risk for developing gestational diabetes (diabetes while pregnant) if you:

- had gestational diabetes during a previous pregnancy
- have given birth to a baby who weighed more than nine pounds
- are overweight
- are more than 25 years old
- have a family history of type 2 diabetes
- have a hormone disorder called polycystic ovary syndrome (PCOS)
- are African American, Hispanic/Latino American, American Indian, Alaska Native, Native Hawaiian, or Pacific Islander

Gestational diabetes usually goes away after your baby is born but increases your risk for type 2 diabetes later in life. Your baby is more likely to become obese as a child or teen, and is more likely to develop type 2 diabetes later in life too.

Before you get pregnant, you may be able to prevent gestational diabetes by losing weight if you're overweight, eating healthier, and getting regular physical activity.

Chapter 13

Family History—A Potential Risk Factor for Diabetes

If you have a mother, father, sister, or brother with diabetes, you are more likely to get diabetes yourself. You are also more likely to have prediabetes. Talk to your doctor about your family health history of diabetes. Your doctor can help you take steps to prevent or delay diabetes, and reverse prediabetes if you have it.

Over 30 million people have diabetes. People with diabetes have levels of blood sugar that are too high. The different types of diabetes include type 1 diabetes, type 2 diabetes, and gestational diabetes. Diabetes can cause serious health problems, including heart disease, kidney problems, stroke, blindness, and the need for lower leg amputations.

People with prediabetes have levels of blood sugar that are higher than normal, but not high enough for them to be diagnosed with diabetes. People with prediabetes are more likely to get type 2 diabetes. About 84 million people in the United States have prediabetes, but most of them don't know they have it. If you have prediabetes, you can take steps to reverse it and prevent or delay diabetes—but not if you

This chapter contains text excerpted from the following sources: Text in this chapter begins with excerpts from "Family Health History and Diabetes," Centers for Disease Control and Prevention (CDC), July 18, 2017; Text beginning with the heading "How to Collect Your Family Health History" is excerpted from "Knowing Is Not Enough—Act on Your Family Health History," Centers for Disease Control and Prevention (CDC), November 15, 2017.

don't know that you have it. Could you have prediabetes? Take a test (www.doihaveprediabetes.org) to find out.

If you have a family health history of diabetes, you are more likely to have prediabetes and develop diabetes. You are also more likely to get type 2 diabetes if you have had gestational diabetes, are overweight or obese, or are African American, American Indian, Asian American, Pacific Islander, or Hispanic. Learning about your family health history of diabetes is an important step in finding out if you have prediabetes and knowing if you are more likely to get diabetes. Be sure to let your doctor know about your family health history of diabetes, especially if you have a mother, father, sister, or brother with diabetes. Your doctor might recommend that you have screening for diabetes earlier.

Even if you have a family health history of diabetes, you can prevent or delay type 2 diabetes by eating healthier, being physically active, and maintaining or reaching a healthy weight. This is especially important if you have prediabetes, and taking these steps can reverse prediabetes.

How to Collect Your Family Health History

Talk to Your Family

Write down the names of your close relatives from both sides of the family—parents, siblings, grandparents, aunts, uncles, nieces, and nephews. Talk to these family members about what conditions they have or had, and at what age the conditions were first diagnosed. You might think you know about all of the conditions in your parents or siblings, but you might find out more information if you ask.

Ask Questions

To find out about your risk for chronic diseases, ask your relatives about which of these diseases they have had and when they were diagnosed. Questions can include:

- Do you have any chronic diseases, such as heart disease, or diabetes, or health conditions, such as high blood pressure or high cholesterol?

- Have you had any other serious diseases, such as cancer or stroke? What type of cancer?

- How old were you when each of these diseases or health conditions was diagnosed? (If your relative doesn't remember the exact age, knowing the approximate age is still useful.)

- What is your family's ancestry? From what countries or regions did your ancestors come to the United States?

- What were the causes and ages of death for relatives who have died?

Record the Information and Keep Updating

Record the information and update it whenever you learn new family health history information. My Family Health Portrait (familyhistory.hhs.gov/FHH/html/index.html), a free web-based tool from the Surgeon General, is helpful in organizing the information in your family health history. It allows you to share this information easily with your doctor and other family members.

Share Your Family Health History

Share family health history information with your doctor and other family members. If you are concerned about diseases that are common in your family, talk with your doctor at your next visit. Even if you don't know all of your family health history information, share what you do know. Family health history information, even if incomplete, can help your doctor decide which screening tests you need and when those tests should start.

If you have a medical condition, such as cancer, heart disease, or diabetes, be sure to let your family members know about your diagnosis. If you have had genetic testing done, share your results with your family members. If you are one of the older members of your family, you may know more about diseases and health conditions in your family, especially in relatives who are no longer living. Be sure to share this information with your younger relatives so that you may all benefit from knowing this family health history information.

How to Act on Your Family Health History

Knowing about your family health history of a disease can motivate you to take steps to lower your chances of getting the disease. You can't change your family health history, but you can change unhealthy behaviors, such as smoking, not exercising or being active, and poor eating habits. Talk with your doctor about steps that you can take, including whether you should consider early screening for the disease. If you have a family health history of disease, you may have the most to gain from lifestyle changes and screening tests.

What you can do if you have a family health history of:

- **Colorectal cancer.** If you have a mother, father, sister, brother, or other close family member who had colorectal cancer before age 50 or have multiple close family members with colorectal cancer, talk to your doctor about whether you should have screening starting at a young age, being done more frequently, and using colonoscopy only instead of other tests. In some cases, your doctor may recommend that you have genetic counseling, and a genetic counselor may recommend genetic testing based on your family health history.

- **Breast or ovarian cancer.** If you have a parent, sibling, or child with breast cancer, talk to your doctor about when you should start mammography screening. If your relative was diagnosed with breast cancer before age 50, if you have a close relative with ovarian cancer, or if you have a male relative with breast cancer, your doctor might refer you for cancer genetic counseling to find out if genetic testing is right for you. In some cases, your doctor might recommend taking tamoxifen or raloxifene, drugs that can decrease risk of developing breast cancer in some women.

- **Heart disease.** If you have a family health history of heart disease, you can take steps to lower your chances of getting heart disease. These steps can include eating a healthy diet, being physically active, maintaining a healthy weight, not smoking, limiting your alcohol use, having any screening tests that your doctor recommends, and, in some cases, taking medication.

- **Osteoporosis.** This is a medical condition where bones become weak and are more likely to break. A family health history of osteoporosis is one of a number of factors that make you more likely to develop osteoporosis. For example, if you are a white woman whose mother or father fractured their hip, talk to your doctor about screening for osteoporosis earlier (at about age 55, compared with age 65 for most women).

- **Diabetes.** If your mother, father, brother, or sister has type 2 diabetes, you could have prediabetes and are more likely to get type 2 diabetes yourself. But there are important steps you can take to prevent type 2 diabetes and reverse prediabetes if you have it. Take this test (www.doihaveprediabetes.org) to find out if you could have prediabetes. Ask your doctor whether you need earlier screening for diabetes.

Chapter 14

Metabolic Syndrome and Diabetes Risk

Metabolic syndrome is a group of conditions that put you at risk for heart disease and diabetes. These conditions are:

- high blood pressure

- high blood glucose, or blood sugar, levels

- high levels of triglycerides, a type of fat, in your blood

- low levels of high-density lipoprotein (HDL), the good cholesterol, in your blood

- too much fat around your waist

Not all doctors agree on the definition or cause of metabolic syndrome. The cause might be insulin resistance. Insulin is a hormone your body produces to help you turn sugar from food into energy for your body. If you are insulin resistant, too much sugar builds up in your blood, setting the stage for disease.

This chapter contains text excerpted from the following sources: Text in this chapter begins with excerpts from "Metabolic Syndrome," MedlinePlus, National Institutes of Health (NIH), April 17, 2018; Text beginning with the heading "Causes of Metabolic Syndrome" is excerpted from "Metabolic Syndrome," National Heart, Lung, and Blood Institute (NHLBI), August 22, 2012. Reviewed September 2018.

Causes of Metabolic Syndrome

Metabolic syndrome has several causes that act together. You can control some of the causes, such as overweight and obesity, an inactive lifestyle, and insulin resistance.

You can't control other factors that may play a role in causing metabolic syndrome, such as growing older. Your risk for metabolic syndrome increases with age.

You also can't control genetics (ethnicity and family history), which may play a role in causing the condition. For example, genetics can increase your risk for insulin resistance, which can lead to metabolic syndrome.

People who have metabolic syndrome often have two other conditions:

1. excessive blood clotting

2. constant, low-grade inflammation throughout the body

Researchers don't know whether these conditions cause metabolic syndrome or worsen it.

Researchers continue to study conditions that may play a role in metabolic syndrome, such as:

- a fatty liver (excess triglycerides and other fats in the liver)

- polycystic ovarian syndrome (PCOS), a tendency to develop cysts on the ovaries

- gallstones

- breathing problems during sleep (such as sleep apnea)

Risk Factors for Metabolic Syndrome

People at greatest risk for metabolic syndrome have these underlying causes:

- abdominal obesity (a large waistline)

- an inactive lifestyle

- insulin resistance

Some people are at risk for metabolic syndrome because they take medicines that cause weight gain or changes in blood pressure, blood cholesterol, and blood sugar levels. These medicines most often are used to treat inflammation, allergies, human immunodeficiency virus (HIV), and depression and other types of mental illness.

Populations Affected by Metabolic Syndrome

Some racial and ethnic groups in the United States are at higher risk for metabolic syndrome than others. Mexican Americans have the highest rate of metabolic syndrome, followed by whites and blacks.

Other groups at increased risk for metabolic syndrome include:

- people who have a personal history of diabetes

- people who have a sibling or parent who has diabetes

- women when compared with men

- women who have a personal history of PCOS

Metabolic Syndrome and Heart Disease Risk

Metabolic syndrome increases your risk for coronary heart disease. Other risk factors, besides metabolic syndrome, also increase your risk for heart disease. For example, a high low-density lipoprotein (LDL) ("bad") cholesterol level and smoking are major risk factors for heart disease.

Even if you don't have metabolic syndrome, you should find out your short-term risk for heart disease. The National Cholesterol Education Program (NCEP) divides short-term heart disease risk into four categories. Your risk category depends on which risk factors you have and how many you have.

Your risk factors are used to calculate your 10-year risk of developing heart disease. The NCEP has an online calculator (www.nhlbi. nih.gov/health-topics/assessing-cardiovascular-risk) that you can use to estimate your 10-year risk of having a heart attack.

- **High risk.** You're in this category if you already have heart disease or diabetes, or if your 10-year risk score is more than 20 percent.

- **Moderately high risk.** You're in this category if you have two or more risk factors and your 10-year risk score is 10–20 percent.

- **Moderate risk.** You're in this category if you have two or more risk factors and your 10-year risk score is less than 10 percent.

- **Lower risk.** You're in this category if you have zero or one risk factor.

Even if your 10-year risk score isn't high, metabolic syndrome will increase your risk for coronary heart disease (CHD) over time.

Signs, Symptoms, and Complications of Metabolic Syndrome

Metabolic syndrome is a group of risk factors that raises your risk for heart disease and other health problems, such as diabetes and stroke. These risk factors can increase your risk for health problems even if they're only moderately raised (borderline-high risk factors).

Most of the metabolic risk factors have no signs or symptoms, although a large waistline is a visible sign.

Some people may have symptoms of high blood sugar if diabetes—especially type 2 diabetes—is present. Symptoms of high blood sugar often include increased thirst; increased urination, especially at night; fatigue (tiredness); and blurred vision.

High blood pressure usually has no signs or symptoms. However, some people in the early stages of high blood pressure may have dull headaches, dizzy spells, or more nosebleeds than usual.

Chapter 15

How to Prevent Type 2 Diabetes

Perhaps you have learned that you have a high chance of developing type 2 diabetes, the most common type of diabetes. You might be overweight or have a parent, brother, or sister with type 2 diabetes. Maybe you had gestational diabetes, which is diabetes that develops during pregnancy. These are just a few examples of factors that can raise your chances of developing type 2 diabetes.

Diabetes can cause serious health problems, such as heart disease, stroke, and eye and foot problems. Prediabetes also can cause health problems. The good news is that type 2 diabetes can be delayed or even prevented. The longer you have diabetes, the more likely you are to develop health problems, so delaying diabetes by even a few years will benefit your health. You can help prevent or delay type 2 diabetes by losing a modest amount of weight by following a reduced-calorie eating plan and being physically active most days of the week. Ask your doctor if you should take the diabetes drug metformin to help prevent or delay type 2 diabetes.

This chapter includes text excerpted from "Preventing Type 2 Diabetes," National Institute of Diabetes and Digestive and Kidney Diseases (NIDDK), November 2016.

How Can You Lower Your Chances of Developing Type 2 Diabetes?

Research such as the Diabetes Prevention Program (DPP) shows that you can do a lot to reduce your chances of developing type 2 diabetes. Here are some things you can change to lower your risk:

- **Lose weight and keep it off.** You may be able to prevent or delay diabetes by losing five to seven percent of your starting weight. For instance, if you weigh 200 pounds, your goal would be to lose about 10–14 pounds.

- **Move more.** Get at least 30 minutes of physical activity five days a week. If you have not been active, talk with your healthcare professional about which activities are best. Start slowly to build up to your goal.

- **Eat healthy foods most of the time.** Eat smaller portions to reduce the amount of calories you eat each day and help you lose weight. Choosing foods with less fat is another way to reduce calories. Drink water instead of sweetened beverages.

Ask your healthcare professional about what other changes you can make to prevent or delay type 2 diabetes.

What Should You Do If Your Healthcare Professional Told You That You Have Prediabetes?

Prediabetes is when your blood glucose, also called blood sugar, levels are higher than normal, but not high enough to be called diabetes. Having prediabetes is serious because it raises your chance of developing type 2 diabetes. Many of the same factors that raise your chance of developing type 2 diabetes put you at risk for prediabetes.

Other names for prediabetes include impaired fasting glucose or impaired glucose tolerance.

About one in three Americans has prediabetes, according to a diabetes statistics from the Centers for Disease Control and Prevention (CDC). You won't know if you have prediabetes unless you are tested.

If you have prediabetes, you can lower your chance of developing type 2 diabetes. Lose weight if you need to, become more physically active, and follow a reduced-calorie eating plan.

If You Had Gestational Diabetes When You Were Pregnant, How Can You Lower Your Chances of Developing Type 2 Diabetes?

Gestational diabetes is a type of diabetes that develops during pregnancy. Most of the time, gestational diabetes goes away after your baby is born. Even if your gestational diabetes goes away, you still have a greater chance of developing type 2 diabetes within 5–10 years. Your child may also be more likely to become obese and develop type 2 diabetes later in life. Making healthy choices helps the whole family and may protect your child from becoming obese or developing diabetes.

Here are steps you should take for yourself and your child if you had gestational diabetes:

- Get tested for diabetes 6–12 weeks after your baby is born. If your blood glucose is still high, you may have type 2 diabetes. If your blood glucose is normal, you should get tested every three years to see if you have developed type 2 diabetes.

- Be more active and make healthy food choices to get back to a healthy weight

- Breastfeed your baby. Breastfeeding gives your baby the right balance of nutrients and helps you burn calories.

- Ask your doctor if you should take the diabetes drug metformin to help prevent type 2 diabetes.

Chapter 16

Tests Used to Diagnose Diabetes

Chapter Contents

Section 16.1

Diabetes Tests and Diagnosis: An Overview

This section includes text excerpted from "Diabetes Tests and Diagnosis," National Institute of Diabetes and Digestive and Kidney Diseases (NIDDK), November 2016.

Your healthcare professional can diagnose diabetes, prediabetes, and gestational diabetes through blood tests. The blood tests show if your blood glucose, also called blood sugar, is too high.

Do not try to diagnose yourself if you think you might have diabetes. Testing equipment that you can buy over-the-counter (OTC), such as a blood glucose meter (BGM), cannot diagnose diabetes.

Who Should Be Tested for Diabetes?

Anyone who has symptoms of diabetes should be tested for the disease. Some people will not have any symptoms but may have risk factors for diabetes and need to be tested. Testing allows healthcare professionals to find diabetes sooner and work with their patients to manage diabetes and prevent complications.

Testing also allows healthcare professionals to find prediabetes. Making lifestyle changes to lose a modest amount of weight if you are overweight may help you delay or prevent type 2 diabetes.

Type 1 Diabetes

Most often, testing for type 1 diabetes occurs in people with diabetes symptoms. Doctors usually diagnose type 1 diabetes in children and young adults. Because type 1 diabetes can run in families, a study called TrialNet (www.trialnet.org) offers free testing to family members of people with the disease, even if they don't have symptoms.

Type 2 Diabetes

Experts recommend routine testing for type 2 diabetes if you:

- are age 45 or older

- are between the ages of 19–44, are overweight or obese, and have one or more other diabetes risk factors

- are a woman who had gestational diabetes

Medicare covers the cost of diabetes tests for people with certain risk factors for diabetes. If you have Medicare, find out if you qualify for coverage. If you have different insurance, ask your insurance company if it covers diabetes tests.

Though type 2 diabetes most often develops in adults, children also can develop type 2 diabetes. Experts recommend testing children between the ages of 10–18 who are overweight or obese and have at least two other risk factors for developing diabetes.

- low birthweight

- a mother who had diabetes while pregnant with them

- any risk factor for Type 2 Diabetes

Gestational Diabetes

All pregnant women who do not have a prior diabetes diagnosis should be tested for gestational diabetes. If you are pregnant, you will take a glucose challenge test between 24–28 weeks of pregnancy.

What Tests Are Used to Diagnose Diabetes and Prediabetes?

Healthcare professionals most often use the fasting plasma glucose (FPG) test or the A1C test to diagnose diabetes. In some cases, they may use a random plasma glucose (RPG) test.

Fasting Plasma Glucose Test

The FPG blood test measures your blood glucose level at a single point in time. For the most reliable results, it is best to have this test in the morning, after you fast for at least eight hours. Fasting means having nothing to eat or drink except sips of water.

A1C Test

The A1C test is a blood test that provides your average levels of blood glucose over the past 3 months. Other names for the A1C test are hemoglobin A1C, HbA1C, glycated hemoglobin, and glycosylated hemoglobin test. You can eat and drink before this test. When it comes to using the A1C to diagnose diabetes, your doctor will consider factors such as your age and whether you have anemia or another problem with your blood. The A1C test is not accurate in people with anemia.

If you're of African, Mediterranean, or Southeast Asian descent, your A1C test results may be falsely high or low. Your healthcare professional may need to order a different type of A1C test.

Your healthcare professional will report your A1C test result as a percentage, such as an A1C of seven percent. The higher the percentage, the higher your average blood glucose levels.

People with diabetes also use information from the A1C test to help manage their diabetes.

Random Plasma Glucose Test

Sometimes healthcare professionals use the RPG test to diagnose diabetes when diabetes symptoms are present and they do not want to wait until you have fasted. You do not need to fast overnight for the RPG test. You may have this blood test at any time.

What Tests Are Used to Diagnose Gestational Diabetes?

Pregnant women may have the glucose challenge test, the oral glucose tolerance test, or both. These tests show how well your body handles glucose.

Glucose Challenge Test

If you are pregnant and a healthcare professional is checking you for gestational diabetes, you may first receive the glucose challenge test. Another name for this test is the glucose screening test. In this test, a healthcare professional will draw your blood 1 hour after you drink a sweet liquid containing glucose. You do not need to fast for this test. If your blood glucose is too high—135 to 140 or more—you may need to return for an oral glucose tolerance test while fasting.

Oral Glucose Tolerance Test

The oral glucose tolerance test (OGTT) measures blood glucose after you fast for at least eight hours. First, a healthcare professional will draw your blood. Then you will drink the liquid containing glucose. For diagnosing gestational diabetes, you will need your blood drawn every hour for 2–3 hours.

High blood glucose levels at any two or more blood test times during the OGTT—fasting, one hour, two hours, or three hours—mean you have gestational diabetes. Your healthcare team will explain what your OGTT results mean.

Healthcare professionals also can use the OGTT to diagnose type 2 diabetes and prediabetes in people who are not pregnant. The OGTT helps healthcare professionals detect type 2 diabetes and prediabetes better than the FPG test. However, the OGTT is a more expensive test and is not as easy to give. To diagnose type 2 diabetes and prediabetes, a healthcare professional will need to draw your blood one hour after you drink the liquid containing glucose and again after two hours.

What Test Numbers Tell You If You Have Diabetes or Prediabetes?

Each test to detect diabetes and prediabetes uses a different measurement. Usually, the same test method needs to be repeated on a second day to diagnose diabetes. Your doctor may also use a second test method to confirm that you have diabetes.

The following table helps you understand what your test numbers mean if you are not pregnant.

Table 16.1. Pregnancy Test Numbers

Diagnosis	A1C (Percent)	Fasting Plasma Glucose (FPG)[a]	Oral Glucose Tolerance Test (OGTT)[ab]	Random Plasma Glucose Test (RPG)[a]
Normal	below 5.7	99 or below	139 or below	
Prediabetes	5.7–6.4	100–125	140–199	
Diabetes	6.5 or above	126 or above	200 or above	200 or above

[a] Glucose values are in milligrams per deciliter, or mg/dL.
[b] At 2 hours after drinking 75 grams of glucose. To diagnose gestational diabetes, healthcare professionals give more glucose to drink and use different numbers as cutoffs.

Which Tests Help You Healthcare Professional Know What Kind of Diabetes You Have?

Even though the tests described here can confirm that you have diabetes, they can't identify what type you have. Sometimes healthcare professionals are unsure if diabetes is type 1 or type 2. A rare type of diabetes that can occur in babies, called monogenic diabetes, can also be mistaken for type 1 diabetes. Treatment depends on the type of diabetes, so knowing which type you have is important.

To find out if your diabetes is type 1, your healthcare professional may look for certain autoantibodies. Autoantibodies are antibodies that mistakenly attack your healthy tissues and cells. The presence of one or more of several types of autoantibodies specific to diabetes is common in type 1 diabetes, but not in type 2 or monogenic diabetes. A healthcare professional will have to draw your blood for this test.

If you had diabetes while you were pregnant, you should get tested no later than 12 weeks after your baby is born to see if you have type 2 diabetes.

Section 16.2

Blood Glucose Test

This section includes text excerpted from "Blood Glucose Test," MedlinePlus, National Institutes of Health (NIH), July 12, 2018.

What Is a Blood Glucose Test?

A blood glucose test measures the glucose levels in your blood. Glucose is a type of sugar. It is your body's main source of energy. A hormone called insulin helps move glucose from your bloodstream into your cells. Too much or too little glucose in the blood can be a sign of a serious medical condition. High blood glucose levels (hyperglycemia) may be a sign of diabetes, a disorder that can cause heart disease, blindness, kidney failure, and other complications. Low blood glucose levels (hypoglycemia) can also lead to major health problems, including brain damage, if not treated.

Other name for this test includes: blood sugar, self-monitoring of blood glucose (SMBG), fasting plasma glucose (FPG), fasting blood sugar (FBS), fasting blood glucose (FBG), glucose challenge test, and oral glucose tolerance test (OGTT).

What Is It Used For?

A blood glucose test is used to find out if your blood sugar levels are in the healthy range. It is often used to help diagnose and monitor diabetes.

Why Do You Need a Blood Glucose Test?

Your healthcare provider may order a blood glucose test if you have symptoms of high glucose levels (hyperglycemia) or low glucose levels (hypoglycemia).

Symptoms of high blood glucose levels include:

- Increased thirst
- More frequent urination
- Blurred vision
- Fatigue
- Wounds that are slow to heal

Symptoms of low blood glucose levels include:

- Anxiety
- Sweating
- Trembling
- Hunger
- Confusion

You may also need a blood glucose test if you have certain risk factors for diabetes. These include:

- Being overweight
- Lack of exercise
- Family member with diabetes
- High blood pressure
- Heart disease

If you are pregnant, you will likely get a blood glucose test between the 24th and 28th week of your pregnancy to check for gestational diabetes. Gestational diabetes is a form of diabetes that happens only during pregnancy.

What Happens during a Blood Glucose Test?

A healthcare professional will take a blood sample from a vein in your arm, using a small needle. After the needle is inserted, a small amount of blood will be collected into a test tube or vial. You may feel a little sting when the needle goes in or out. For some types of glucose blood tests, you will need to drink a sugary drink before your blood is drawn.

If you have diabetes, your healthcare provider may recommend a kit to monitor your blood sugar at home. The kit will include a device to prick your finger. You will use this to collect a drop of blood for testing. Read the kit instructions carefully and talk to your healthcare provider to make sure you collect and test your blood correctly.

Will You Need to Do Anything to Prepare for the Test?

You will probably need to fast (not eat or drink) for eight hours before the test. If you are pregnant and are being checked for gestational diabetes

- you will drink a sugary liquid one hour before your blood is drawn;
- you won't need to fast for this test; and
- if your results show higher than normal blood glucose levels, you may need another test, which requires fasting.

Talk to your health provider about specific preparations needed for your glucose test.

Are There Any Risks to the Test?

There is very little risk to having a blood test. You may have slight pain or bruising at the spot where the needle was put in, but most symptoms go away quickly.

What Do the Results Mean?

If your results show higher than normal glucose levels, it may mean you have or are at risk for getting diabetes. High glucose levels may also be a sign of:

- Kidney disease
- Hyperthyroidism

- Pancreatitis

- Pancreatic cancer

If your results show lower than normal glucose levels, it may be a sign of:

- Hypothyroidism

- Too much insulin or other diabetes medicine

- Liver disease

If your glucose results are not normal, it doesn't necessarily mean you have a medical condition needing treatment. High stress and certain medicines can affect glucose levels.

Is There Anything Else That You Should Know about a Blood Glucose Test?

Many people with diabetes need to check blood glucose levels every day. If you have diabetes, be sure to talk to your healthcare provider about the best ways to manage your disease.

Section 16.3

Glucose in Urine Test

This section includes text excerpted from "Glucose in Urine Test," MedlinePlus, National Institutes of Health (NIH), October 17, 2017.

What Is a Glucose in Urine Test?

A glucose in urine test measures the amount of glucose in your urine. Glucose is a type of sugar. It is your body's main source of energy. A hormone called insulin helps move glucose from your bloodstream into your cells. If too much glucose gets into the blood, the extra glucose will be eliminated through your urine. A urine glucose test can be used to help determine if blood glucose levels are too high, which may be a sign of diabetes.

What Is It Used For?

A glucose in urine test may be part of a urinalysis, a test that measures different cells, chemicals, and other substances in your urine. Urinalysis is often included as part of a routine exam. A glucose in urine test may also be used to screen for diabetes. However, a urine glucose test is not as accurate as a blood glucose test. It may be ordered if blood glucose testing is difficult or not possible. Some people can't get blood drawn because their veins are too small or too scarred from repeated punctures. Other people avoid blood tests due to extreme anxiety or fear of needles.

Why Do You Need a Glucose in Urine Test?

You may get a glucose in urine test as part of your regular checkup or if you have symptoms of diabetes and cannot take a blood glucose test. Symptoms of diabetes include:

- Increased thirst
- More frequent urination
- Blurred vision
- Fatigue

You may also need a urinalysis, which includes a glucose in urine test, if you are pregnant. If high levels of glucose in urine are found, it may indicate gestational diabetes. Gestational diabetes is form of diabetes that happens only during pregnancy. Blood glucose testing can be used to confirm a diagnosis of gestational diabetes. Most pregnant women are tested for gestational diabetes with a blood glucose test, between their 24th and 28th weeks of pregnancy.

What Happens during a Glucose in Urine Test?

If your urine glucose test is part of a urinalysis, you will need to provide a sample of your urine. During your office visit, you will receive a container in which to collect the urine and special instructions to ensure the sample is sterile. These instructions are often referred to as the "clean-catch method." The clean-catch method includes the following steps:

1. Wash your hands.

2. Clean your genital area with a cleansing pad. Men should wipe the tip of their penis. Women should open their labia and clean from front to back.

3. Start to urinate into the toilet.

4. Move the collection container under your urine stream.

5. Collect at least an ounce or two of urine into the container, which should have markings to indicate the amount.

6. Finish urinating into the toilet.

7. Return the sample container as instructed by your healthcare provider.

Your healthcare provider may ask you to monitor your urine glucose at home with a test kit. He or she will provide you with either a kit or a recommendation of which kit to buy. Your urine glucose test kit will include instructions on how to perform the test and a package of strips for testing. Be sure to follow the kit instructions carefully, and talk to your healthcare provider if you have any questions.

Will You Need to Do Anything to Prepare for the Test?

You don't need any special preparations for this test.

Are There Any Risks to the Test?

There is no known risk to having a glucose in urine test.

What Do the Results Mean?

Glucose is not normally found in urine. If results show glucose, it may be a sign of:

- Diabetes
- Pregnancy. As many half of all pregnant women have some glucose in their urine during pregnancy. Too much glucose may indicate gestational diabetes.
- A kidney disorder

A urine glucose test is only a screening test. If glucose is found in your urine, your provider will order a blood glucose test to help make a diagnosis.

Chapter 17

Steps to Manage Your Diabetes for Life

You are the most important member of your healthcare team. You are the one who manages your diabetes day by day. Talk to your doctor about how you can best care for your diabetes to stay healthy. Some others who can help are:

- dentist
- diabetes doctor
- diabetes educator
- dietitian
- eye doctor
- foot doctor
- friends and family
- mental health counselor
- nurse
- nurse practitioner

This chapter includes text excerpted from "4 Steps to Manage Your Diabetes for Life," National Institute of Diabetes and Digestive and Kidney Diseases (NIDDK), January 2016.

- pharmacist
- social worker

How to Learn More about Diabetes

- Take classes to learn more about living with diabetes. To find a class, check with your healthcare team, hospital, or area health clinic. You can also search online.
- Join a support group—in-person or online—to get peer support with managing your diabetes.

Take Diabetes Seriously

You may have heard people say they have "a touch of diabetes" or that their "sugar is a little high." These words suggest that diabetes is not a serious disease. That is not correct. Diabetes is serious, but you can learn to manage it.

People with diabetes need to make healthy food choices, stay at a healthy weight, move more every day, and take their medicine even when they feel good. It's a lot to do. It's not easy, but it's worth it!

Why Take Care of Your Diabetes?

Taking care of yourself and your diabetes can help you feel good today and in the future. When your blood sugar (glucose) is close to normal, you are likely to:

- have more energy
- be less tired and thirsty
- need to pass urine less often
- heal better
- have fewer skin or bladder infections

You will also have less chance of having health problems caused by diabetes such as:

- heart attack or stroke
- eye problems that can lead to trouble seeing or going blind
- pain, tingling, or numbness in your hands and feet, also called nerve damage

- kidney problems that can cause your kidneys to stop working
- teeth and gum problems

Actions You Can Take

- Ask your healthcare team what type of diabetes you have.
- Learn where you can go for support.
- Learn how caring for your diabetes helps you feel good today and in the future.

How to Learn More about Diabetes

- Take classes to learn more about living with diabetes. To find a class, check with your healthcare team, hospital, or area health clinic. You can also search online.
- Join a support group—in-person or online—to get peer support with managing your diabetes.

Take Diabetes Seriously

You may have heard people say they have "a touch of diabetes" or that their "sugar is a little high." These words suggest that diabetes is not a serious disease. That is not correct. Diabetes is serious, but you can learn to manage it.

People with diabetes need to make healthy food choices, stay at a healthy weight, move more every day, and take their medicine even when they feel good. It's a lot to do. It's not easy, but it's worth it!

Why Take Care of Your Diabetes?

Taking care of yourself and your diabetes can help you feel good today and in the future. When your blood sugar (glucose) is close to normal, you are likely to:

- have more energy
- be less tired and thirsty
- need to pass urine less often
- heal better
- have fewer skin or bladder infections

You will also have less chance of having health problems caused by diabetes such as:

- heart attack or stroke

- eye problems that can lead to trouble seeing or going blind

- pain, tingling, or numbness in your hands and feet, also called nerve damage

- kidney problems that can cause your kidneys to stop working

- teeth and gum problems

Actions You Can Take

- Ask your healthcare team what type of diabetes you have.

- Learn where you can go for support.

- Learn how caring for your diabetes helps you feel good today and in the future.

Know Your Diabetes ABCs

Talk to your healthcare team about how to manage your A1C, Blood pressure, and Cholesterol. This can help lower your chances of having a heart attack, stroke, or other diabetes problems.

A for the A1C test

What Is It?

The A1C is a blood test that measures your average blood sugar level over the past three months. It is different from the blood sugar checks you do each day.

Why Is It Important?

You need to know your blood sugar levels over time. You don't want those numbers to get too high. High levels of blood sugar can harm your heart, blood vessels, kidneys, feet, and eyes.

What Is the A1C Goal?

The A1C goal for many people with diabetes is below 7. It may be different for you. Ask what your goal should be.

B for Blood Pressure

What Is It?

Blood pressure is the force of your blood against the wall of your blood vessels.

Why Is It Important?

If your blood pressure gets too high, it makes your heart work too hard. It can cause a heart attack, stroke, and damage your kidneys and eyes.

What Is the Blood Pressure Goal?

The blood pressure goal for most people with diabetes is below 140/90. It may be different for you. Ask what your goal should be.

C for Cholesterol

What Is It?

There are two kinds of cholesterol in your blood: LDL and HDL.
LDL or "bad" cholesterol can build up and clog your blood vessels. It can cause a heart attack or stroke.
HDL or "good" cholesterol helps remove the "bad" cholesterol from your blood vessels.

What Are the LDL and HDL Goals?

Ask what your cholesterol numbers should be. Your goals may be different from other people. If you are over 40 years of age, you may need to take a statin drug for heart health.

Actions You Can Take

- Ask your healthcare team:
  - What your A1C, blood pressure, and cholesterol numbers are and what they should be. Your ABC goals will depend on how long you have had diabetes, other health problems, and how hard your diabetes is to manage.
  - What you can do to reach your ABC goals
- Write down your numbers on the record at the back of this chapter to track your progress.

Learn How to Live with Diabetes

It is common to feel overwhelmed, sad, or angry when you are living with diabetes. You may know the steps you should take to stay healthy, but have trouble sticking with your plan over time. This chapter has tips on how to cope with your diabetes, eat well, and be active.

Cope with Your Diabetes

- Stress can raise your blood sugar. Learn ways to lower your stress. Try deep breathing, gardening, taking a walk, meditating, working on your hobby, or listening to your favorite music.

- Ask for help if you feel down. A mental health counselor, support group, member of the clergy, friend, or family member who will listen to your concerns may help you feel better.

Eat Well

- Make a diabetes meal plan with help from your healthcare team.

- Choose foods that are lower in calories, saturated fat, trans fat, sugar, and salt.

- Eat foods with more fiber, such as whole grain cereals, breads, crackers, rice, or pasta.

- Choose foods such as fruits, vegetables, whole grains, bread and cereals, and low-fat or skim milk and cheese.

- Drink water instead of juice and regular soda.

- When eating a meal, fill half of your plate with fruits and vegetables, one quarter with a lean protein, such as beans, or chicken or turkey without the skin, and one quarter with a whole grain, such as brown rice or whole wheat pasta.

Be Active

- Set a goal to be more active most days of the week. Start slow by taking 10 minute walks, 3 times a day.

- Twice a week, work to increase your muscle strength. Use stretch bands, do yoga*, heavy gardening (digging and planting with tools), or try push-ups.

A mind and body practice with origins in ancient Indian philosophy.

- Stay at or get to a healthy weight by using your meal plan and moving more.

Know What to Do Every Day

- Take your medicines for diabetes and any other health problems even when you feel good. Ask your doctor if you need aspirin to prevent a heart attack or stroke. Tell your doctor if you cannot afford your medicines or if you have any side effects.
- Check your feet every day for cuts, blisters, red spots, and swelling. Call your healthcare team right away about any sores that do not go away.
- Brush your teeth and floss every day to keep your mouth, teeth, and gums healthy.
- Stop smoking. Ask for help to quit. Call 800-QUITNOW (800-784-8669).
- Keep track of your blood sugar. You may want to check it one or more times a day.
- Check your blood pressure if your doctor advises and keep a record of it.

Talk to Your Healthcare Team

- Ask your doctor if you have any questions about your diabetes.
- Report any changes in your health.

Actions You Can Take

- Ask for a healthy meal plan.
- Ask about ways to be more active.
- Ask how and when to test your blood sugar and how to use the results to manage your diabetes.
- Use these tips to help with your self-care.
- Discuss how your diabetes plan is working for you each time you visit your healthcare team.

Get Routine Care to Stay Healthy

See your healthcare team at least twice a year to find and treat any problems early.

At each visit, be sure you have a:

- blood pressure check
- foot check
- weight check
- review of your self-care plan

Two times each year, have an:

- A1C test. It may be checked more often if it is over 7.

Once each year, be sure you have a:

- cholesterol test
- complete foot exam
- dental exam to check teeth and gums
- dilated eye exam to check for eye problems
- flu shot
- urine and a blood test to check for kidney problems

At least once in your lifetime, get a:

- pneumonia shot
- hepatitis B shot

If you have Medicare, check to see how your plan covers diabetes care. Medicare covers some of the costs for:

- diabetes education
- diabetes supplies
- diabetes medicine
- visits with a dietitian
- special shoes, if you need them

Actions You Can Take

- Ask your healthcare team about these and other tests you may need. Ask what your results mean.
- Write down the date and time of your next visit.
- If you have Medicare, check your plan.

Chapter 18

The Diabetes Treatment Team

Managing Diabetes

A team approach to diabetes care can effectively help people cope with the vast array of complications that can arise from diabetes. People with diabetes can lower their risk for microvascular complications, such as eye disease and kidney disease; macrovascular complications, such as heart disease and stroke; and other diabetes complications, such as nerve damage, by:

- controlling their ABCs (A1C, blood pressure, cholesterol, and smoking cessation)

- following an individualized meal plan

- engaging in regular physical activity

- avoiding tobacco use

- taking medicines as prescribed

- coping effectively with the demands of a complex chronic disease

Patients who increase their use of effective behavioral interventions to lower the risk of diabetes—and treatments to improve glycemic

This chapter includes text excerpted from "Team Care Approach for Diabetes," Centers for Disease Control and Prevention (CDC), June 15, 2011. Reviewed September 2018.

control and cardiovascular risk profiles—can prevent or delay progression to kidney failure, vision loss, nerve damage, lower extremity amputation, and cardiovascular disease (CVD). This in turn can lead to increased patient satisfaction with care, better quality of life, improved health outcomes, and ultimately, lower healthcare costs.

The challenge is to broaden delivery of care by expanding the healthcare team to include several types of healthcare professionals. Collaborative teams vary according to patients' needs, patient load, organizational constraints, resources, clinical setting, geographic location, and professional skills.

Pharmacy, Podiatry, Optometry, and Dentistry and the Team Approach

You and other pharmacy, podiatry, optometry, and dentistry (PPOD) providers play an integral role in the team care approach to diabetes care. When you are educated about the complications of diabetes care issues in your own and other PPOD disciplines, you can better recognize symptomatic concerns warranting timely referral and reinforce annual screening recommendations that are proven to lower the risk of serious complications for diabetic patients. Below you will find information and resources to promote this comprehensive, team-based diabetes care for patients. A multidisciplinary team approach is critical to success in diabetes care and complications prevention. Evidence indicates that a team approach:

- Can facilitate diabetes management
- Can lower the risk for chronic disease complications
- Helps educate about ways to reduce risk factors for type 2 diabetes in your patients' family members

Healthcare Team for People with Diabetes

There are many other possible members of the healthcare team in addition to physicians (e.g., primary care, endocrinologist, obstetrician-gynecologist, ophthalmologist). This team could include (but is not limited to):

- Pharmacists
- Podiatrists
- Optometrists
- Dental care professionals

- Primary care physicians

- Physician assistants

- Nurse practitioners

- Dietitians

- Certified diabetes educators

- Community health workers

- Mental health professionals

Other Valuable Team Members. Clinical care teams can be augmented by including the resources and support of community partners such as:

- School nurses

- Trained peer leaders

Nontraditional approaches to healthcare can expand access to team care and, if used effectively, can build team care practices. These approaches include telehealth, shared medical appointments, and group education. For instance, pharmacist-directed telehealth programs have improved outcomes in blood pressure and diabetes medication management. There are also opportunities to partner with primary care providers in shared group appointments (SGAs). These shared group visits allow time for learning and integration of new knowledge and skills. A literature review showed that SGAs build synergy between healthcare providers and patients while using group interactions to increase knowledge and self-care skills. All of these team members play important roles in the delivery of care for people with diabetes. When you work together using a team care approach, you can:

- Minimize patients' health risks through assessment, intervention, and surveillance

- Identify problems early and initiate timely treatment

Promoting Team Interaction

Below are some tools and resources you can use to promote interaction among PPOD professionals and other providers:

- The National Diabetes Education Program's (NDEP) Redesigning the Healthcare Team illustrates how teams can work together effectively. Examples from the peer-reviewed literature and case studies that show the diversity and effectiveness of healthcare professional teams working with people who have diabetes include:

- Community-based primary care providers who involve a pharmacist and dietitian in implementing treatment algorithms, nurse and dietitian case managers, and educators who help to improve patients' weight loss and A1C values.

- A nurse practitioner-physician team that manages patients with diabetes and hypertension

- Healthcare professionals who use telehealth to improve eye care, nutrition counseling, and diabetes self-management education

- Pharmacists who work with company employees who have diabetes and their physicians to improve clinical measures and lower healthcare costs. Trained community health workers who bridge the gap among traditional healthcare teams to improve access to diabetes healthcare, complications assessment, and education in underserved communities.

- Podiatrists and other healthcare professionals who help reduce lower-extremity amputation rates in foot care clinics

- Dental and eye care professionals who help prevent and manage diabetes complications

- The NDEP's comprehensive *Diabetes Head to Toe Checklist Examination Report* was developed by the NDEP healthcare Providers Stakeholders' Group (comprised of physicians, nurses, physician assistants, and diabetes educators), and the PPOD Providers Stakeholders' Group (comprised of providers in all four of the PPOD fields—pharmacy, podiatry, optometry, and dentistry)—to foster collaboration. The groups developed the checklist to support coordination of care and to recognize the following variables:

  - Coordination will help ensure patients understand and can implement the intended treatment plan and can identify drug and disease management and psychosocial problems in a timely manner.

- Coordination of care presents many challenges when delivered by multiple providers in a variety of settings.

- PPOD professionals are often a primary point of care for people with type 2 diabetes. You have an important role in ensuring that diabetes care is continuous and patient-centered.

The checklist was pilot-tested by a range of healthcare providers and was found to be useful in a real-world clinical setting. They indicated that they were likely to change their practice to more of a team approach, incorporating the members of the team, or to adopt a referral approach. The providers also reported that the checklist helped them educate their patients about how preventive care can decrease the risk of diabetes complications. Further, 30 percent indicated that the checklist has useful application in electronic medical record/electronic health record systems.

Chapter 19

Glucose Monitoring

Chapter Contents

Section 19.1

Blood Glucose Monitoring Devices

This section includes text excerpted from "Blood
Glucose Monitoring Devices," U.S. Food and Drug
Administration (FDA), March 26, 2018.

Glucose is a sugar that your body uses as a source of energy. Unless you have diabetes, your body regulates the amount of glucose in your blood. People with diabetes may need special diets and medications to control blood glucose.

What Does Blood Glucose Monitoring Devices Do?

This is a quantitative test system for use at home or in healthcare settings to measure the amount of sugar (glucose) in your blood.

Why Should You Take This Test?

You should take this test if you have diabetes and you need to monitor your blood sugar (glucose) levels. You and your doctor can use the results to:

- determine your daily adjustments in treatment
- know if you have dangerously high or low levels of glucose
- understand how your diet and exercise change your glucose levels

How Often Should You Test Your Glucose?

Follow your doctor's recommendations about how often you test your glucose. You may need to test yourself several times each day to determine adjustments in your diet or treatment.

What Should Your Glucose Levels Be?

According to the American Diabetes Association (ADA) (*Standards of Medical Care in Diabetes—2017*. Diabetes Care, January 2017, vol. 40, Supplement 1, S11–S24) the blood glucose levels for an adult without diabetes are below 100 mg/dL before meals and fasting and are less than 140 mg/dL two hours after meals.

People with diabetes should consult their doctor or healthcare provider to set appropriate blood glucose goals. You should treat your low or high blood glucose as recommended by your healthcare provider.

How Accurate Is This Test?

The accuracy of this test depends on many factors including:

- The quality of your meter

- The quality of your test strips

- How well you perform the test. For example, you should wash and dry your hands before testing and closely follow the instructions for operating your meter.

- Your hematocrit (the amount of red blood cells (RBCs) in the blood). If you are severely dehydrated or anemic, your test results may be less accurate. Your healthcare provider can tell you if your hematocrit is low or high, and can discuss with you how it may affect your glucose testing.

- Interfering substances (some substances, such as vitamin C, Tylenol, and uric acid, may interfere with your glucose testing). Check the instructions for your meter and test strips to find out what substances may affect the testing accuracy.

- Altitude, temperature, and humidity (high altitude, low and high temperatures, and humidity can cause unpredictable effects on glucose results). Check the meter manual and test strip package insert for more information.

- Store and handle the meter and strips according to manufacturer's instructions. It is important to store test strip vials closed.

How Do You Take This Test?

Before you test your blood glucose, you must read and understand the instructions for your meter. In general, you prick your finger with a lancet to get a drop of blood. Then you place the blood on a disposable "test strip" that is inserted in your meter. The test strip contains chemicals that react with glucose. Some meters measure the amount of electricity that passes through the test strip. Others measure how much light reflects from it. In the United States, meters report results in milligrams of glucose per deciliter of blood, or mg/dl.

You can get information about your meter and test strips from several different sources, including the toll-free number in the manual that comes with your meter or on the manufacturer's website. If you have an urgent problem, always contact your healthcare provider or a local emergency room for advice.

How Do You Choose a Glucose Meter?

There are many different types of meters available for purchase that differ in several ways, including:

- accuracy
- amount of blood needed for each test
- how easy it is to use
- pain associated with using the product
- testing speed
- overall size
- ability to store test results in memory
- likelihood of interferences
- ability to transmit data to a computer
- cost of the meter
- cost of the test strips used
- doctor's recommendation
- technical support provided by the manufacturer
- special features such as automatic timing, error codes, large display screen, or spoken instructions or results

Talk to your healthcare provider about the right glucose meter for you, and how to use it.

How Can You Check Your Meter's Performance?

There are three ways to make sure your meter works properly:

1. Use liquid control solutions:
    - every time you open a new container of test strips
    - occasionally as you use the container of test strips

- if you drop the meter

- whenever you get unusual results

To test a liquid control solution, you test a drop of these solutions just like you test a drop of your blood. The value you get should match the value written on the test strip vial label.

2. Use electronic checks. Every time you turn on your meter, it does an electronic check. If it detects a problem it will give you an error code. Look in your meter's manual to see what the error codes mean and how to fix the problem. If you are unsure if your meter is working properly, call the toll-free number in your meter's manual, or contact your healthcare provider.

3. Compare your meter with a blood glucose test performed in a laboratory. Take your meter with you to your next appointment with your healthcare provider. Ask your provider to watch your testing technique to make sure you are using the meter correctly. Ask your healthcare provider to have your blood tested with a laboratory method. If the values you obtain on your glucose meter match the laboratory values, then your meter is working well and you are using good technique.

What should you do if your meter malfunctions? If your meter malfunctions, you should tell your healthcare provider and contact the company that made your meter and strips.

Can You Test Blood Glucose from Sites Other than Your Fingers?

Some meters allow you to test blood from sites other than the fingertip. Examples of such alternative sampling sites are your palm, upper arm, forearm, thigh, or calf. Alternative site testing (AST) should not be performed at times when your blood glucose may be changing rapidly, as these alternative sampling sites may provide inaccurate results at those times. You should use only blood from your fingertip to test if any of the following applies:

- you have just taken insulin

- you think your blood sugar is low

- you are not aware of symptoms when you become hypoglycemic

- the results do not agree with the way you feel

- you have just eaten

- you have just exercised

- you are ill

- you are under stress

Also, you should never use results from an alternative sampling site to calibrate a continuous glucose monitor (CGM), or in insulin dosing calculations.

Section 19.2

Continuous Glucose Monitoring

This section includes text excerpted from "Continuous Glucose Monitoring," National Institute of Diabetes and Digestive and Kidney Diseases (NIDDK), June 2017.

What Is Continuous Glucose Monitoring?

Continuous glucose monitoring (CGM) automatically tracks blood glucose levels, also called blood sugar, throughout the day and night. You can see your glucose level anytime at a glance. You can also review how your glucose changes over a few hours or days to see trends. Seeing glucose levels in real time can help you make more informed decisions throughout the day about how to balance your food, physical activity, and medicines.

How Does a Continuous Glucose Monitor Work?

- A CGM works through a tiny sensor inserted under your skin, usually on your belly or arm. The sensor measures your interstitial glucose level, which is the glucose found in the fluid between the cells. The sensor tests glucose every few minutes. A transmitter wirelessly sends the information to a monitor.

- The monitor may be part of an insulin pump or a separate device, which you might carry in a pocket or purse. Some CGMs send information directly to a smartphone or tablet.

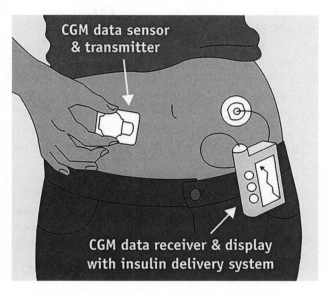

Figure 19.1. *Continuous Glucose Monitor (CGM) Data Sensor and Transmitter*

Special Features of a Continuous Glucose Monitor

CGMs are always on and recording glucose levels—whether you're showering, working, exercising, or sleeping. Many CGMs have special features that work with information from your glucose readings:

An alarm can sound when your glucose level goes too low or too high

You can note your meals, physical activity, and medicines in a CGM device, too, alongside your glucose levels

You can download data to a computer or smart device to more easily see your glucose trends

Some models can send information right away to a second person's smartphone—perhaps a parent, partner, or caregiver. For example, if a child's glucose drops dangerously low overnight, the CGM could be set to wake a parent in the next room.

As of now, one CGM model is approved for treatment decisions, the Dexcom G5 Mobile. That means you can make changes to your diabetes care plan based on CGM results alone. With other models, you must first confirm a CGM reading with a finger-stick blood glucose test before you take insulin or treat hypoglycemia.

Special Requirements Needed to Use a Continuous Glucose Monitor

Twice a day, you may need to check the CGM itself. You'll test a drop of blood on a standard glucose meter. The glucose reading should be similar on both devices.

You'll also need to replace the CGM sensor every 3–7 days, depending on the model.

For safety it's important to take action when a CGM alarm sounds about high or low blood glucose. You should follow your treatment plan to bring your glucose into the target range, or get help.

Who Can Use a Continuous Glucose Monitor?

Most people who use CGMs have type 1 diabetes. Research is underway to learn how CGMs might help people with type 2 diabetes.

CGMs are approved for use by adults and children with a doctor's prescription. Some models may be used for children as young as age 2. Your doctor may recommend a CGM if you or your child:

- are on intensive insulin therapy (IIT), also called tight blood sugar control (TBSC)

- have hypoglycemia unawareness

- often have high or low blood glucose

Your doctor may suggest using a CGM system all the time or only for a few days to help adjust your diabetes care plan.

What Are the Benefits of a Continuous Glucose Monitor?

Compared with a standard blood glucose meter, using a CGM system can help you:

- better manage your glucose levels every day

- have fewer low blood glucose emergencies

- need fewer finger sticks

A graphic on the CGM screen shows whether your glucose is rising or dropping—and how quickly—so you can choose the best way to reach your target glucose level.

Over time, good management of glucose greatly helps people with diabetes stay healthy and prevent complications of the disease. People who gain the largest benefit from a CGM are those who use it every day or nearly every day.

What Are the Limits of a Continuous Glucose Monitor?

Researchers are working to make CGMs more accurate and easier to use. But you still need a finger-stick glucose test twice a day to check the accuracy of your CGM against a standard blood glucose meter.

In 2016, the U.S. Food and Drug Administration (FDA) approved a type of artificial pancreas system called a hybrid closed-loop system. This system tests your glucose level every five minutes throughout the day and night through a CGM, and automatically gives you the right amount of basal insulin, a long-acting insulin, through a separate insulin pump. You will still need to test your blood with a glucose meter a few times a day. And you'll manually adjust the amount of insulin the pump delivers at mealtimes and when you need a correction dose.

The hybrid closed-loop system may free you from some of the daily tasks needed to keep your blood glucose stable—or help you sleep through the night without the need to wake and test your glucose or take medicine. Talk with your healthcare provider about whether this system might be right for you. The devices may also help people with type 2 diabetes and gestational diabetes.

Chapter 20

Routine Medical Examinations and Recommended Vaccinations

Chapter Contents

119

Section 20.1

A1C Testing

This section includes text excerpted from "The A1C Test and Diabetes," National Institute of Diabetes and Digestive and Kidney Diseases (NIDDK), April 2018.

What Is the A1C Test?

The A1C test is a blood test that provides information about your average levels of blood glucose, also called blood sugar, over the past three months. The A1C test can be used to diagnose type 2 diabetes and prediabetes. The A1C test is also the primary test used for diabetes management.

The A1C test is sometimes called the hemoglobin A1C, HbA1c, glycated hemoglobin, or glycohemoglobin test. Hemoglobin is the part of a red blood cell (RBC) that carries oxygen to the cells. Glucose attaches to or binds with hemoglobin in your blood cells, and the A1C test is based on this attachment of glucose to hemoglobin.

The higher the glucose level in your bloodstream, the more glucose will attach to the hemoglobin. The A1C test measures the amount of hemoglobin with attached glucose and reflects your average blood glucose levels over the past three months.

The A1C test result is reported as a percentage. The higher the percentage, the higher your blood glucose levels have been. A normal A1C level is below 5.7 percent.

Why Should a Person Get the A1C Test?

Testing can help healthcare professionals:

- find prediabetes and counsel you about lifestyle changes to help you delay or prevent type 2 diabetes

- find type 2 diabetes

- work with you to monitor the disease and help make treatment decisions to prevent complications

If you have risk factors for prediabetes or diabetes, talk with your doctor about whether you should be tested.

How Is the A1C Test Used to Diagnose Type 2 Diabetes and Prediabetes?

Healthcare professionals can use the A1C test alone or in combination with other diabetes tests to diagnose type 2 diabetes and prediabetes. You don't have to fast before having your blood drawn for an A1C test, which means that blood can be drawn for the test at any time of the day.

If you don't have symptoms but the A1C test shows you have diabetes or prediabetes, you should have a repeat test on a different day using the A1C test or one of the other diabetes tests to confirm the diagnosis.

Table 20.1. A1C Test Results

Diagnosis*	A1C Level
Normal	below 5.7 percent
Prediabetes	5.7–6.4 percent
Diabetes	6.5 percent or above

* Any test used to diagnose diabetes requires confirmation with a second measurement, unless there are clear symptoms of diabetes.

When using the A1C test for diagnosis, your doctor will send your blood sample taken from a vein to a lab that uses a National Glycohemoglobin Standardization Program (NGSP)-certified method. The NGSP certifies that makers of A1C tests provide results that are consistent and comparable with those used in the Diabetes Control and Complications Trial (DCCT).

Blood samples analyzed in a doctor's office or clinic, known as point-of-care tests, should not be used for diagnosis.

The A1C test should not be used to diagnose type 1 diabetes, gestational diabetes, or cystic fibrosis-related diabetes. The A1C test may give false results in people with certain conditions.

Having prediabetes is a risk factor for developing type 2 diabetes. Within the prediabetes A1C range of 5.7–6.4 percent, the higher the A1C, the greater the risk of diabetes.

Is the A1C Test Used during Pregnancy?

Healthcare professionals may use the A1C test early in pregnancy to see if a woman with risk factors had undiagnosed diabetes before becoming pregnant. Since the A1C test reflects your average blood glucose levels over the past three months, testing early in pregnancy may include values reflecting time before you were pregnant. The glucose challenge test or the oral glucose tolerance test (OGTT) are used to check for gestational diabetes, usually between 24–28 weeks of pregnancy. If you had gestational diabetes, you should be tested for diabetes no later than 12 weeks after your baby is born. If your blood glucose is still high, you may have type 2 diabetes. Even if your blood glucose is normal, you still have a greater chance of developing type 2 diabetes in the future and should get tested every three years.

Can Other Blood Glucose Tests Be Used to Diagnose Type 2 Diabetes and Prediabetes?

Yes. Healthcare professionals also use the fasting plasma glucose (FPG) test and the OGTT to diagnose type 2 diabetes and prediabetes. For these blood glucose tests used to diagnose diabetes, you must fast at least eight hours before you have your blood drawn. If you have symptoms of diabetes, your doctor may use the random plasma glucose test, which doesn't require fasting. In some cases, healthcare professionals use the A1C test to help confirm the results of another blood glucose test.

Can the A1C Test Result in a Different Diagnosis than the Blood Glucose Tests?

Yes. In some people, a blood glucose test may show diabetes when an A1C test does not. The reverse can also occur—an A1C test may indicate diabetes even though a blood glucose test does not. Because of these differences in test results, healthcare professionals repeat tests before making a diagnosis.

People with differing test results may be in an early stage of the disease, when blood glucose levels have not risen high enough to show up on every test. In this case, healthcare professionals may choose to follow the person closely and repeat the test in several months.

Why Do Diabetes Blood Test Results Vary?

Lab test results can vary from day to day and from test to test. This can be a result of the following factors:

Blood Glucose Levels Move Up and Down

Your results can vary because of natural changes in your blood glucose level. For example, your blood glucose level moves up and down when you eat or exercise. Sickness and stress also can affect your blood glucose test results. A1C tests are less likely to be affected by short-term changes than FPG or OGTT tests.

Figure 20.1. shows how multiple blood glucose measurements over four days compare with an A1C measurement.

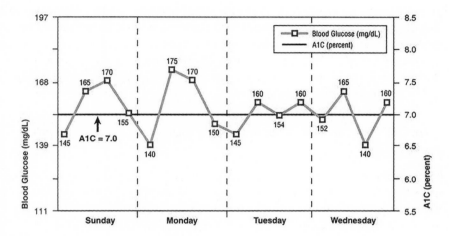

Figure 20.1. *Blood Glucose Measurements Compared with A1C Measurements over Four Days*

Blood glucose (mg/dL) measurements were taken four times per day (fasting or pre-breakfast, prelunch, predinner, and bedtime).

The straight black line shows an A1C measurement of 7.0 percent. The zigzag line shows an example of how blood glucose test results might look from self-monitoring four times a day over a four-day period.

A1C Tests Can Be Affected by Changes in Red Blood Cells or Hemoglobin

Conditions that change the lifespan of RBCs, such as recent blood loss, sickle cell disease (SCD), erythropoietin treatment, hemodialysis, or transfusion, can change A1C levels.

A falsely high A1C result can occur in people who are very low in iron; for example, those with iron-deficiency anemia. Other causes of false A1C results include kidney failure or liver disease.

If you're of African, Mediterranean, or Southeast Asian descent or have family members with sickle cell anemia (SCA) or a thalassemia, an A1C test can be unreliable for diagnosing or monitoring diabetes and prediabetes. People in these groups may have a different type of hemoglobin, known as a hemoglobin variant, which can interfere with some A1C tests. Most people with a hemoglobin variant have no symptoms and may not know that they carry this type of hemoglobin. healthcare professionals may suspect interference—a falsely high or low result—when your A1C and blood glucose test results don't match.

Not all A1C tests are unreliable for people with a hemoglobin variant. People with false results from one type of A1C test may need a different type of A1C test to measure their average blood glucose level. The NGSP provides information for healthcare professionals about which A1C tests are appropriate to use for specific hemoglobin variants.

Small Changes in Temperature, Equipment, or Sample Handling

Even when the same blood sample is repeatedly measured in the same lab, the results may vary because of small changes in temperature, equipment, or sample handling. These factors tend to affect glucose measurements—fasting and OGTT—more than the A1C test.

Healthcare professionals understand these variations and repeat lab tests for confirmation. Diabetes develops over time, so even with variations in test results, healthcare professionals can tell when overall blood glucose levels are becoming too high.

How Precise Is the A1C Test?

When repeated, the A1C test result can be slightly higher or lower than the first measurement. This means, for example, an A1C reported as 6.8 percent on one test could be reported in a range from 6.4–7.2 percent on a repeat test from the same blood sample. In the past, this range was larger but updated, stricter quality-control standards mean more precise A1C test results.

How Is the A1C Test Used after Diagnosis of Diabetes?

Your healthcare professional may use the A1C test to set your treatment goals, modify therapy, and monitor your diabetes management. Experts recommend that people with diabetes have an A1C test at least twice a year. Healthcare professionals may check your A1C more often if you aren't meeting your treatment goals.

What A1C Goal Should You Have?

People will have different A1C targets, depending on their diabetes history and their general health. You should discuss your A1C target with your healthcare professional. Studies have shown that some people with diabetes can reduce the risk of diabetes complications by keeping A1C levels below seven percent.

Managing blood glucose early in the course of diabetes may provide benefits for many years to come. However, an A1C level that is safe for one person may not be safe for another. For example, keeping an A1C level below seven percent may not be safe if it leads to problems with hypoglycemia, also called low blood glucose.

Less strict blood glucose control, or an A1C between 7–8 percent— or even higher in some circumstances—may be appropriate in people who have:

- limited life expectancy

- long-standing diabetes and trouble reaching a lower goal

- severe hypoglycemia or inability to sense hypoglycemia (also called hypoglycemia unawareness)

- advanced diabetes complications such as chronic kidney disease (CKD), nerve problems, or cardiovascular disease

How Does A1C Relate to Estimated Average Glucose?

Estimated average glucose (eAG) is calculated from your A1C. Some laboratories report eAG with A1C test results. The eAG number helps you relate your A1C to daily glucose monitoring levels. The eAG calculation converts the A1C percentage to the same units used by home glucose meters—milligrams per deciliter (mg/dL).

The eAG number will not match daily glucose readings because it's a long-term average—rather than your blood glucose level at a single time, as is measured with a home glucose meter.

Will the A1C Test Show Short-Term Changes in Blood Glucose Levels?

Large changes in your blood glucose levels over the past month will show up in your A1C test result, but the A1C test doesn't show sudden, temporary increases or decreases in blood glucose levels. Even though

A1C results represent a long-term average, blood glucose levels within the past 30 days have a greater effect on the A1C reading than those in previous months.

Section 20.2

Ketone Testing

This section includes text excerpted from "Ketones in Urine," MedlinePlus, National Institutes of Health (NIH), September 22, 2017.

What Is a Ketones in Urine Test?

The test measures ketone levels in your urine. Normally, your body burns glucose (sugar) for energy. If your cells don't get enough glucose, your body burns fat for energy instead. This produces a substance called ketones, which can show up in your blood and urine. High ketone levels in urine may indicate diabetic ketoacidosis (DKA), a complication of diabetes that can lead to a coma or even death. Ketones in urine test can prompt you to get treatment before a medical emergency occurs.

This test is also known by names ketones urine test, ketone test, urine ketones, and ketone bodies.

What Is It Used For?

The test is often used to help monitor people at a higher risk of developing ketones. These include people with type 1 or type 2 diabetes. If you have diabetes, ketones in urine can mean that you are not getting enough insulin. If you don't have diabetes, you may still be at risk for developing ketones if you:

- experience chronic vomiting and/or diarrhea

- have a digestive disorder

- participate in strenuous exercise

- are on a very low-carbohydrate diet
- have an eating disorder
- are pregnant

Why Do You Need a Ketones in Urine Test?

Your healthcare provider may order a ketones in urine test if you have diabetes or other risk factors for developing ketones. You may also need this test if you have symptoms of ketoacidosis. These include:

- nausea or vomiting
- abdominal pain
- confusion
- trouble breathing
- feeling extremely sleepy

People with type 1 diabetes are at a higher risk for ketoacidosis.

What Happens during a Ketones in Urine Test?

instructions to provide a "clean catch" sample. The clean catch method generally includes the following seven steps:

- **Step 1.** Wash your hands.
- **Step 2.** Clean your genital area with a cleansing pad. Men should wipe the tip of their penis. women should open their labia and clean from front to back.
- **Step 3.** Start to urinate into the toilet.
- **Step 4.** Move the collection container under your urine stream.
- **Step 5.** Collect at least an ounce or two of urine into the container, which should have markings to indicate the amount.
- **Step 6.** Finish urinating into the toilet.
- **Step 7.** Return the sample container as instructed by your healthcare provider.

If you do the test at home, follow the instructions that are in your test kit. Your kit will include a package of strips for testing. You will either be instructed to provide a clean-catch sample in a container as described above or to put the test strip directly in the stream of your urine. Talk to your healthcare provider about specific instructions.

Will You Need to Do Anything to Prepare for the Test?

You may have to fast (not eat or drink) for a certain period of time before taking a ketones in urine test. Ask your healthcare provider if you need to fast or do any other type of preparation before your test.

Are There Any Risks to the Test?

There is no known risk to having a ketones in urine test.

What Do the Results Mean?

Your test results may be a specific number or listed as a "small," "moderate," or "large" amount of ketones. Normal results can vary, depending on your diet, activity level, and other factors. Because high ketone levels can be dangerous, be sure to talk to your healthcare provider about what is normal for you and what your results mean.

Is There Anything Else That You Need to Know about a Ketones in Urine Test?

Ketone test kits are available at most pharmacies without a prescription. If you are planning to test for ketones at home, ask your healthcare provider for recommendations on which kit would be best for you. At-home urine tests are easy to perform and can provide accurate results as long as you carefully follow all instructions.

Section 20.3

Recommended Vaccinations for Diabetes

This section contains text excerpted from the following sources:
Text in this section begins with excerpts from "Vaccine Information
for Adults—Diabetes Type 1 and Type 2 and Adult Vaccination,"
Centers for Disease Control and Prevention (CDC), May 2, 2016; Text
under the heading "Vaccines You Need" is excerpted from "Healthy
Living with Diabetes: Getting the Vaccines You Need," Centers for
Disease Control and Prevention (CDC), May 2018.

Each year thousands of adults in the United States get sick from
diseases that could be prevented by vaccines—some people are hospi-
talized, and some even die. People with diabetes (both type 1 and type
2) are at higher risk for serious problems from certain vaccine-pre-
ventable diseases. Getting vaccinated is an important step in staying
healthy. If you have diabetes, talk with your doctor about getting your
vaccinations up-to-date.

Why Vaccines Are Important for You

Diabetes, even if well managed, can make it harder for your immune
system to fight infections, so you may be at risk for more serious complications from an illness compared to people without diabetes.

- Some illnesses, like influenza, can raise your blood glucose to
  dangerously high levels

- People with diabetes have higher rates of hepatitis B than the
  rest of the population. Outbreaks of hepatitis B associated with
  blood glucose monitoring procedures have happened among
  people with diabetes.

- People with diabetes are at increased risk for death from
  pneumonia (lung infection), bacteremia (blood infection), and
  meningitis (infection of the lining of the brain and spinal
  cord).

Immunization provides the best protection against vaccine-pre-
ventable diseases.

Vaccines are one of the safest ways for you to protect your health,
even if you are taking prescription medications. Vaccine side effects
are usually mild and go away on their own. Severe side effects are
very rare.

Vaccines You Need

Influenza Vaccine

- Flu is a contagious respiratory illness caused by influenza viruses.

- People with diabetes are at high risk of serious flu complications, such as pneumonia, bronchitis, sinus infections, and ear infections, often resulting in hospitalization and sometimes, even death.

- A flu shot every year is the single best way to protect yourself from the flu.

Tdap Vaccine

- The Tdap vaccine protects against three serious diseases caused by bacteria:

- Tetanus causes painful muscle tightening and stiffness. It kills about 1 out of 10 people who are infected, even after receiving medical care.

- Diphtheria causes a thick coating to form in the back of the throat and can lead to breathing problems, heart failure, paralysis, and death.

- Pertussis (whooping cough) causes severe coughing spells, which can cause difficulty breathing, vomiting, and disturbed sleep.

CDC recommends all adults get the Tdap vaccine once, and a Td vaccine booster dose every 10 years, to protect against tetanus, diphtheria, and pertussis.

Zoster Vaccine

- Shingles is a painful rash caused by the same virus that causes chickenpox. After a person recovers from chickenpox, the virus stays in the body. Years later, it may cause shingles.

- For some people the pain can last for months or even years after the rash goes away—known as postherpetic neuralgia (PHN).

- Zoster vaccine reduces the risk of developing shingles and PHN in people who have been vaccinated.

Herpes zoster vaccine is approved for people age 50 years and older. CDC recommends vaccination. People with very weak immune systems should not get the zoster vaccine.

Pneumococcal Vaccine

- Pneumococcal disease is an infection caused by pneumococcus bacteria.

- People with diabetes are at increased risk for death from pneumococcal infections, which include pneumonia (lung infection), bacteremia (blood infection), meningitis (infection of the lining of the brain and spinal cord), and ear infections.

CDC recommends people with diabetes get pneumococcal vaccines once as an adult before 65 years of age and then two more doses at 65 years or older.

Hepatitis B Vaccine

- Hepatitis B is a liver infection caused by the hepatitis B virus (HBV) and transmitted through blood or other body fluid. Chronic hepatitis B can lead to serious health issues, such as cirrhosis or liver cancer.

- People with type 1 or type 2 diabetes have a higher risk of hepatitis B virus infection.

- Hepatitis B can be spread through sharing of blood sugar meters, finger stick devices, or other diabetes care equipment, such as insulin pens. To prevent hepatitis B infection, never share diabetes care equipment.

CDC recommends hepatitis B vaccination for all unvaccinated adults with diabetes who are younger than 60 years of age. Many people have had the hepatitis B vaccine as a child, so check with your doctor to see if you have been vaccinated already. If you are 60 years or older, talk to your doctor to see if you should get the hepatitis B vaccine.

Part Three

Medications and Diabetes Care

Chapter 21

Diabetes Medicines: What You Need to Know

Diabetes can make it hard to control how much sugar (called glucose) is in your blood.

There is hope! Some people with diabetes can take medicines to help keep their blood sugar at a healthy level. This chapter gives some basic facts about the medicines used to treat people with diabetes. Use this chapter to help you talk to your doctor, nurse, or pharmacist about the kind of medicine that is right for you.

Do not wait. Diabetes is a serious illness. Diabetes can cause a heart attack, stroke, blindness, kidney disease, nerve damage, and other serious health problems. This is why it is so important for you to get treatment for your diabetes. Treatment can help prevent or slow some of these serious health problems.

You can control your diabetes. There are a few kinds of medicines used to treat diabetes. Each kind affects your body in a different way. Some diabetes medicines are taken as pills that you swallow. There are other medicines that you inject. Some people with diabetes need to use medicines every day. What you need depends on your health and the type of diabetes you have. Your healthcare provider can tell you if you need to use medicine to treat your diabetes.

This chapter includes text excerpted from "Diabetes Medicines," U.S. Food and Drug Administration (FDA), February 19, 2015.

Do You Need to Take Diabetes Medicines?

Some people with diabetes need to use medicines every day. What you need depends on your health and the type of diabetes you have. Your doctor can tell you if you need to use medicine to treat your diabetes.

Type 1 Diabetes

People with type 1 diabetes make very little or no insulin in their bodies. They must take insulin every day to stay alive.

Type 2 Diabetes

People with type 2 diabetes do not make enough insulin or do not use it well enough. Some people with type 2 diabetes can use pills or other medicines that are injected into the body. Other people with type 2 diabetes need insulin to help control their diabetes.

Gestational Diabetes

Some women develop diabetes for the first time when they become pregnant. This is called gestational diabetes. Some women with gestational diabetes need to use insulin to control their blood sugar.

What You Can Do about Side Effects

Diabetes medicines affect each person differently. These medicines can sometimes cause side effects. The side effects will depend on your body and the type of medicine you are taking. Follow these tips to help you learn how to handle the side effects.

- **Get the facts.** Ask your healthcare provider for the side effects, warnings, and other facts for the medicines you are taking. This chapter does not give all facts for each kind of diabetes medicine.

- **Speak up.** Tell someone about any problems you may be having with your medicines. Your doctor may change your medicine or give you tips to help you deal with the side effects.

- **Check the U.S. Food and Drug Administration (FDA) website.** You can find up-to-date safety information about your medicine at report serious problems with your medicines. You or your doctor can tell the FDA about serious problems with your medicines. Call 800-FDA-1088 (800-332-1088) to request a form.

Diabetes Medicines

The different kinds of diabetes medicines are listed below. These medicines are most often used to treat type 2 diabetes. The brand names and other names are given for each drug. There are also some general tips about each kind of diabetes medicine. Ask your doctor, nurse, or pharmacist to tell you the side effects and warnings for the medicines you are taking.

Meglitinides

How Do They Work?

These pills help your body make more insulin around mealtime.

Table 21.1. Meglitinides

Brand Name	Other Name
Prandin	Repaglinide
Starlix	Nateglinide

Some Things to Think About

Before you start taking these medicines, tell your healthcare provider if:

- you have liver or kidney problems
- you are pregnant or breastfeeding

Common Side Effects

Hypoglycemia (blood sugar that is too low)

Alpha-Glucosidase Inhibitors

How Do They Work?

These pills help your body digest sugar more slowly.

Table 21.2. Alpha-Glucosidase Inhibitors

Brand Name	Other Name
Glyset	Miglitol
Precose	Acarbose

Some Things to Think About

Before you start taking these medicines, tell your healthcare provider if:

- you have heart, liver, or kidney problems

- you are pregnant or breastfeeding.

These medicines are not likely to cause low blood sugar or weight gain.
These pills help your body digest sugar more slowly.

Common Side Effects

- stomach pain

- diarrhea

- gas

- abnormal liver tests

Thiazolidinediones

How Do They Work?

These pills help the cells in your body use glucose.

Table 21.3. Thiazolidinediones

Brand Name	Other Name
Actos	Pioglitazone
Avandia	Rosiglitazone

Some Things to Think About

- Before you start taking these drugs, tell your doctor if you have heart failure.

- Before you take Actos, tell your doctor if you are a pre-menopausal woman (before the "change of life") who does not have periods regularly or at all. Actos may increase your chance of becoming pregnant. Talk to your doctor about birth control choices while taking Actos.

- These medicines may raise your chance of having a broken bone (fracture).

Common Side Effects

- fluid retention
- weight gain
- heart failure (heart cannot pump blood well)
- anemia (low red blood cell counts)
- upper respiratory tract infection

Dipeptidyl Peptidase-4 Inhibitors

How Do They Work?

These pills help your body release more insulin.

Table 21.4. DPP-4 Inhibitors

Brand Name	Other Name
Januvia	Sitagliptin
Onglyza Saxagliptin	Saxagliptin
Nesina	Alogliptin
Tradjenta	Linagliptin

Some Things to Think About

- Call your doctor right away if you have severe stomach pain or vomiting. This may be a sign of a serious side effect.

Common Side Effects

- upper respiratory infection (URI)
- headache

Sulfonylureas

How Do They Work?

These pills help your body make more insulin.

Table 21.5. Sulfonylureas

Brand Name	Other Name
Amaryl	Glimepiride

Table 21.5. Continued

Brand Name	Other Name
Diabeta Glynase	Glyburide
Diabinese	Chlorpropamide
Glucotrol, Glucotrol XL (extended release)	Glipizide
No brand name	Tolbutamide
No brand name	Tolazamide

Some Things to Think About

- Before you start taking these drugs, tell your doctor you have heart, liver, or kidney problems.

- Older adults and people with kidney or liver problems may be more likely to have low blood sugar when taking these medicines.

Common Side Effects

- hypoglycemia (blood sugar that is too low)

- weight gain

- headache

- dizziness

Biguanides

How Do They Work?

- These pills stop your liver from making too much sugar (glucose).

- They also help the sugar get into your cells.

Table 21.6. Biguanides

Brand Name	Other Name
Fortamet	Metformin
Glucophage	Metformin
Glucophage XR (long-lasting extended release)	Metformin
Glumetza	Metformin
Riomet	Metformin

Some Things to Think About

- Talk to your doctor about your kidney health before you start and while you are taking this type of medicine.

- These medicines are not likely to cause low blood sugar or weight gain.

- People who drink a lot of alcohol and people with kidney problems may have a rare side effect called lactic acidosis (acid buildup in the blood).

Common Side Effects

- diarrhea

- gas

- indigestion

- feeling weak

- nausea and vomiting

- headache

Dopamine Receptor Agonists

How Do They Work?

This pill affects a chemical called dopamine in your cells. It is not clear how this pill works for diabetes.

Table 21.7. Dopamine Receptor Agonists

Brand Name	Other Name
Cycloset	Bromocriptine

Some Things to Think About

- Do not take this medicine if you are breastfeeding.

Common Side Effects

- nausea

- headache

- feel very tired

- feel dizzy

- vomiting

Bile Acid Sequestrants

How Do They Work?

It is not clear how this pill works for diabetes.

Table 21.8. Bile Acid Sequestrants

Brand Name	Other Name
Welchol	Colesevelam

Some Things to Think About

- This medicine is also used to treat high cholesterol.

- Tell your doctor if you are taking other cholesterol medicines.

Common Side Effects

- constipation

- dyspepsia (upset stomach/indigestion)

- nausea

Sodium-Dependent Glucose Cotransporters (SGLT2) Inhibitors

How Do They Work?

These pills affect the kidney to increase the amount of sugar that goes out in the urine.

Table 21.9. Bile Acid Sequestrants

Brand Name	Other Name
Farxiga	Dapagliflozin
Invokana	Canagliflozin
Jardiance	Empagliflozin

Some Things to Think About

- Do not take these drugs if you have severe kidney problems or are on dialysis.

- Before you take these drugs, tell your doctor if you have kidney or liver problems.

Common Side Effects

- vaginal yeast infections

- urinary tract infections (UTI)

- changes in urination

Combination Medicines

These combinations are made up of two kinds of medicines. Ask your doctor for the facts about the combination drug you are taking.

Table 21.10. Combination Medicines

Brand Name	Other Name
ActoPlus Met	Pioglitazone and Metformin
ActoPlus Met XR (extended release)	Pioglitazone and Metformin
Avandamet	Rosiglitazone and Metformin
Avandaryl	Rosiglitazone and Glimepiride
Duetact	Pioglitazone and Glimepiride
Glucovance	Glyburide and Metformin
Invokamet	Canagliflozin and Metformin
Janumet	Sitagliptin and Metformin
Janumet XR (extended release)	Sitagliptin and Metformin
Kazano	Alogliptin and Metformin
Kombiglyze	Saxagliptin and Metformin
Kombiglyze XR (extended release)	Saxagliptin and Metformin
Metaglip	Glipizide and Metformin
Oseni	Alogliptin and Pioglitazone
PrandiMet	Repaglinide and Metformin
Xigduo XR	Dapagliflozin and Metformin

Glucagon-Like Peptide (GLP-1) Receptor Agonists

These are medicines that you inject under your skin. These medicines should not be used instead of insulin.

Table 21.11. GLP-1 Receptor Agonists

Brand Name	Other Name
Byetta	Exenatide
Bydureon	Exenatide
Tanzeum	Albiglutide
Trulicity	Dulaglutide
Victoza	Liraglutide

Some Things to Think About

- These medicines are not the same as insulin.

- Some people feel nauseous when they first start taking these medicines.

Amylin Analog

This is a medicine that you inject under your skin. This medicine should not be used instead of insulin.

Table 21.12. Amylin Analog

Brand Name	Other Name
Symlin	Pramlintide Acetate

Some Things to Think About

- People who use insulin can also use Symlin.

- People with type 1 diabetes can use Symlin.

- Symlin should be taken in a separate injection. Do not mix Symlin and insulin in the same injection.

- This medicine is usually taken before meals.

- Some people feel nauseous when they first start taking this medicine.

Write down the facts about your diabetes medicines the next time you talk to your doctor, nurse, or diabetes educator.

- How will my medicines affect my blood sugar?
- Will it affect my other medicines?
- What are the side effects?
- What do I do if I start having side effects?
- What should I do if I am pregnant, planning to get pregnant, or breastfeeding?
- What else should I know about my diabetes medicines?

You Can Control Your Diabetes

- **Make a plan.** Work with your doctor, nurse, or diabetes educator to plan how you will manage your diabetes.
- **Use medicines wisely.** Ask your healthcare provider when and how to safely use your diabetes medicines.
- **Check your blood sugar.** Use your glucose meter to test your blood glucose (sugar) level.
- **Watch what you eat.** Work with your healthcare team to come up with a meal plan just for you.
- **Be active and get exercise.** Dance, take a walk, or join an exercise class. Check with your doctor about safe ways to be more active.
- **Monitor your overall mental and physical health.** Work with your healthcare team to keep your feet, eyes, heart, and teeth healthy.

Chapter 22

Guide to Insulin

Insulin helps to take the sugar in your blood to other parts of your body. Diabetes affects how your body makes or uses insulin. Diabetes can make it hard to control how much sugar is in your blood.

There is hope! There are different kinds of insulin that people with diabetes can use every day to help them stay healthy. This chapter gives some basic facts about insulin.

Do not wait. Diabetes is a serious illness. Diabetes can cause a heart attack, stroke, blindness, kidney disease, nerve damage, and other serious health problems. This is why it is so important for you to get treatment for your diabetes. Treatment can help prevent or slow some of these serious health problems. Exercise, eat a balanced diet, and take your diabetes medicines. You can do it.

Your Insulin Guide

Ask your healthcare provider these questions before you start using your insulin.

- How often should I use my insulin?
- Can you show me the right way to inject the insulin?
- Will the insulin affect my other medicines? What about my birth control?

This chapter includes text excerpted from "Insulin," U.S. Food and Drug Administration (FDA), February 16, 2018.

- What are the side effects? What do I do if I start having side effects?

- What is my target blood sugar level?

- How often should I check my blood sugar?

- What should I do if I am pregnant, planning to get pregnant, or breastfeeding?

- How should I store my insulin?

Type 1 Diabetes

People with type 1 diabetes make very little or no insulin in their bodies. They must take insulin every day to stay alive.

Type 2 Diabetes

People with type 2 diabetes do not make enough insulin or do not use it well enough. Some people with type 2 diabetes can use pills or other medicines that are injected into the body. Other people with type 2 also need insulin to help control their diabetes.

Gestational Diabetes

Some women develop diabetes for the first time when they become pregnant. This is called gestational diabetes. Some women with gestational diabetes need to use insulin to control their blood sugar.

How Often Should You Inject Insulin?

Each person is different. Some people need to inject insulin one time each day. Others need to inject insulin more often. Many things affect how much insulin you need each day:

- type of insulin you use

- what you eat

- your activity level

- your other health conditions

Your doctor will tell you how often you should inject your insulin.

Types of Insulin

There are many different types of insulin. The type lets you know how fast the insulin starts working or how long it lasts in your body. Your healthcare provider will help you find the insulin that is best for you.

- **Rapid-acting.** This insulin starts working within 15 minutes after you use it. It is mostly gone out of your body after a few hours. It should be taken just before or just after you eat.

- **Short-acting.** This insulin starts working within 30 minutes to 1 hour after you use it. It is mostly gone out of your body after a few hours. It should be taken 30–45 minutes before you eat.

- **Intermediate-acting.** This insulin starts working within 2–4 hours after you use it. It reaches its highest level in your blood around 6–8 hours after you use it. It is often used to help control your blood sugar between meals. Some people use this type of insulin in the morning, at bedtime, or both.

- **Long-acting.** This insulin starts working within 2–4 hours after you use it. It can last in the body for up to 24 hours. It is often used in the morning or at bedtime to help control your blood sugar throughout the day.

- **Premixed.** This is a mix of two different types of insulin. It includes one type that helps to control your blood sugar at meals and another type that helps between meals.

Table 22.1. Types of Insulin

Brand Name	Other Names	Type of Insulin (How Fast Insulin Works)
Afrezza (inhalation powder)	Insulin Human	Rapid Acting
Apidra Apidra Solostar	Insulin Glulisine	Rapid Acting
Humalog Humalog Pen Humalog Kwikpen	Insulin Lispro	Rapid Acting
Novolog	Insulin Aspart	Rapid Acting
Humulin R Humulin R Pen	Regular Human Insulin	Short Acting

Table 22.1. Continued

Brand Name	Other Names	Type of Insulin (How Fast Insulin Works)
Novolin R	Regular Human Insulin	Short Acting
Humulin N	NPH Human Insulin (Human Insulin Isophane Suspension)	Intermediate Acting
Novolin N	NPH Human Insulin (Human Insulin Isophane Suspension)	Intermediate Acting
Lantus	Insulin Glargine	Long Acting
Levemir	Insulin Detemir	Long Acting
Toujeo	Insulin Glargine	Long Acting
Tresiba	Insulin Analog	Long Acting
Humalog Mix 75/25 Humalog Mix 75/25 Pen	75% Insulin Lispro Protamine Suspension 25% Insulin Lispro Injection	Intermediate and Rapid Acting
Humalog Mix 50/50 Humalog Mix 50/50 Pen	50% Insulin Lispro Protamine Suspension 50% Insulin Lispro Injection	Intermediate and Rapid Acting
Humulin 70/30 Humulin 70/30 Pen	70% NPH Human Insulin 30% Regular Human Insulin Injection	Intermediate and Short Acting
NovoLog Mix 70/30 NovoLog Mix 70/30 FlexPen	70% Insulin Aspart Protamine Suspension 30% Insulin Aspart Injection	Intermediate and Rapid Acting
Novolin 70/30	70% NPH Human Insulin 30% Regular Human Insulin Injection	Intermediate and Short Acting
Ryzodeg 70/30	70% Insulin Degludec 30% Insulin Aspart	Long and Rapid Acting

Insulin Side Effects

Insulin affects each person differently. Insulin can sometimes cause side effects. The side effects will depend on your body and the type of insulin you are taking. Follow these tips to help you learn how to handle side effects.

- **Get the facts.** Ask your healthcare provider for the side effects, warnings, and other facts for your insulin. This chapter does not give all facts for each kind of insulin.

- **Speak up.** Tell someone about any problems you may be having with your insulin. Your doctor may change your prescription or give you tips to help you deal with the side effects.

- **Keep yourself updated.** Check the U.S. Food and Drug Administration (FDA) website. You can find up-to-date safety information about your insulin at: www.fda.gov.

- **Report serious problems with your insulin or device.** You or your doctor can tell the FDA about serious problems with your medicines.

Insulin Safety Tips

For insulin safety follow the tips given below:

- Never drink insulin.

- Do not share insulin needles, pens, or cartridges with anyone else.

- Talk to your doctor before you change or stop using your insulin.

- Do not inject your insulin in the exact same spot each time.

- Throw away needles in a hard container that can be closed like a laundry detergent bottle.

- Check the expiration date on the insulin before you use it.

- Make a plan about how to handle your insulin when you travel and during an emergency.

You Can Control Your Diabetes

- **Make a plan.** Work with your doctor, nurse, or diabetes educator to plan how you will manage your diabetes.

- **Check your blood sugar.** Use your glucose meter to test your blood glucose (sugar) level.

- **Watch what you eat.** Work with your healthcare team to come up with a meal plan just for you.

- **Use medicines wisely.** Ask your healthcare provider when and how to safely use your diabetes medicines.

- **Be active and get exercise.** Dance, take a walk, or join an exercise class. Check with your doctor about safe ways to be more active.

- **Monitor your overall mental and physical health.** Work with your healthcare team to keep your feet, eyes, heart, and teeth healthy.

Chapter 23

Different Ways to Take Insulin

What Are the Different Ways to Take Insulin?

The way you take insulin may depend on your lifestyle, insurance plan, and preferences. You may decide that needles are not for you and prefer a different method. Talk to your doctor about the options and which is best for you. Most people with diabetes use a needle and syringe, pen, or insulin pump. Inhalers, injection ports, and jet injectors are less common.

Needle and Syringe

You'll give yourself insulin shots using a needle and syringe. You will draw up your dose of insulin from the vial, or bottle, into the syringe. Insulin works fastest when you inject it into your belly, but you should rotate spots where you inject insulin. Other injection spots include your thigh, buttocks, or upper arm. Some people with diabetes who take insulin need 2–4 shots a day to reach their blood glucose targets. Others can take a single shot.

This chapter contains text excerpted from the following sources: Text under the heading "What Are the Different Ways to Take Insulin?" is excerpted from "Insulin, Medicines, and Other Diabetes Treatments," National Institute of Diabetes and Digestive and Kidney Diseases (NIDDK), November 2016; Text under the heading "Tips for Insulin Devices" is excerpted from "Insulin," U.S. Food and Drug Administration (FDA), February 16, 2018.

Pen

An insulin pen looks like a pen but has a needle for its point. Some insulin pens come filled with insulin and are disposable. Others have room for an insulin cartridge that you insert and then replace after use. Insulin pens cost more than needles and syringes but many people find them easier to use.

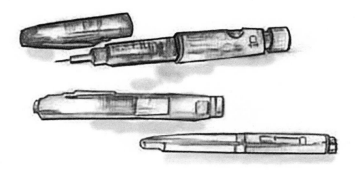

Figure 23.1. *Insulin Pens* (Source: "Alternative Devices for Taking Insulin," National Institute of Diabetes and Digestive and Kidney Diseases (NIDDK).)

Pump

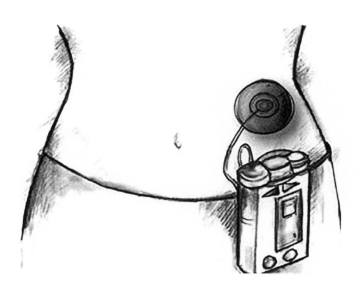

Figure 23.2. *Insulin Pump* (Source: "Alternative Devices for Taking Insulin," National Institute of Diabetes and Digestive and Kidney Diseases (NIDDK).)

An insulin pump is a small machine that gives you small, steady doses of insulin throughout the day. You wear one type of pump outside your body on a belt or in a pocket or pouch. The insulin pump connects to a small plastic tube and a very small needle. You insert the needle under your skin and it stays in place for several days. Insulin then pumps from the machine through the tube into your body 24 hours a day. You also can give yourself doses of insulin through the pump at mealtimes. Another type of pump has no tubes and attaches directly to your skin, such as a self-adhesive pod.

Inhaler

Another way to take insulin is by breathing powdered insulin from an inhaler device into your mouth. The insulin goes into your lungs and moves quickly into your blood. Inhaled insulin is only for adults with type 1 or type 2 diabetes.

Injection Port

An injection port has a short tube that you insert into the tissue beneath your skin. On the skin's surface, an adhesive patch or dressing holds the port in place. You inject insulin through the port with a needle and syringe or an insulin pen. The port stays in place for a few days, and then you replace the port. With an injection port, you no longer puncture your skin for each shot—only when you apply a new port.

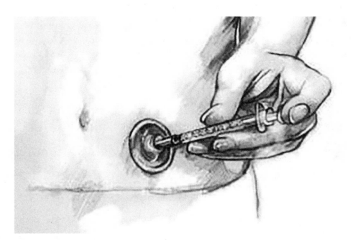

Figure 23.3. *Injection Port* (Source: "Alternative Devices for Taking Insulin," National Institute of Diabetes and Digestive and Kidney Diseases (NIDDK).)

Jet Injector

This device sends a fine spray of insulin into the skin at high pressure instead of using a needle to deliver the insulin.

Tips for Insulin Devices

Each insulin device is different. Find below a list some basic tips about insulin devices. Talk to your healthcare provider to learn everything you should know about your insulin device.

General Tips

- Never share insulin needles (syringes) or devices.

- Ask your doctor or nurse to show you how to inject your insulin.

- Always wash your hands before you inject your insulin.

- Do not inject your insulin in the exact same spot on your body each time.

  - The skin may get thick or thin if you use the same spot.

  - Inject in the same general area of your body.

- Do not use your insulin if it looks cloudy or looks like something is floating in it. Take it back to the drug store for a new one.

- Do not use insulin needles (syringes), pens, and injectors after the expiration date printed on the label or on the box.

How to Throw Away Used Devices

- Follow the directions on when to throw away the needles, pens or injectors.

- You should throw away your used needles in a hard container like an empty laundry detergent bottle or a metal coffee can.

  - Make sure the needles cannot poke through the container.

  - Put a label on the container to warn people that it is dangerous.

  - Keep the container where children cannot get to it.

  - Always put a lid or top on the container.

Chapter 24

New Diabetes Drugs

Chapter Contents

Section 24.1

Adlyxin (Lixisenatide)

This section includes text excerpted from "FDA Approves
Adlyxin to Treat Type 2 Diabetes," U.S. Food and
Drug Administration (FDA), July 28, 2016.

The U.S. Food and Drug Administration (FDA) approved Adlyxin
(lixisenatide), a once-daily injection to improve glycemic control
(blood sugar levels), along with diet and exercise, in adults with type
2 diabetes.

"The FDA continues to support the development of new drug therapies for diabetes management," said Mary Thanh Hai Parks, M.D.,
deputy director, Office of Drug Evaluation (ODE) II in the FDA's Center for Drug Evaluation and Research (CDER). "Adlyxin will add to
the available treatment options to control blood sugar levels for those
with type 2."

Type 2 diabetes affects more than 29 million people and accounts
for more than 90 percent of diabetes cases diagnosed in the United
States. Over time, high blood sugar levels can increase the risk for
serious complications, including heart disease, blindness and nerve
and kidney damage.

Adlyxin is a glucagon-like peptide-1 (GLP-1) receptor agonist, a
hormone that helps normalize blood sugar levels. The drug's safety and
effectiveness were evaluated in 10 clinical trials that enrolled 5,400
patients with type 2 diabetes. In these trials, Adlyxin was evaluated
both as a standalone therapy and in combination with other FDA-approved diabetic medications, including metformin, sulfonylureas, pioglitazone and basal insulin. Use of Adlyxin improved hemoglobin A1c
levels (a measure of blood sugar levels) in these trials.

In addition, more than 6,000 patients with type 2 diabetes at risk for
atherosclerotic cardiovascular disease were treated with either Adlyxin
or a placebo in a cardiovascular outcomes trial. Use of Adlyxin did not
increase the risk of cardiovascular adverse events in these patients.

Adlyxin should not be used to treat people with type 1 diabetes
or patients with increased ketones in their blood or urine (diabetic
ketoacidosis).

The most common side effects associated with Adlyxin are nausea,
vomiting, headache, diarrhea, and dizziness. Hypoglycemia in patients
treated with both Adlyxin and other antidiabetic drugs such as sulfonylurea and/or basal insulin is another common side effect.

Section 24.2

Admelog (Insulin Lispro Injection)

This section includes text excerpted from "FDA Approves Admelog, the First Short-Acting 'Follow-On' Insulin Product to Treat Diabetes," U.S. Food and Drug Administration (FDA), December 11, 2017.

The U.S. Food and Drug Administration (FDA) approved Admelog (insulin lispro injection), a short-acting insulin indicated to improve control in blood sugar levels in adults and pediatric patients aged 3 years and older with type 1 diabetes mellitus and adults with type 2 diabetes mellitus. Admelog is the first short-acting insulin approved as a "follow-on" product (submitted through the agency's 505(b)(2) pathway).

According to the Centers for Disease Control and Prevention (CDC), more than 30 million people in the United States have diabetes, a chronic disease that affects how the body turns food into energy and the body's production of natural insulin. Over time, diabetes increases the risk of serious health complications, including heart disease, blindness, and nerve and kidney damage. Improvement in blood sugar control through treatment with insulin, a common treatment, can reduce the risk of some of these long-term complications.

"One of my key policy efforts is increasing competition in the market for prescription drugs and helping facilitate the entry of lower-cost alternatives. This is particularly important for drugs like insulin that are taken by millions of Americans every day for a patient's lifetime to manage a chronic disease," said FDA Commissioner Scott Gottlieb, M.D. "In the coming months, we'll be taking additional policy steps to help to make sure patients continue to benefit from improved access to lower cost, safe and effective alternatives to brand-name drugs approved through the agency's abbreviated pathways."

Admelog was approved through an abbreviated approval pathway under the Federal Food, Drug, and Cosmetic Act (FD&C Act), called the 505(b)(2) pathway. A new drug application submitted through this pathway may rely on the FDA's finding that a previously approved drug is safe and effective or on published literature to support the safety and/or effectiveness of the proposed product, if such reliance is scientifically justified. The use of abbreviated pathways can reduce drug development costs so products can be offered at a lower price to patients. In the case of Admelog, the manufacturer submitted a 505(b)(2) application that relied, in part, on the FDA's finding of safety and effectiveness for Humalog (insulin lispro injection) to support approval. The applicant demonstrated that reliance on the FDA's finding of safety and effectiveness for Humalog was scientifically justified and provided Admelog-specific data to establish the drug's safety and efficacy for its approved uses. The Admelog-specific data included two phase 3 clinical trials which enrolled approximately 500 patients in each.

Admelog is a short-acting insulin product, which can be used to help patients with diabetes control their blood sugar. Short-acting insulin products are generally, but not always, administered just before meals to help control blood sugar levels after eating. These types of insulin products can also be used in insulin pumps to meet both background insulin needs as well as mealtime insulin needs. This is in contrast to long-acting insulin products, like insulin glargine, insulin degludec, and insulin detemir, which are generally used to provide a background level of insulin to control blood sugars between meals, and are administered once or twice a day. While both types of insulin products can play important roles in the treatment of types 1 and 2 diabetes mellitus, patients with type 1 diabetes require both types of insulin while patients with type 2 diabetes may never need a short-acting insulin product.

"With today's approval, we are providing an important short-acting insulin option for patients that meets our standards for safety and effectiveness," said Mary T. Thanh Hai, M.D., deputy director of the Office of New Drug (OND) Evaluation II in the FDA's Center for Drug Evaluation and Research (CDER).

Admelog can be administered by injection under the skin (subcutaneous), subcutaneous infusion (i.e., via insulin pump), or intravenous infusion. Dosing of Admelog should be individualized based on the route of administration and the patient's metabolic needs, blood glucose monitoring results and glycemic control goal.

The most common adverse reactions associated with Admelog in clinical trials was hypoglycemia, itching, and rash. Other adverse reactions that can occur with Admelog include allergic reactions, injection site reactions, and thickening or thinning of the fatty tissue at the injection site (lipodystrophy).

Admelog should not be used during episodes of hypoglycemia (low blood sugar) or in patients with hypersensitivity to insulin lispro or one of its ingredients. Admelog SoloStar prefilled pens or syringes must never be shared between patients, even if the needle is changed.

Patients or caregivers should monitor blood glucose in all patients treated with insulin products. Insulin regimens should be modified cautiously and only under medical supervision. Admelog may cause low blood sugar (hypoglycemia), which can be life-threatening. Patients should be monitored more closely with changes to insulin dosage, coadministration of other glucose-lowering medications, meal pattern, physical activity and in patients with renal impairment or hepatic impairment or hypoglycemia unawareness.

Accidental mix-ups between insulin products can occur. Patients should check insulin labels before injecting the insulin product.

Severe, life-threatening, generalized allergic reactions, including anaphylaxis, may occur.

Healthcare providers should monitor potassium levels in patients at risk of hyperkalemia, a serious and potentially life-threatening condition in which the amount of potassium in the blood is too low.

Admelog received tentative approval from the FDA on September 1, 2017, and is now being granted final approval.

The approval of Admelog was granted to Sanofi-Aventis U.S.

Chapter 25

Aspirin Therapy for Diabetics

How Is Diabetes Linked with Cardiovascular Disease and Stroke?

Diabetes is one of the major risk factors for cardiovascular disease (CVD) and stroke. Diabetes—type 2 diabetes, in particular—increases blood glucose level and can lead to hypertension, high cholesterol, and obesity. These conditions eventually increase the chances of developing CVD and stroke. Hence, a person with diabetes may encounter cardiovascular events at a relatively young age and the severity may also be high.

The CVD that develops in people with diabetes is called diabetic heart disease (DHD) and it includes:

- Coronary heart disease (CHD)

- Heart failure

- Diabetic cardiomyopathy

CVD is the cause of a high premature mortality rate in people with diabetes. According to the American Heart Association (AHA), adults with diabetes are two to four times more likely to die from CVD than those who do not have diabetes.

"Aspirin Therapy for Diabetics," © 2018 Omnigraphics. Reviewed September 2018.

Aspirin, and How Aspirin Therapy Is Helpful

Aspirin is a pharmaceutical drug that is widely used to prevent and treat CVD and stroke. CVD or stroke usually occur when the blood flow to the heart or brain gets blocked due to plaque formation. Plaque is a waxy substance made up of fat, cholesterol, calcium, cellular wastes, and so on, that builds up in the blood vessels or arteries. The condition in which the plaques build up in the inner lining of the arteries is called atherosclerosis. When these plaques rupture, blood clots occur and the blood flow is blocked. If the block occurs in the arteries carrying blood to the heart, then it causes a heart attack. If the block occurs in the arteries carrying blood to the brain, then it causes a stroke.

Aspirin blocks the secretion of an enzyme called cyclooxygenase, which is responsible for the inflammation of plaques. It also stops the chemicals that trigger the formation of blood clots. Low doses of aspirin, when taken every day, can be effective in preventing the damage to the heart and decrease the risk of stroke. Therefore, doctors recommend aspirin therapy for people with diabetes who are at an increased risk for CVD and stroke.

How Much Aspirin Should Be Taken?

Adults with diabetes with an increased risk of CVD and stroke are usually prescribed low doses of aspirin ranging from 75–162 mg. daily. This is less than half of the standard 325 mg. aspirin. A lower dosage of aspirin is considered safer since a higher dosage may sometimes lead to adverse side effects. Aspirin therapy should be undertaken only under the guidance of a doctor. Check with your doctor to find out which dosage is right for you.

What Are the Side Effects of Aspirin Therapy?

Since aspirin tends to prevent clotting action of the blood, aspirin therapy can be dangerous for people with bleeding or clotting disorders. Even low doses of aspirin may increase bleeding episodes. The major risks and side effects of aspirin therapy include:

- Gastrointestinal hemorrhage
- Stomach ulcers and abdominal bleeding
- Bleeding in the brain during stroke
- Blood in the urine and stool
- Nosebleeds

- Heavy bleeding from cuts and wounds
- Excessive menstrual bleeding in women
- Nausea and vomiting
- Stomach upset
- Headache

Who Should Not Take Aspirin?

Since aspirin can cause several complications, it is always a good idea to check with your doctor before beginning aspirin therapy. Whether diabetic or not, the following people should avoid aspirin therapy.

- People with anemia or renal disease
- People with ulcers
- People with aspirin allergy or hypersensitivity
- Pregnant women (unless prescribed by the doctor)
- Heavy alcohol drinkers
- People about to undergo surgery or dental procedures
- Children below the age of 18 who are recovering from viral infections

What Are Alternate Ways to Stay Healthy without Aspirin?

If you are a person with diabetes and if you wish to stay away from CVD and stroke without undergoing aspirin therapy, a few tips you could follow are:

- **Stay active:** Regular exercise and an active lifestyle can strengthen the heart muscles and reduce the risk of developing CVD.
- **Proper diet:** Limit the intake of salt in your diet to decrease your chances of developing hypertension. Avoid foods that contain saturated fat to reduce cholesterol levels and obesity.
- **Quit smoking:** Smoking is another important risk factor that causes CVD and stroke. Smoking also makes treatment of

diabetes more difficult. Hence, cessation of smoking can reduce the additional risks linked to diabetes.

References

1. "Diabetic Heart Disease," National Heart, Lung, and Blood Institute (NHLBI), March 12, 2013.

2. "Cardiovascular Disease and Diabetes," American Heart Association (AMA), August 30, 2015.

3. "Should You Take Aspirin For Heart Disease?" WebMD, April 26, 2018.

4. "Updated Recommendations on Aspirin Therapy in Diabetic Patients," Diabetes in Control, January 23, 2014.

5. "Should Aspirin Be Included in Your Diabetes Treatment Plan?" Everyday Health, November 15, 2017.

Chapter 26

Alternative and Complementary Therapies for Diabetes

Diabetes is a disease that occurs when your blood glucose, also called blood sugar, is too high. Over time, having too much glucose in your blood can cause health problems. About 9.4 percent of the people in the United States have diabetes, but about one in four people who have diabetes don't know it.

Although diabetes has no cure, people with diabetes can take steps to manage their condition and stay healthy. Taking insulin or other diabetes medicines is often part of treating diabetes, along with healthy food choices and physical activity.

The most common type of diabetes is type 2 diabetes, in which your body does not make or use insulin well. This type of diabetes occurs most often in middle-aged and older people, but it can develop at any age, even in childhood.

You are more likely to develop type 2 diabetes if you are 45 years old or older, have a family history of diabetes, or are overweight. Physical inactivity, race, certain health problems such as high blood pressure, having prediabetes, or having had gestational diabetes while pregnant also affect your likelihood of developing type 2 diabetes.

This chapter includes text excerpted from "Diabetes and Dietary Supplements," National Center for Complementary and Integrative Health (NCCIH), May 2018.

What the Science Says about the Effectiveness and Safety of Dietary Supplements for Diabetes

Alpha-Lipoic Acid

Alpha-lipoic acid (ALA) is being studied for its effect on complications of diabetes, including diabetic macular edema (an eye condition that can cause vision loss) and diabetic neuropathy (nerve damage caused by diabetes).

- In a 2011 study of 235 people with type 2 diabetes, 2 years of supplementation with alpha-lipoic acid did not help to prevent macular edema.

- A 2016 assessment of treatments for symptoms of diabetic neuropathy that included two studies of oral alpha-lipoic acid, with a total of 205 participants, indicated that alpha-lipoic acid may be helpful.

Safety

High doses of alpha-lipoic acid supplements can cause stomach problems.

Chromium

Found in many foods, chromium is an essential trace mineral. If you have too little chromium in your diet, your body can't use glucose efficiently.

- Taking chromium supplements, along with conventional care, slightly improved blood sugar control in people with diabetes (primarily type 2) who had poor blood sugar control, a 2014 review concluded. The review included 25 studies with about 1,600 participants.

Safety

Chromium supplements may cause stomach pain and bloating, and there have been a few reports of kidney damage, muscular problems, and skin reactions following large doses. The effects of taking chromium long term haven't been well investigated.

Herbal Supplements

There is no reliable evidence that any herbal supplements can help to control diabetes or its complications.

- There are no clear benefits of cinnamon for people with diabetes

- Other herbal supplements studied for diabetes include bitter melon, various Chinese herbal medicines, fenugreek, ginseng, milk thistle, and sweet potato. Studies haven't proven that any of these are effective, and some may have side effects.

Safety

- There is little conclusive information on the safety of herbal supplements for people with diabetes.

- Cassia cinnamon, the most common type of cinnamon sold in the United States and Canada, contains varying amounts of a chemical called coumarin, which might cause or worsen liver disease. In most cases, cassia cinnamon doesn't have enough coumarin to make you sick. However, for some people, such as those with liver disease, taking a large amount of cassia cinnamon might worsen their condition.

- Using herbs such as St. John's wort, prickly pear cactus, aloe, or ginseng with conventional diabetes drugs can cause unwanted side effects.

Magnesium

Found in many foods, including in high amounts in bran cereal, certain seeds and nuts, and spinach, magnesium is essential to the body's ability to process glucose.

- Magnesium deficiency may increase the risk of developing diabetes. A number of studies have looked at whether taking magnesium supplements helps people who have diabetes or who are at risk of developing it. However, the studies are generally small and their results aren't conclusive.

Safety

Large doses of magnesium in supplements can cause diarrhea and abdominal cramping. Very large doses—more than 5,000 mg per day—can be deadly

Omega-3s

Taking omega-3 fatty acid supplements, such as fish oil, hasn't been shown to help people who have diabetes control their blood sugar levels or reduce their risk of heart disease.

Fish and other seafood, especially cold-water fatty fish such as salmon and tuna contain omega-3 fatty acids. Studies on the effects of eating fish have had conflicting results, according to two 2012 research reviews with hundreds of thousands of participants, and a 2017 review. Some research from the United States and Europe found that people who ate more fish had a higher incidence of diabetes. Research from Asia and Australia found the opposite—eating more fish was associated with a lower risk of diabetes. There's no strong evidence explaining these differences.

Safety

Omega-3 supplements don't usually have side effects. When side effects do occur, they typically consist of minor symptoms, such as bad breath, indigestion, or diarrhea. It may interact with drugs that affect blood clotting.

Selenium

An assessment of four studies involving more than 20,000 total participants found that selenium supplementation did not reduce the likelihood that people would develop type 2 diabetes.

Safety

Long-term intake of too much selenium can have harmful effects, including hair and nail loss, gastrointestinal symptoms, and nervous system abnormalities

Vitamins

Studies generally show that taking vitamin C doesn't improve blood sugar control or other conditions in people with diabetes. However, a 2017 research review of 22 studies with 937 participants found weak evidence that vitamin C helps with blood sugar in people with type 2 diabetes when they took it for longer than 30 days.

Having low levels of vitamin D is associated with an increased risk of developing a metabolic disorder, such as type 2 diabetes, metabolic syndrome, or insulin resistance, studies and research reviews have found. However, taking vitamin D doesn't appear to help prevent diabetes or improve blood sugar levels for adults with normal levels, prediabetes, or type 2 diabetes, a 2014 research review of 35 studies with 43,407 participants showed.

Safety

Taking too much vitamin D can cause nausea, constipation, weakness, kidney damage, disorientation, and problems with your heart rhythm. You're unlikely to get too much vitamin D from food or the sun.

Other Supplements

The evidence is still very preliminary on how supplements or foods rich in polyphenols—antioxidants found in tea, coffee, wine, fruits, grains, and vegetables—might affect diabetes.

Nutrition and Physical Activity for People with Diabetes

Nutrition and physical activity are important parts of a healthy lifestyle for people with diabetes. Eating well and being physically active can help you

- keep your blood glucose level, blood pressure, and cholesterol in your target ranges;

- lose weight or stay at a healthy weight;

- prevent or delay diabetes problems; and

- feel good and have more energy.

Chapter 27

Beware of Diabetes Treatment Fraud

As the number of people diagnosed with diabetes continues to grow, illegally marketed products promising to prevent, treat, and even cure diabetes are flooding the marketplace.

The U.S. Food and Drug Administration (FDA) is advising consumers not to use such products—for many reasons. For example, they may contain harmful ingredients or may improperly be marketed as over-the-counter (OTC) products when they should be marketed as prescription products. Illegally marketed products carry an additional risk if they cause people to delay or discontinue effective treatments for diabetes. Without proper disease management, people with diabetes are at a greater risk for developing serious health complications.

More than 30 million people in the United States have diabetes, and one out of four don't know they have it, according to the Centers for Disease Control and Prevention (CDC). Millions more have prediabetes, meaning they have higher than normal blood sugar levels and can reduce their risks of developing diabetes through healthy lifestyle changes, including diet and exercise.

"People with chronic or incurable diseases may feel desperate and become easy targets. Bogus products for diabetes are particularly troubling because there are effective options available to help manage this serious disease rather than exposing patients to unproven and

This chapter includes text excerpted from "Beware of Illegally Marketed Diabetes Treatments," U.S. Food and Drug Administration (FDA), November 15, 2017.

unreasonably risky products," said Jason Humbert, a captain with the U.S. Public Health Service (PHS) who is with FDA's Office of Regulatory Affairs (ORA). "Failure to follow well-established treatment plans can lead to, among other things, amputations, kidney disease, blindness, and death."

To protect the public health, the FDA surveys the marketplace for illegally marketed products promising to treat diabetes and its complications, and investigates consumer complaints.

Unapproved Diabetes Drugs

The FDA has issued warning letters to various companies that market products for diabetes in violation of federal law. These products were marketed as dietary supplements; alternative medicines, such as ayurvedic medicines; prescription drugs; OTC drugs; and homeopathic products. Some of the companies also promoted the same unapproved drugs for other serious diseases, including cancer, sexually transmitted diseases (STDs), and macular degeneration.

FDA laboratory analysis has found "all-natural" products for diabetes to contain undeclared active ingredients found in approved prescription drugs intended for treatment of diabetes. Undeclared active ingredients can cause serious harm. If consumers and their healthcare professionals are unaware of the actual active ingredients in the products they are taking, these products may interact in dangerous ways with other medications. One possible complication: Patients may end up taking a larger combined dose of the diabetic drugs than they intended. This may cause a significant and unsafe drop in blood sugar levels, a condition known as hypoglycemia.

The FDA also looks at illegal marketing of prescription drugs by fraudulent online pharmacies. Signs that may indicate an online pharmacy is legitimate include: requiring that patients have a valid prescription, providing a physical address in the United States, being licensed by a state pharmacy board, and providing a state-licensed pharmacist to answer questions.

Some fraudulent online pharmacies illegally market drugs that are not approved in the United States, or sell otherwise approved prescription drug products without meeting necessary requirements. Although some of these websites may offer for sale what appear to be FDA-approved prescription drugs, the FDA cannot be certain that the manufacture or the handling of these drugs follows U.S. regulations or that the drugs are safe and effective for their intended uses. Also, there is a risk the drugs may be counterfeit, contaminated, expired, or otherwise unsafe.

Sound Too Good to Be True?

Then it's probably a scam. Watch out for these and similar red flags:

- "Lowers your blood sugar naturally!"
- "Inexpensive therapy to fight and eliminate type II diabetes!"
- "Protects your eyes, kidneys, and blood vessels from damage!"
- "Replaces your diabetes medicine!"
- "Effective treatment to relieve all symptoms of diabetes!"
- "Natural diabetes cure!"

A Far-Reaching Problem

"Products that promise an easy fix might be alluring, but consumers are gambling with their health. In general, diabetes is a chronic disease, but it is manageable. And people can lower their risk for developing complications by following treatments prescribed by healthcare professionals, carefully monitoring blood sugar levels, and sticking to an appropriate diet and exercise program," Humbert said.

Healthcare professionals and consumers should report any problems or reactions—often referred to as potential adverse reactions—to the FDA's MedWatch program at www.fda.gov/Medwatch/report.htm. Or, you can call 800-FDA-1088 (800-332-1088), send a fax to 800-FDA-0178 (800-332-0178), or e-mail FDA form 3500 (available on the MedWatch "Download Forms" page (www.fda.gov/Safety/MedWatch/HowToReport/DownloadForms/default.htm)) to the address on the preaddressed form.

Part Four

Dietary and Other Lifestyle Issues Important for Diabetes Control

Chapter 28

Diabetes Meal Planning

Chapter Contents

Section 28.1

Healthy Eating with Diabetes

This section includes text excerpted from "Eat-Well!"
Centers for Disease Control and Prevention (CDC),
May 17, 2018.

When you have diabetes, deciding what, when, and how much to eat may seem challenging. So, what can you eat, and how can you fit the foods you love into your meal plan? Eating healthy food at home and choosing healthy food when eating out are important in managing your diabetes.

The first step is to work with your doctor or dietitian to make a meal plan just for you. As soon as you find out you have diabetes, ask for a meeting with your doctor or dietitian to discuss how to make and follow a meal plan. During this meeting, you will learn how to choose healthier foods—a variety of vegetables and fruits, whole grains, fat-free or low-fat dairy foods, lean meats, and other proteins. You will also learn to watch your portion sizes and what to drink while staying within your calorie, fat, and carbohydrate (carbs) limits.

You can still enjoy food while eating healthily. But how do you do that? Here are a few tips to help you when eating at home and away from home.

Eating Healthy Portions

An easy way to know portion sizes is to use the "plate method."

• Fill the largest section with nonstarchy vegetables, like salad, green beans, broccoli, cauliflower, cabbage, and carrots.

• In one of the smaller sections, put a grain or starchy food such as bread, noodles, rice, corn, or potatoes.

• In the other smaller section, put your protein, like fish, chicken, lean beef, tofu, or cooked dried beans.

Eating Out

American adults eat out at least three times a week on average. Restaurant portion sizes and how foods are prepared will affect the management of your diabetes. How can you eat out, manage your diabetes, and follow your meal plan? Here are some ideas.

- Talk to the server before you order. Don't be shy about asking questions about the food and, if it is not obvious, ask how foods are prepared.

- Choose meat or fish dishes that are baked, broiled, grilled, or poached instead of fried.

- If you see that portions are large, ask your server at the beginning of the meal to box half of your meal to-go and only serve the other half.

- Look at the menu for meals that are lower in fat or calories; many restaurants will mark healthier items.

- Remember that sugar-sweetened drinks can be a major source of calories. For low-calorie options, drink water, low-fat milk, unsweetened tea, black coffee, or diet drinks.

- If you drink alcohol, women should have no more than one drink per day. Men should have no more than two drinks per day. Avoid high-calorie mixed drinks.

- Skip dessert or share one with a friend. Or choose fruit for dessert. It will save calories and money!

Eating from a buffet presents its own challenges for people with diabetes.

Grocery Shopping

When you go grocery shopping, you are surrounded by foods and drinks that have a lot of fat, sugar, and salt. Avoid impulse buying; make a checklist of foods in your meal plan before you shop to help you focus on healthy foods for you and your family. Here are a few things to keep in mind.

- Your cart should look like the plate method outlined above.

- Half of your food items should be nonstarchy vegetables like lettuce, asparagus, broccoli, cauliflower, cucumber, spinach, mushrooms, onions, and peppers.

- The rest of the cart should have lean proteins, whole grains, fruit, dairy, beans, and starchy vegetables such as corn, peas, parsnips, potatoes, pumpkin, squash, zucchini, and yams.

- You may be able to have a treat occasionally (check with your dietitian, if unsure). Instead of treats high in calories, fat, and sugar, consider buying a healthier option such as fruit as a treat.

Try to stay in the outside aisles where stores usually have fruits, vegetables, meat, fish, and dairy. Spend less time in the inside aisles.

Nutrition Facts	
2 servings per container	
Serving size 1 1/2 cup (208g)	
Amount per serving	
Calories	**240**
	% Daily Value*
Total Fat 4g	**5%**
Saturated Fat 1.5g	**8%**
Trans Fat 0g	
Cholesterol 5mg	**2%**
Sodium 430mg	**19%**
Total Carbohydrate 46g	**17%**
Dietary Fiber 7g	**25%**
Total Sugars 4g	
Includes 2g Added Sugars	**4%**
Protein 11g	
Vitamin D 2mcg	10%
Calcium 260mg	20%
Iron 6mg	35%
Potassium 240mg	6%

* The % Daily Value (DV) tells you how much a nutrient in a serving of food contributes to a daily diet. 2,000 calories a day is used for general nutrition advice.

Figure 28.1. *Nutrition Facts Label*

Checking Labels on Packaged Foods

One way to make sure you are buying packaged foods that are lower in calories, sugar, and fat is to look at the updated Nutrition Facts label. Here is some advice on the information you will find on the label:

- Look at serving size first. It gives you important information for understanding the rest of the label. On the label pictured here, all the other numbers are for a 1½ cup serving. So, a 1½ cup of this food has 240 calories and 4 grams of total fat.

- The top of the label also lists how many servings are in a package. For example, this label is for a package with two servings. If you eat the whole package, you'll have eaten twice as many calories, carbs, fats, and other nutrients as are listed on the label.

- Total carbohydrate on the label includes all types of carbs— sugar, starch, and fiber.

- Choose foods with lower calories, saturated fat, trans fat, added sugars, and sodium. These numbers are listed near the top of the label.

- Try to choose foods with more dietary fiber, which is listed lower on the label under total carbohydrates.

Getting Help from Family and Friends

Remember, eating healthily is not just for people with diabetes. Healthy foods benefit everyone in your family and can help prevent those who don't have the disease from developing it.

- Talk to friends and family about diabetes. Thank them for being concerned about you.

- Ask your family to support your efforts to manage the disease by providing healthy options in regular meal planning and at special occasions.

- Teach them what you've learned about foods and how foods affect you. Tell them you have to choose when, what, and how much to eat.

Section 28.2

Meal Plan Methods

This section contains text excerpted from the following
sources: Text in this section begins with excerpts from "Diabetes
Diet, Eating, and Physical Activity," National Institute of Diabetes
and Digestive and Kidney Diseases (NIDDK), November 2016; Text
under the heading "How Can Carbohydrate Counting Help Me?" is
excerpted from "Carbohydrate Counting and Diabetes," National
Institute of Diabetes and Digestive and Kidney Diseases (NIDDK),
June 2014. Reviewed September 2018.

Two common ways to help you plan how much to eat if you have
diabetes are the plate method and carbohydrate counting, also called
carb counting. Check with your healthcare team about the method
that's best for you.

Plate Method

The plate method helps you control your portion sizes. You don't
need to count calories. The plate method shows the amount of each
food group you should eat. This method works best for lunch and
dinner.

Use a nine-inch plate. Put nonstarchy vegetables on half of the
plate; a meat or other protein on one-fourth of the plate; and a grain or
other starch on the last one-fourth. Starches include starchy vegetables
such as corn and peas. You also may eat a small bowl of fruit or a piece
of fruit, and drink a small glass of milk as included in your meal plan.

Your daily eating plan also may include small snacks between
meals.

Portion Sizes

You can use everyday objects or your hand to judge the size of a
portion:

- One serving of meat or poultry is the palm of your hand or a
  deck of cards.

- One three-ounce serving of fish is a checkbook.

- One serving of cheese is six dice.

- Half a cup of cooked rice or pasta is a rounded handful or a
  tennis ball.

- One serving of a pancake or waffle is a DVD.

- Two tablespoons of peanut butter is a ping-pong ball.

Carbohydrate Counting

Carbohydrate counting involves keeping track of the amount of carbohydrates you eat and drink each day. Because carbohydrates turn into glucose in your body, they affect your blood glucose level more than other foods do. Carb counting can help you manage your blood glucose level. If you take insulin, counting carbohydrates can help you know how much insulin to take.

The right amount of carbohydrates varies by how you manage your diabetes, including how physically active you are and what medicines you take, if any. Your healthcare team can help you create a personal eating plan based on carbohydrate counting.

The amount of carbohydrates in foods is measured in grams. To count carbohydrate grams in what you eat, you'll need to:

- learn which foods have carbohydrates

- read the Nutrition Facts food label, or learn to estimate the number of grams of carbohydrate in the foods you eat

- add the grams of carbohydrate from each food you eat to get your total for each meal and for the day

Most carbohydrates come from starches, fruits, milk, and sweets. Try to limit carbohydrates with added sugars or those with refined grains, such as white bread and white rice. Instead, eat carbohydrates from fruit, vegetables, whole grains, beans, and low-fat or nonfat milk.

How Can Carbohydrate Counting Help Me?

Carbohydrate counting can help keep your blood glucose levels close to normal. Keeping your blood glucose levels as close to normal as possible may help you:

- stay healthy longer

- prevent or delay diabetes problems such as kidney disease, blindness, nerve damage, and blood vessel disease that can lead to heart attacks, strokes, and amputations—surgery to remove a body part

- feel better and more energetic

You may also need to take diabetes medicines or have insulin shots to control your blood glucose levels. Discuss your blood glucose targets with your doctor. Targets are numbers you aim for. To meet your targets, you will need to balance your carbohydrate intake with physical activity and diabetes medicines or insulin shots.

Section 28.3

Exchange Lists

This section includes text excerpted from "Food Exchange Lists," National Heart, Lung, and Blood Institute (NHLBI), May 10, 2005. Reviewed September 2018.

You can use the American Dietetic Association food exchange lists to check out serving sizes for each group of foods and to see what other food choices are available for each group of foods.

Vegetables contain 25 calories and 5 grams of carbohydrate. One serving equals:

Measurement	Ingredient
½ C	Cooked vegetables (carrots, broccoli, zucchini, cabbage, etc.)
1 C	Raw vegetables or salad greens
½ C	Vegetable juice

If you're hungry, eat more fresh or steamed vegetables.

Fat-Free and Very Low-Fat Milk contain 90 calories per serving. One serving equals:

Measurement	Ingredient
1 C	Milk, fat-free or 1% fat
¾ C	Yogurt, plain, nonfat, or low-fat
1 C	Yogurt, artificially sweetened

Very Lean Protein choices have 35 calories and 1 gram of fat per serving. One serving equals:

Measurement	Ingredient
1 oz.	Turkey breast or chicken breast, skin removed
1 oz.	Fish fillet (flounder, sole, scrod, cod, etc.)
1 oz.	Canned tuna in water
1 oz.	Shellfish (clams, lobster, scallop, shrimp)
¾ C	Cottage cheese, nonfat or low-fat
2	Egg whites
¼ C	Egg substitute
1 oz.	Fat-free cheese
½ C	Beans, cooked (black beans, kidney, chickpeas or lentils): count as 1 starch/bread and 1 very lean protein

Fruits contain 15 grams of carbohydrate and 60 calories. One serving equals:

Measurement	Ingredient
1 small	Apple, banana, orange, nectarine
1 med.	Fresh peach
1	Kiwi
½	Grapefruit
½	Mango
1 C	Fresh berries (strawberries, raspberries, or blueberries)
1 C	Fresh melon cubes
⅛ C	Honeydew melon
4 oz.	Unsweetened juice
4 tsp.	Jelly or jam

Lean Protein choices have 55 calories and 2–3 grams of fat per serving. One serving equals:

Measurement	Ingredient
1 oz.	Chicken—dark meat, skin removed
1 oz.	Turkey—dark meat, skin removed
1 oz.	Salmon, swordfish, herring
1 oz.	Lean beef (flank steak, London broil, tenderloin, roast beef)*
1 oz.	Veal, roast or lean chop*
1 oz.	Lamb, roast or lean chop*

1 oz.	Pork, tenderloin or fresh ham*
1 oz.	Low-fat cheese (with 3 grams or less of fat per ounce)
1 oz.	Low-fat luncheon meats (with 3 grams or less of fat per ounce)
¼ C	4.5% cottage cheese
2 med.	Sardines

Limit to 1–2 times per week

Medium-Fat Proteins have 75 calories and 5 grams of fat per serving. One serving equals:

Measurement	Ingredient
1 oz.	Beef (any prime cut), corned beef, ground beef**
1 oz.	Pork chop
1	Whole egg (medium)**
1 oz.	Mozzarella cheese
¼ C	Ricotta cheese
4 oz.	Tofu (note this is a heart-healthy choice)

** *Choose these very infrequently*

Starches contain 15 grams of carbohydrate and 80 calories per serving. One serving equals:

Measurement	Ingredient
1 slice	Bread (white, pumpernickel, whole wheat, rye)
2 slices	Reduced-calorie or "lite" bread
¼ (1 oz.)	Bagel (varies)
½ C	English muffin
½ C	Hamburger bun
¾ C	Cold cereal
1/3 C	Rice, brown or white, cooked
1/3 C	Barley or couscous, cooked
1/3 C	Legumes (dried beans, peas or lentils), cooked
½ C	Pasta, cooked
½ C	Bulgar, cooked
½ C	Corn, sweet potato, or green peas
3 oz.	Baked sweet or white potato
¾ oz.	Pretzels
3 C	Popcorn, hot air popped or microwave (80% light)

Fats contain 45 calories and 5 grams of fat per serving. One serving equals:

Measurement	Ingredient
1 tsp.	Oil (vegetable, corn, canola, olive, etc.)
1 tsp.	Butter
1 tsp.	Stick margarine
1 tsp.	Mayonnaise
1 Tbsp.	Reduced-fat margarine or mayonnaise
1 Tbsp.	Salad dressing
1 Tbsp.	Cream cheese
2 Tbsp.	Lite cream cheese
1/8 C	Avocado
8 large	Black olives
10 large	Stuffed green olives
1 slice	Bacon

Chapter 29

Alcohol and Tobacco Can Increase Diabetes Problems

Chapter Contents

Section 29.1

Alcohol and Diabetes: A Dangerous Mix

This section includes text excerpted from "Diabetes, Drinking,
and Smoking: A Dangerous Combination," U.S.
Department of Veterans Affairs (VA), April 27, 2017.

A healthy lifestyle can help control diabetes. For instance, regular
physical activity and a good diet play a big role in managing the disease. But unhealthy habits, such as smoking and drinking too much
alcohol, can make diabetes and its complications worse.

Everything in Moderation

Consuming alcohol when you have diabetes poses another danger
to your health. For instance, if you take insulin or diabetes medicine
by mouth, too much alcohol may lower your blood sugar for up to 12
hours after drinking, especially if you drink on an empty stomach or
increase your physical activity.

"When you drink too much, your liver stops every other job it does,
including making blood sugar, to work on getting rid of the alcohol,
which it sees as a toxin," said Dr. Sharon Watts, a Nurse Practitioner
and Certified Diabetes Educator for the VA. "People think too much
alcohol will increase their blood sugar, but actually the opposite is
true."

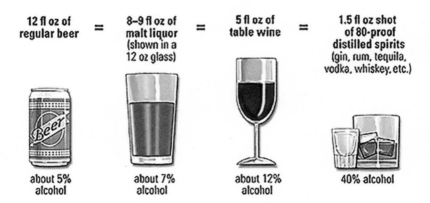

Figure 29.1. *Standard Drink* (Source: "Alcohol Overdose: The Dangers of
Drinking Too Much," National Institute on Alcohol Abuse and Alcoholism
(NIAAA).)

Alcohol can also worsen nerve pain caused by diabetes and cause weight gain. Being obese or overweight can cause diabetes or make it worse if you already have it.

If you drink and have diabetes, do it in moderation. For a man, moderate drinking is up to two drinks per day; for a woman, one drink. A drink is a 12-ounce beer, 5-ounce glass of wine, or 1.5 ounces of distilled spirits (such as vodka, gin, or rum).

If you have diabetes and plan to drink:

- Always eat some form of carbohydrate with your drink, such as crackers, bread, or pretzels.

- Avoid sweet wines, drinks, and liqueurs.

- Check your blood sugar more often.

- Always have a ready source of sugar on hand, such as pieces of hard candy.

- Talk to your healthcare provider.

- Always carry identification that says that you have diabetes.

Section 29.2

Smoking and Diabetes

This section includes text excerpted from "Smoking and Diabetes," Centers for Disease Control and Prevention (CDC), March 22, 2018.

How Is Smoking Related to Diabetes?

We now know that smoking causes type 2 diabetes. In fact, smokers are 30–40 percent more likely to develop type 2 diabetes than nonsmokers. And people with diabetes who smoke are more likely than nonsmokers to have trouble with insulin dosing and with controlling their disease. The more cigarettes you smoke, the higher your risk for type 2 diabetes. No matter what type of diabetes you have, smoking makes your diabetes harder to control. If you have diabetes and you smoke, you are more likely to have serious health problems from diabetes. Smokers with diabetes have higher risks for serious complications, including:

- Heart and kidney disease

- Poor blood flow in the legs and feet that can lead to infections, ulcers, and possible amputation (removal of a body part by surgery, such as toes or feet)

- Retinopathy (an eye disease that can cause blindness)

- Peripheral neuropathy (damaged nerves to the arms and legs that causes numbness, pain, weakness, and poor coordination)

If you are a smoker with diabetes, quitting smoking will benefit your health right away. People with diabetes who quit have better control of their blood sugar levels. For free help to quit, call 800-QUIT NOW (800-784-8669).

How Can Diabetes Be Prevented?

Don't smoke. Smoking increases your chance of having type 2 diabetes.

Lose weight. If you are overweight or obese, lose weight.

Stay active. Physical activity can prevent or delay type 2 diabetes in adults who are at high risk for the disease.

Chapter 30

Physical Activity and Diabetes

Why Should You Be Physically Active If You Have Diabetes?

Physical activity is an important part of managing your blood glucose level and staying healthy. Being active has many health benefits. Physical activity

- lowers blood glucose levels;

- lowers blood pressure;

- improves blood flow;

- burns extra calories so you can keep your weight down if needed;

- improves your mood;

- can prevent falls and improve memory in older adults; and

- may help you sleep better.

If you are overweight, combining physical activity with a reduced-calorie eating plan can lead to even more benefits. In the Look AHEAD: Action for Health in Diabetes study, overweight adults with type 2

This chapter includes text excerpted from "Diabetes Diet, Eating, and Physical Activity," National Institute of Diabetes and Digestive and Kidney Diseases (NIDDK), November 2016.

diabetes who ate less and moved more had greater long-term health benefits compared to those who didn't make these changes. These benefits included improved cholesterol levels, less sleep apnea, and being able to move around more easily.

Even small amounts of physical activity can help. Experts suggest that you aim for at least 30 minutes of moderate or vigorous physical activity five days of the week. Moderate activity feels somewhat hard, and vigorous activity is intense and feels hard. If you want to lose weight or maintain weight loss, you may need to do 60 minutes or more of physical activity five days of the week.

Be patient. It may take a few weeks of physical activity before you see changes in your health.

How Can You Be Physically Active Safely If You Have Diabetes?

Be sure to drink water before, during, and after exercise to stay well hydrated. The following are some other tips for safe physical activity when you have diabetes.

Plan Ahead

Talk with your healthcare team before you start a new physical activity routine, especially if you have other health problems. Your healthcare team will tell you a target range for your blood glucose level and suggest how you can be active safely.

Your healthcare team also can help you decide the best time of day for you to do physical activity based on your daily schedule, meal plan, and diabetes medicines. If you take insulin, you need to balance the activity that you do with your insulin doses and meals so you don't get low blood glucose.

Prevent Low Blood Glucose

Because physical activity lowers your blood glucose, you should protect yourself against low blood glucose levels (BGL), also called hypoglycemia. You are most likely to have hypoglycemia if you take insulin or certain other diabetes medicines, such as a sulfonylurea. Hypoglycemia also can occur after a long intense workout or if you have skipped a meal before being active. Hypoglycemia can happen during or up to 24 hours after physical activity.

Planning is key to preventing hypoglycemia. For instance, if you take insulin, your healthcare provider might suggest you take less insulin or eat a small snack with carbohydrates before, during, or after physical activity, especially intense activity.

You may need to check your blood glucose level before, during, and right after you are physically active.

Stay Safe When Blood Glucose Is High

If you have type 1 diabetes, avoid vigorous physical activity when you have ketones in your blood or urine. Ketones are chemicals your body might make when your blood glucose level is too high, a condition called hyperglycemia, and your insulin level is too low. If you are physically active when you have ketones in your blood or urine, your blood glucose level may go even higher. Ask your healthcare team what level of ketones are dangerous for you and how to test for them. Ketones are uncommon in people with type 2 diabetes.

Take Care of Your Feet

People with diabetes may have problems with their feet because of poor blood flow and nerve damage that can result from high blood glucose levels. To help prevent foot problems, you should wear comfortable, supportive shoes and take care of your feet before, during, and after physical activity.

What Physical Activities Should You Do If You Have Diabetes?

- Most kinds of physical activity can help you take care of your diabetes. Certain activities may be unsafe for some people, such as those with low vision or nerve damage to their feet. Ask your healthcare team what physical activities are safe for you. Many people choose walking with friends or family members for their activity.

- Doing different types of physical activity each week will give you the most health benefits. Mixing it up also helps reduce boredom and lower your chance of getting hurt. Try these options for physical activity.

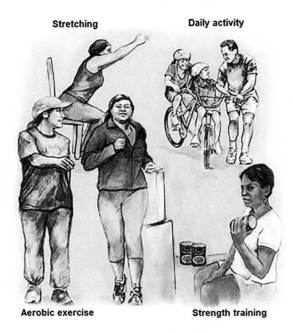

Figure 30.1. *Four Kinds of Physical Activities for People with Diabetes* (Source: "Be Active When You Have Diabetes," National Institute of Diabetes and Digestive and Kidney Diseases (NIDDK).)

Add Extra Activity to Your Daily Routine

If you have been inactive or you are trying a new activity, start slowly, with 5–10 minutes a day. Then add a little more time each week. Increase daily activity by spending less time in front of a television (TV) or other screens. Try these simple ways to add physical activities in your life each day:

- Walk around while you talk on the phone, or during TV commercials.

- Do chores, such as work in the garden, rake leaves, clean the house, or wash the car.

- Park at the far end of the shopping center parking lot and walk to the store.

- Take the stairs instead of the elevator.

- Make your family outings active, such as a family bike ride or a walk in a park.

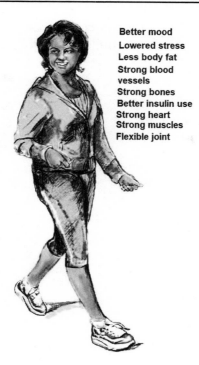

Better mood
Lowered stress
Less body fat
Strong blood vessels
Strong bones
Better insulin use
Strong heart
Strong muscles
Flexible joint

Figure 30.2. *Benefits of Regular Physical Activities for People with Diabetes* (Source: "Be Active When You Have Diabetes," National Institute of Diabetes and Digestive and Kidney Diseases (NIDDK).)

- If you are sitting for a long time, such as working at a desk or watching TV, do some light activity for three minutes or more every half hour. Light activities include:
  - leg lifts or extensions
  - overhead arm stretches
  - desk chair swivels
  - torso twists
  - side lunges
  - walking in place

Do Aerobic Exercise

Aerobic exercise is an activity that makes your heart beat faster and makes you breathe harder. You should aim for doing aerobic exercise

199

for 30 minutes a day most days of the week. You do not have to do all the activity at one time. You can split up these minutes into a few times throughout the day.

To get the most out of your activity, exercise at a moderate to vigorous level. Try:

- walking briskly or hiking

- climbing stairs

- swimming or a water aerobics class

- dancing

- riding a bicycle or a stationary bicycle

- taking an exercise class

- playing basketball, tennis, or other sports

Talk with your healthcare team about how to warm up and cool down before and after you exercise.

Do Strength Training to Build Muscle

Strength training is a light or moderate physical activity that builds muscle and helps keep your bones healthy. Strength training is important for both men and women. When you have more muscle and less body fat, you'll burn more calories. Burning more calories can help you lose and keep off extra weight.

You can do strength training with hand weights, elastic bands, or weight machines. Try to do strength training two to three times a week. Start with a light-weight. Slowly increase the size of your weights as your muscles become stronger.

Do Stretching Exercises

Stretching exercises are light or moderate physical activity. When you stretch, you increase your flexibility, lower your stress, and help prevent sore muscles.

You can choose from many types of stretching exercises. Yoga is a type of stretching that focuses on your breathing and helps you relax. Even if you have problems moving or balancing, certain types of yoga can help. For instance, chair yoga has stretches you can do when sitting in a chair or holding onto a chair while standing. Your healthcare team can suggest whether yoga is right for you.

Chapter 31

Weight Management and Diabetes

Overweight and obesity may increase the risk of many health problems, including diabetes, heart disease, and certain cancers. If you are pregnant, excess weight may lead to short- and long-term health problems for you and your child.

This chapter tells you more about the links between excess weight and many health conditions. It also explains how reaching and maintaining a normal weight may help you and your loved ones stay healthier as you grow older.

What Kinds of Health Problems Are Linked to Overweight and Obesity?

Excess weight may increase the risk for many health problems, including:

- type 2 diabetes

- high blood pressure

- heart disease and strokes

- certain types of cancer

This chapter includes text excerpted from "Health Risks of Being Overweight," National Institute of Diabetes and Digestive and Kidney Diseases (NIDDK), February 2015.

- sleep apnea

- osteoarthritis (OA)

- fatty liver disease

- kidney disease

- pregnancy problems, such as high blood sugar during pregnancy, high blood pressure, and increased risk for cesarean delivery (C-section)

How Is Type 2 Diabetes Linked to Being Overweight?

More than 87 percent of adults with diabetes are overweight or obese. It isn't clear why people who are overweight are more likely to develop this disease. It may be that being overweight causes cells to change, making them resistant to the hormone insulin. Insulin carries sugar from blood to the cells, where it is used for energy. When a person is insulin resistant, blood sugar cannot be taken up by the cells, resulting in high blood sugar. In addition, the cells that produce insulin must work extra hard to try to keep blood sugar normal. This may cause these cells to gradually fail.

How Can Weight-Loss Help?

If you are at risk for type 2 diabetes, losing weight may help prevent or delay the onset of diabetes. If you have type 2 diabetes, losing weight and becoming more physically active can help you control your blood sugar levels and prevent or delay health problems. Losing weight and exercising more may also allow you to reduce the amount of diabetes medicine you take.

How Much Weight Loss May Prevent or Delay Diabetes?

The National Institutes of Health (NIH) sponsored a large clinical study named the Diabetes Prevention Program (DPP) to look at ways to prevent type 2 diabetes in adults who were overweight.

The DPP found that losing just 5–7 percent of your body weight and doing moderately intense exercise (like brisk walking) for 150 minutes a week may prevent or delay the onset of type 2 diabetes.

How Can You Lower Your Risk of Having Health Problems Related to Being Overweight and Obese?

If you are considered to be overweight, losing as little as five percent of your body weight may lower your risk for several diseases, including heart disease and type 2 diabetes. If you weigh 200 pounds, this means losing 10 pounds. Slow and steady weight loss of 1/2–2 pounds per week, and not more than three pounds per week, is the safest way to lose weight.

Federal guidelines on physical activity recommend that you get at least 150 minutes a week of moderate aerobic activity (like biking or brisk walking). To lose weight, or to maintain weight loss, you may need to be active for up to 300 minutes per week. You also need to do activities to strengthen muscles (like push-ups or sit-ups) at least twice a week.

Federal dietary guidelines (FDG) and the MyPlate website recommend many tips for healthy eating that may also help you control your weight. Here are a few examples:

• Make half of your plate fruits and vegetables.

• Replace unrefined grains (white bread, pasta, white rice) with whole-grain options (whole wheat bread, brown rice, oatmeal).

• Enjoy lean sources of protein, such as lean meats, seafood, beans and peas, soy, nuts, and seeds.

For some people who have obesity and related health problems, bariatric (weight-loss) surgery may be an option. Bariatric surgery has been found to be effective in promoting weight loss and reducing the risk for many health problems.

Chapter 32

Diabetes and Daily Challenges

Chapter Contents

Section 32.1

Driving

This section includes text excerpted from "Driving
When You Have Diabetes," National Highway Traffic
Safety Administration (NHTSA), January 6, 2015.

You have been a safe driver for years. For you, driving means freedom and control. As you get older, changes in your body and your mind can affect how safely you drive. When you have diabetes, your body is unable to keep your blood sugar (glucose) levels in your normal range. This means your levels may be too high or too low. But you may not recognize early symptoms of this disease. Without proper treatment, diabetes can make it harder for you to drive safely.

How Can Diabetes Affect the Way You Drive?

Diabetes can make you:

- feel sleepy or dizzy
- feel tired or irritable
- feel confused or disoriented
- have blurry vision
- lose consciousness
- have a seizure

Uncontrolled diabetes also can cause nerve damage. This will make it hard for you to feel your legs, feet, hands, or arms. You may not be able to press the brake pedal fast enough to avoid a crash. In severe cases, diabetes can even cause blindness or result in amputation.

What Should You Do If You Have Any of These Signs?

The first thing you should do is talk with your family and your healthcare provider. Together, you can find the best treatment plan that will allow you to continue to drive safely.

Do not drive if your blood sugar (glucose) level is dangerously low, a condition called hypoglycemia.

- Low blood sugar can make it hard to make good choices, focus on your driving, or control your car. Work with your healthcare provider to figure out when and how often you should check your blood sugar level before you drive.

- Always keep your blood glucose testing meter and plenty of snacks with you. As soon as you feel any signs that your blood sugar has dropped, pull your car over and check your level. If your blood glucose level is too low, eat or drink a snack that contains sugar, such as juice, soda (not diet), hard candy, or sugar tablets. Wait 15 minutes, and then check your level again. If it is in your normal range, eat a nourishing snack or meal that contains protein.

- Do not start driving again until your blood sugar has returned to your normal level.

- If you have hypoglycemia but do not have any warning signs, do not drive. Talk with your healthcare provider.

Do not drive if your blood sugar (glucose) level is dangerously high, a condition called hyperglycemia.

- If you had very high glucose levels in the past, talk with your healthcare provider. Your provider can determine when and how your high levels can affect your ability to drive safely.

- Very high blood sugar can prevent you from thinking clearly and making sound judgments.

- Hyperglycemia can cause a seizure.

Diabetes Can Cause Eye Problems

Diabetes also can cause eye problems. To help prevent these problems:

- control your blood glucose levels

- control your blood pressure (BP)

- take care of your eyes

- get a yearly eye examination

What Can You Do When Diabetes Affects Your Driving Safety?

It is important to know how diabetes is changing your driving safety. If you have long-term complications of diabetes, such as vision or sensation problems, or if you have had an amputation, two types of specialists can help you:

- A driver rehabilitation specialist can test how well you drive on and off the road. This specialist also can help you decide when you need to stop driving. To find a driver rehabilitation specialist, go to www.aota.org/olderdriver.

- An occupational therapist with special training in driving skills assessment and remediation. To find an occupational therapist in your area, contact local hospitals and rehabilitation facilities.

What Can You Do If You Have to Limit or Stop Driving?

Even if you have to limit or give up driving, you can stay active and do the things you like to do. First, plan ahead. Talk with family and friends about how you can shift from driver to passenger. Below are some ways to get where you want to go and see the people you want to see:

- Rides with family and friends
- Taxis
- Shuttle buses or vans
- Public buses, trains, and subways
- Walking
- Paratransit services (special transportation services for people with disabilities). Some offer door-to-door service.

Take someone with you. You may want to have a family member or friend go with you when you use public transportation or when you walk. Having someone with you can help you get where you want to go without confusion.

Find out about transportation services in your area. Some areas offer low-cost bus or taxi service for older people. Many community-based volunteer programs offer free or low-cost transportation.

Where Can You Get Help with Transportation?

To find transportation services in your area, visit www.eldercare. gov or call the national ElderCare Locator at 800-677-1116, and ask for your local Office on Aging. If you have a disability, check out Easter Seals Project ACTION at www.projectaction.org, or call 800-659-6428. This project works with the transportation industry and the disability community to give people with disabilities more ways to get around.

Section 32.2

Eating Out

This section includes text excerpted from "Food Safety for People with Diabetes," U.S. Food and Drug Administration (FDA), June 22, 2018.

Food Safety: It's Especially Important for You

As a person with diabetes, you are not alone—there are many people in the United States with this chronic disease. Diabetes can affect various organs and systems of your body, causing them not to function properly, and making you more susceptible to infection. For example:

- Your immune system, when functioning properly, readily fights off harmful bacteria and other pathogens that cause infection. With diabetes, your immune system may not readily recognize harmful bacteria or other pathogens. This delay in the body's natural response to foreign invasion places a person with diabetes at increased risk for infection.

- Your gastrointestinal tract, when functioning properly, allows the foods and beverages you consume to be digested normally. Diabetes may damage the cells that create stomach acid and the nerves that help your stomach and intestinal tract move the food throughout the intestinal tract. Because of this damage, your stomach may hold on to the food and beverages you consume for a longer period of time, allowing harmful bacteria and other pathogens to grow.

- Additionally, your kidneys, which work to cleanse the body, may not be functioning properly and may hold on to harmful bacteria, toxins, and other pathogens.

- A consequence of having diabetes is that it may leave you more susceptible to developing infections—like those that can be brought on by disease-causing bacteria and other pathogens that cause foodborne illness. Should you contract a foodborne illness, you are more likely to have a lengthier illness, undergo hospitalization, or even die.

- To avoid contracting a foodborne illness, you must be vigilant when handling, preparing, and consuming foods.

Make safe handling a lifelong commitment to minimize your risk of foodborne illness. Be aware that as you age, your immunity to infection naturally is weakened.

Being Smart When Eating Out

Eating out can be lots of fun—so make it an enjoyable experience by following some simple guidelines to avoid foodborne illness. Remember to observe your food when it is served, and don't ever hesitate to ask questions before you order. Waiters and waitresses can be quite helpful if you ask how a food is prepared. Also, let them know you don't want any food item containing raw meat, poultry, seafood, sprouts, or eggs.

- Ask whether the food contains uncooked ingredients such as eggs, sprouts, meat, poultry, or seafood. If so, choose something else.

- Ask how these foods have been cooked. If the server does not know the answer, ask to speak to the chef to be sure your food has been cooked to a safe minimum internal temperature.

- If you plan to get a "doggy bag" or save leftovers to eat at a later time, refrigerate perishable foods as soon as possible— and always within two hours after purchase or delivery. If the leftover is in air temperatures above 90°F, refrigerate within 1 hour.

If in doubt, make another selection!

Table 32.1. Smart Menu Choices

Higher Risk	Lower Risk
Soft cheese made from unpasteurized (raw) milk	Hard or processed cheeses. Soft cheeses only if they are made from pasteurized milk

Table 32.1. Continued

Higher Risk	Lower Risk
Refrigerated smoked seafood and raw or undercooked seafood	Fully cooked fish or seafood
Cold or improperly heated hot dogs	Hot dogs reheated to steaming hot. If the hot dogs are served cold or lukewarm, ask to have them reheated until steaming, or choose something else
Sandwiches with cold deli or luncheon meat	Grilled sandwiches in which the meat or poultry is heated until steaming
Raw or undercooked fish, such as sashimi, nonvegetarian sushi or ceviche	Fully cooked fish that is firm and flaky
Soft-boiled or "over-easy" eggs, as the yolks are not fully cooked	Fully cooked eggs with firm yolk and whites
Salads, wraps, or sandwiches containing raw (uncooked) or lightly cooked sprouts	Salads, wraps, or sandwiches containing cooked sprouts

Section 32.3

Sick Days

This section includes text excerpted from "Sick Days,"
Centers for Disease Control and Prevention (CDC),
September 25, 2015.

Being sick can make blood sugars hard to control. Here are some things you can do to speed up your recovery.

Ahead of Time

Ask your medical team about handling sick days before you get ill. Also train one or two family members or friends in blood glucose monitoring and other ways to help when you are sick.

Keep a box filled with medicines and easy-to-fix foods. If you wait until you are sick, you may not have the energy to collect all the things you need.

Good choices are:

- Milk of magnesia

- A pain reliever

- Medicine to control diarrhea

- A thermometer

- Antacids

- Suppositories for vomiting

If you cannot eat meals, you will need about 50 grams of carbohydrate every four hours.

Foods you may want to keep on hand are:

- Sports drinks

- Instant cooked cereals

- Small juice containers

- Crackers

- Canned soup

- Instant pudding

- Regular gelatin

- Canned applesauce

- Regular soft drinks

You can add other, more perishable, foods like toast, yogurt, ice cream, or milk when you are sick.

While You Are Sick

Even if you cannot eat normally, you will need to take your diabetes medicine. In fact, you may need to increase or change your medicine because your blood sugar may go higher. While you are sick, your medical team may ask you to test your blood sugar more often. Keep good written records about your blood sugar levels, medicines, temperature, and weight. You may need to test your urine for ketones if your blood sugar goes very high.

Drink plenty of fluids to prevent dehydration. Keep a pitcher of water or other noncaloric drink by your bed, so that you can drink 4–6 ounces every half hour. You may also need to drink beverages with sugar if you cannot get 50 grams of carbohydrate through other food choices. The portions of these sweet beverages must be controlled, as you don't want your blood sugar to get too high.

When to Call the Doctor

Call your healthcare provider if any of the following occurs:

- You have moderate to high ketone levels in your urine
- You have not eaten normally for more than 24 hours
- You have a fever over 101 degrees for 24 hours
- You can't keep any liquids down for more than four hours
- You have vomiting and/or diarrhea for more than six hours
- You lose five pounds or more during the illness
- Your blood glucose reading is under 60 mg/dl or over 300 mg/dl
- You have trouble breathing
- You can't stay awake or think clearly

If you cannot think clearly or feel too sleepy, have someone else call your healthcare provider or take you to the emergency room.

Questions to Ask

1. Do I have a written plan from my medical team to guide me on sick days?

2. Have I made a sick day box with needed medicines and foods?

3. Have I trained at least two persons who can help me if I am sick?

Section 32.4

Sleep Problems

This section contains text excerpted from the following sources: Text beginning with the heading "Sleep Can Lead to Chronic Diseases" is excerpted from "Sleep and Chronic Diseases," Centers for Disease Control and Prevention (CDC), August 8, 2018; Text under the heading "Sleep Apnea and Diabetes" is excerpted from "Diabetes," U.S. Department of Veterans Affairs (VA), December 27, 2017.

Sleep Can Lead to Chronic Diseases

As chronic diseases have assumed an increasingly common role in premature death and illness, interest in the role of sleep health in the development and management of chronic diseases has grown. Notably, insufficient sleep has been linked to the development and management of a number of chronic diseases and conditions, including type 2 diabetes, cardiovascular disease (CVD), obesity, and depression.

Insufficient Sleep and Diabetes

Research has found that insufficient sleep is linked to an increased risk for the development of type 2 diabetes. Specifically, sleep duration and quality have emerged as predictors of levels of Hemoglobin A1C, an important marker of blood sugar control. Research suggests that optimizing sleep duration and quality may be important means of improving blood sugar control in persons with type 2 diabetes.

Sleep Apnea and Diabetes

Sleep apnea and poor sleep quality—A study conducted by researchers at the Veteran Affairs (VA) Puget Sound Healthcare System that was part of the joint VA-U.S. Department of Defense (DoD) Millennium Cohort Study (MCS) on the health of service members and veterans, found that sleep apnea and poor sleep quality predicted diabetes, independent of other diabetes risk factors or mental health status.

Sleep apnea increased the risk of diabetes by 78 percent, and simply having trouble sleeping increased the risk of diabetes by 21 percent. The study included more than 47,000 service members and veterans who were an average age of about 49.

Statin use—Researchers at the VA North Texas Health System and their colleagues examined the health records of tens of thousands of Tricare beneficiaries for a nearly 10-year period. Their study, published in 2015, found that the use of statins to lower cholesterol is associated with a significantly higher risk of new-onset diabetes—even in a very healthy population.

They also found that statin use is associated with a very high risk of diabetes complications in this healthy population, and with a higher risk of obesity. High-intensity statin therapy was associated with greater risks for all outcomes.

Section 32.5

Depression

This section contains text excerpted from the following sources: Text under the heading "Depression and Medical Comorbidities" is excerpted from "Adult Depression in Primary Care: Percentage of Patients with Type 2 Diabetes with Documentation of Screening for Major Depression or Persistent Depressive Disorder Using Either PHQ-2 or PHQ-9," Agency for Healthcare Research and Quality (AHRQ), U.S. Department of Health and Human Services (HHS), March 2016; Text under the heading "People with Depression Are at Higher Risk for Other Medical Conditions" is excerpted from "Chronic Illness and Mental Health," National Institute of Mental Health (NIMH), December 2015.

Depression and Medical Comorbidities

The importance of the interplay between depression and many medical comorbidities cannot be overstated. A long list of medical conditions has been associated with increased risk for depression; these include diabetes, chronic pain, cancer, human immunodeficiency virus (HIV), Parkinson disease (PD), cardiovascular and cerebrovascular disease, and multiple sclerosis (MS).

Individuals with diabetes have two to threefold higher odds of depression than those without diabetes. Additionally, depression earlier in life increases the risk of developing diabetes. Depressive symptom severity is associated with poor self-care and medication compliance in addition to higher healthcare-related costs. Patient physical and mental quality of life is also decreased.

Major depression was second only to back and neck pain for having the greatest effect on disability days, at 386.6 million United States (U.S.) days per year. In a World Health Organization (WHO) study of more than 240,000 people across 60 countries, depression was shown to produce the greatest decrease in quality of health compared to several other chronic diseases. Health scores worsened when depression was a comorbid condition, and the most disabling combination was depression and diabetes.

Depression in the elderly is widespread, often undiagnosed, and usually untreated. It is a common misperception that it is a part of normal aging. Losses, social isolation, and chronic medical problems that older patients experience can contribute to depression.

The rate of depression in adults older than 65 years of age treated in primary care settings ranges from 17–37 percent and is between 14 percent and 42 percent in patients who live in long-term care facilities. Comorbidities are more common in the elderly. The highest rates of depression are found in those with strokes (30% to 60%), coronary artery disease (up to 44%), cancer (up to 40%), Parkinson disease (40%), Alzheimer disease (AD) (20% to 40%), and dementia (17% to 31%). The recurrence rate is also extremely high at 40 percent.

Between 14 percent and 23 percent of pregnant women and 10–15 percent of postpartum women will experience a depressive disorder. A study cites a point prevalence of 13 percent at three months after delivery and an average of 9 percent during each trimester of pregnancy. According to a large-scale epidemiological study depression during the postpartum period may be more common than at other times in a woman's life.

With growing understanding of the systemic impact of perinatal stressors, there is a new body of research examining paternal depression. A meta-analysis shows a 10–14 percent incidence of paternal depression during the perinatal period, with a moderate positive correlation with maternal depression.

From 50–85 percent of people who suffer an episode of major depression will have a recurrence, usually within two or three years. Patients who have had three or more episodes of major depression are at 90 percent risk of having another episode.

Depression Is Treatable

Major depression is a treatable cause of pain, suffering, disability and death, yet primary care clinicians detect major depression in only one-third to one-half of their patients with major depression. Additionally, more than 80 percent of patients with depression have a medical comorbidity. Usual care for depression in the primary care setting has resulted in only about half of depressed adults getting treated and only 20–40 percent showing substantial improvement over 12 months. Approximately 70–80 percent of antidepressants are prescribed in primary care, making it critical that clinicians know how to use them and have a system that supports best practices.

People with Depression Are at Higher Risk for Other Medical Conditions

It may have come as no surprise that people with a medical illness or condition are more likely to suffer from depression. The reverse is also true: the risk of developing some physical illnesses is higher in people with depression.

People with depression have an increased risk of diabetes, cardiovascular disease, stroke, and Alzheimer disease, for example. Research also suggests that people with depression are at higher risk for osteoporosis relative to others. The reasons are not yet clear. One factor with some of these illnesses is that many people with depression may have less access to good medical care. They may have a harder time caring for their health, for example, seeking care, taking prescribed medication, eating well, and exercising.

Ongoing research is also exploring whether physiological changes seen in depression may play a role in increasing the risk of physical illness. In people with depression, scientists have found changes in the way several different systems in the body function, all of which can have an impact on physical health:

- Signs of increased inflammation

- Changes in the control of heart rate and blood circulation

- Abnormalities in stress hormones

- Metabolic changes typical of those seen in people at risk for diabetes

Section 32.6

Traveling

This section includes text excerpted from "Tips to
Care for Your Diabetes While on Vacation," Centers for
Disease Control and Prevention (CDC), July 2, 2017.

Are you counting the days until your vacation? Or are you just
starting to plan one? As you get ready for your time away, make sure
you plan ahead to take care of your diabetes.

Getting Ready to Travel

Before you leave, make sure you have everything that you need
to take care of your diabetes. First, talk to your doctor about your
vacation plans to learn what you need to do before, during, and after
your trip.

Things to think about and discuss:

- Will you be more physically active or less active on your
  vacation? Ask your doctor about how your planned activities
  could affect your diabetes.

- Will you be walking a lot or going to the beach? Find out how to
  take care of your feet.

- When should you take your medicine if you change time zones?

- Will your meals be at different times from your usual schedule
  at home? Ask how this will affect your diabetes.

- How should you adjust your diabetes medicines based on your
  glucose (sugar) readings?

- Are your immunizations up to date? Do you need any special
  ones for where you're going?

- Where can you get medical care if needed when away from
  home? What do you need to do to let your health insurance
  company know about your travel plans?

Are You Going on a Road Trip?

If you are traveling by car, you often have more control of the items
you can take and have access to them at any time during your trip.

- Pack a small cooler with foods such as:
  - Fresh fruit and sliced raw vegetables that may be difficult to find during your trip
  - Dried fruit, nuts, and seeds. Keep in mind that these foods can be high in calories, so measure out small portions (¼ cup) in advance.
- Don't forget to take enough bottles of water or a large water container for the road.
- If you need to take insulin, don't forget to include it in your bag. Don't store insulin in direct sunlight or in a hot car. Put it in a cooler instead, but don't place it directly on ice or on a gel pack as it may get damaged.
- Make sure you add a few stops throughout the trip to walk or move around every hour or two. This will help you reduce your risk for blood clots.

Are You Traveling by Plane?

- Keep in mind the hours you will spend in airports and the length of flights.
- Plan when and where you will get meals.
- If the airline serves a meal during your flight, you can call ahead to ask for a special diabetic, low fat, or low cholesterol meal. If they do not offer a special meal, you will need to bring a healthy meal or buy it separately. Take some snacks with you in case there are any delays.
- Plan to walk or at least get up and move between and during flights whenever possible to reduce your risk for blood clots.
- Be sure to pack all your medicines and diabetes supplies in your carry-on luggage, and keep them with you for easy access during the flight. If your carry-on luggage is checked at the gate, remove your medications and diabetes supplies and take them with you onto the plane.

Tips for Airport Security Screening

- If you can, bring prescription labels for your medicines and medical devices. Although airport security doesn't specifically require them, having them available may make the security process go more quickly.

- Put medicines and other diabetes supplies in your carry-on luggage and take them on the plane with you.

- Pack medications in a separate clear, resealable bag. Bags of medicines in your carry-on luggage need to be removed and separated from your other belongings for screening.

- If you use an insulin pump, you can be screened without disconnecting from the pump. Tell the officer conducting the screening about the pump before you start the screening process. You can be screened with advanced imaging technology (AIT), metal detectors, or thorough pat down.

- If you wear an insulin pump and continuous glucose monitor (CGM), you may go through the airport metal detector. It is not recommended you go through an airport scanner (AIT). If you disconnect your sensors for screening, do not send them through the baggage X-ray machine. Put them in a separate bag and show it to the screening officer. If you do not wish to disconnect your devices, you may ask for a pat-down screening. If you choose a full pat down, or if the officers say you need pat-down screening, you have a right to have this screening done in private and with a witness of your choice.

- You can get an information card about insulin pumps to show to the screener and get more information about airport screening and traveling with a pump and/or CGM from the manufacturer's website.

Chapter 33

Diabetes in the Workplace: Know Your Rights

The Americans with Disabilities Act (ADA), which was amended by the ADA Amendments Act of 2008 ("Amendments Act" or "ADAAA"), is a federal law that prohibits discrimination against qualified individuals with disabilities. Individuals with disabilities include those who have impairments that substantially limit a major life activity, have a record (or history) of a substantially limiting impairment, or are regarded as having a disability.

Title I of the ADA covers employment by private employers with 15 or more employees as well as state and local government employers. Section 501 of the Rehabilitation Act (RA) provides similar protections related to federal employment. In addition, most states have their own laws prohibiting employment discrimination on the basis of disability. Some of these state laws may apply to smaller employers and may provide protections in addition to those available under the ADA.

The U.S. Equal Employment Opportunity Commission (EEOC) enforces the employment provisions of the ADA. This chapter explains how the ADA applies to job applicants and employees who have or had diabetes. In particular, this document explains:

- when an employer may ask an applicant or employee questions about her diabetes and how it should treat voluntary disclosures;

This chapter includes text excerpted from "Questions and Answers about Diabetes in the Workplace and the Americans with Disabilities Act (ADA)," U.S. Equal Employment Opportunity Commission (EEOC), May 15, 2013. Reviewed September 2018.

- what types of reasonable accommodations employees with diabetes may need;

- how an employer should handle safety concerns about applicants and employees with diabetes; and

- how an employer can ensure that no employee is harassed because of diabetes or any other disability.

With nearly two million cases diagnosed each year, diabetes is becoming more prevalent in the United States and is the most common endocrine disease. As of now an estimated 18.8 million adults in the United States have diabetes.

As a result of changes made by the ADAAA, individuals who have diabetes should easily be found to have a disability within the meaning of the first part of the ADA's definition of disability because they are substantially limited in the major life activity of endocrine function. Additionally, because the determination of whether an impairment is a disability is made without regard to the ameliorative effects of mitigating measures, diabetes is a disability even if insulin, medication, or diet controls a person's blood glucose levels. An individual with a past history of diabetes (for example, gestational diabetes) also has a disability within the meaning of the ADA. Finally, an individual is covered under the third ("regarded as") prong of the definition of disability if an employer takes a prohibited action (for example, refuses to hire or terminates the individual) because of diabetes or because the employer believes the individual has diabetes.

Obtaining, Using, and Disclosing Medical Information

Title I of the ADA limits an employer's ability to ask questions related to diabetes and other disabilities and to conduct medical examinations at three stages: preoffer, postoffer, and during employment.

Job Applicants—Before an Offer of Employment Is Made

May an Employer Ask a Job Applicant whether He / She Has or Had Diabetes or about Him / Her Treatment Related to Diabetes before Making a Job Offer?

No. An employer may not ask questions about an applicant's medical condition or require an applicant to have a medical examination before it makes a conditional job offer. This means that an employer cannot legally ask an applicant questions such as:

- whether he/she has diabetes or has been diagnosed with diabetes (for example, gestational diabetes) in the past;

- whether he/she uses insulin or other prescription drugs or has ever done so in the past; or,

- whether he/she ever has taken leave for medical treatment, or how much sick leave he/she has taken in the past year.

Of course, an employer may ask questions pertaining to the qualifications for, or performance of, the job, such as:

- whether the applicant has a commercial driver's license; or

- whether he/she can work rotating shifts

Does the Americans with Disabilities Act Require an Applicant to Disclose That He / She Has or Had Diabetes or Some Other Disability before Accepting a Job Offer?

No. The ADA does not require applicants to voluntarily disclose that they have or had diabetes or another disability unless they will need a reasonable accommodation for the application process (for example, a break to eat a snack or monitor their glucose levels). Some individuals with diabetes, however, choose to disclose their condition because they want their coworkers or supervisors to know what to do if they faint or experience other symptoms of hypoglycemia (low blood sugar), such as weakness, shakiness, or confusion.

Sometimes, the decision to disclose depends on whether an individual will need a reasonable accommodation to perform the job (for example, breaks to take medication or a place to rest until blood sugar levels become normal). A person with diabetes, however, may request an accommodation after becoming an employee even if he/she did not do so when applying for the job or after receiving the job offer.

May an Employer Ask Any Follow-up Questions If an Applicant Voluntarily Reveals That He / She Has or Had Diabetes?

No. An employer generally may not ask an applicant who has voluntarily disclosed that he/she has diabetes any questions about her diabetes, its treatment, or its prognosis. However, if an applicant voluntarily discloses that he/she has diabetes and the employer reasonably believes that she will require an accommodation to perform the job because of her diabetes or treatment, the employer may ask whether the applicant will need an accommodation and what type. The employer must keep any information an applicant discloses about his/her medical condition confidential.

Job Applicants—After an Offer of Employment Is Made

After making a job offer, an employer may ask questions about the applicant's health (including questions about the applicant's disability) and may require a medical examination, as long as all applicants for the same type of job are treated equally (that is, all applicants are asked the same questions and are required to take the same examination). After an employer has obtained basic medical information from all individuals who have received job offers, it may ask specific individuals for more medical information if it is medically related to the previously obtained medical information. For example, if an employer asks all applicants postoffer about their general physical and mental health, it can ask individuals who disclose a particular illness, disease, or impairment for more medical information or require them to have a medical examination related to the condition disclosed.

What May an Employer Do When It Learns That an Applicant Has or Had Diabetes after He / She Has Been Offered a Job but before He / She Starts Working?

When an applicant discloses after receiving a conditional job offer that he/she has diabetes, an employer may ask the applicant additional questions such as how long he/she has had diabetes; whether he/she uses insulin or oral medication; whether and how often he/she experiences hypoglycemic episodes; and/or whether he/she will need assistance if his/her blood sugar level drops while at work. The employer also may send the applicant for a follow-up medical examination or ask him/her to submit documentation from his/her doctor answering questions specifically designed to assess his/her ability to perform the job functions safely. Permissible follow-up questions at this stage differ from those at the preoffer stage when an employer only may ask an applicant who voluntarily discloses a disability whether he/she needs an accommodation to perform the job and what type.

An employer may not withdraw an offer from an applicant with diabetes if the applicant is able to perform the essential functions of the job, with or without reasonable accommodation, without posing a direct threat (that is, a significant risk of substantial harm) to the health or safety of himself or others that cannot be eliminated or reduced through reasonable accommodation.

Employees

The ADA strictly limits the circumstances under which an employer may ask questions about an employee's medical condition or require the employee to have a medical examination. Once an employee is on the job, his/her actual performance is the best measure of ability to do the job.

When May an Employer Ask an Employee Whether Diabetes, or Some Other Medical Condition, May Be Causing His/Her Performance Problems?

Generally, an employer may ask disability-related questions or require an employee to have a medical examination when it knows about a particular employee's medical condition, has observed performance problems, and reasonably believes that the problems are related to a medical condition. At other times, an employer may ask for medical information when it has observed symptoms, such as extreme fatigue or irritability, or has received reliable information from someone else (for example, a family member or coworker) indicating that the employee may have a medical condition that is causing performance problems. Often, however, poor job performance is unrelated to a medical condition and generally should be handled in accordance with an employer's existing policies concerning performance.

May an Employer Require an Employee on Leave Because of Diabetes to Provide Documentation or Have a Medical Examination before Allowing Him/Her to Return to Work?

Yes. If the employer has a reasonable belief that the employee may be unable to perform his/her job or may pose a direct threat to himself/herself or others, the employer may ask for medical information. However, the employer may obtain only the information needed to make an assessment of the employee's present ability to perform his/her job and to do so safely.

Are There Any Other Instances When an Employer May Ask an Employee with Diabetes about His/Her Condition?

Yes. An employer also may ask an employee about diabetes when it has a reasonable belief that the employee will be unable to safely perform the essential functions of his/her job because of diabetes. In addition, an employer may ask an employee about his/her diabetes to the extent the information is necessary:

- to support the employee's request for a reasonable accommodation needed because of his/her diabetes;

- to verify the employee's use of sick leave related to his/her diabetes if the employer requires all employees to submit a doctor's note to justify their use of sick leave; or

- to enable the employee to participate in a voluntary wellness program.

Keeping Medical Information Confidential

With limited exceptions, an employer must keep confidential any medical information it learns about an applicant or employee. Under the following circumstances, however, an employer may disclose that an employee has diabetes:

- to supervisors and managers in order to provide a reasonable accommodation or to meet an employee's work restrictions;

- to first aid and safety personnel if an employee may need emergency treatment or require some other assistance because, for example, her blood sugar level is too low;

- to individuals investigating compliance with the ADA and similar state and local laws; and

- where needed for workers' compensation or insurance purposes (for example, to process a claim).

May an Employer Tell Employees Who Ask Why Their Coworker Is Allowed to Do Something That Generally Is Not Permitted (Such as Eat at His/Her Desk or Take More Breaks) That She Is Receiving a Reasonable Accommodation?

No. Telling coworkers that an employee is receiving a reasonable accommodation amounts to a disclosure that the employee has a disability. Rather than disclosing that the employee is receiving a reasonable accommodation, the employer should focus on the importance of maintaining the privacy of all employees and emphasize that its policy is to refrain from discussing the work situation of any employee with coworkers. Employers may be able to avoid many of these kinds of questions by training all employees on the requirements of equal employment opportunity laws, including the ADA.

Additionally, an employer will benefit from providing information about reasonable accommodations to all of its employees. This can be done in a number of ways, such as through written reasonable accommodation procedures, employee handbooks, staff meetings, and periodic training. This kind of proactive approach may lead to fewer questions from employees who misperceive coworker accommodations as "special treatment."

If an Employee Experiences an Insulin Reaction at Work, May an Employer Explain to Other Employees or Managers That the Employee Has Diabetes?

No. Although the employee's coworkers and others in the workplace who witness the reaction naturally may be concerned, an employer may not reveal that the employee has diabetes. Rather, the employer should assure everyone present that the situation is under control. An employee, however, may voluntarily choose to tell his/her coworkers that he/she has diabetes and provide them with helpful information, such as how to recognize when his/her blood sugar may be low, what to do if he/she faints or seems shaky or confused (for example, offer a piece of candy or gum), or where to find his/her glucose monitoring kit. However, even when an employee voluntarily discloses that he/she has diabetes, the employer must keep this information confidential consistent with the ADA. An employer also may not explain to other employees why an employee with diabetes has been absent from work if the absence is related to his/her diabetes or another disability.

Accommodating Employees with Diabetes

The ADA requires employers to provide adjustments or modifications—called reasonable accommodations—to enable applicants and employees with disabilities to enjoy equal employment opportunities unless doing so would be an undue hardship (that is, a significant difficulty or expense). Accommodations vary depending on the needs of the individual with a disability. Not all employees with diabetes will need an accommodation or require the same accommodations, and most of the accommodations a person with diabetes might need will involve little or no cost. An employer must provide a reasonable accommodation that is needed because of the diabetes itself, the effects of medication, or both. For example, an employer may have to accommodate an employee who is unable to work while learning to manage his/her diabetes or adjusting to medication. An employer, however, has no obligation to monitor an employee to make sure that he/she is regularly checking his/her blood sugar levels, eating, or taking medication as prescribed.

Reasonable Accommodations

What Other Types of Reasonable Accommodations May Employees with Diabetes Need?

Some employees may need one or more of the following accommodations:

- a private area to test their blood sugar levels or to administer insulin injections

- a place to rest until their blood sugar levels become normal

- breaks to eat or drink, take medication, or test blood sugar levels

How Does an Employee with Diabetes Request a Reasonable Accommodation?

There are no "magic words" that a person has to use when requesting a reasonable accommodation. A person simply has to tell the employer that she needs an adjustment or change at work because of his/her diabetes. A request for a reasonable accommodation also can come from a family member, friend, health professional, or other representative on behalf of a person with diabetes.

May an Employer Request Documentation When an Employee Who Has Diabetes Requests a Reasonable Accommodation?

Yes. An employer may request reasonable documentation where a disability or the need for reasonable accommodation is not known or obvious. An employer, however, is entitled only to documentation sufficient to establish that the employee has diabetes and to explain why an accommodation is needed. A request for an employee's entire medical record, for example, would be inappropriate as it likely would include information about conditions other than the employee's diabetes.

Does an Employer Have to Grant Every Request for a Reasonable Accommodation?

No. An employer does not have to provide an accommodation if doing so will be an undue hardship. Undue hardship means that providing the reasonable accommodation will result in significant difficulty or expense. An employer also does not have to eliminate an essential function of a job as a reasonable accommodation, tolerate performance that does not meet its standards, or excuse violations of conduct rules that are job-related and consistent with business necessity and that the employer applies consistently to all employees (such as rules prohibiting violence, threatening behavior, theft, or destruction of property).

If more than one accommodation will be effective, the employee's preference should be given primary consideration, although the employer is not required to provide the employee's first choice of reasonable accommodation. If a requested accommodation is too difficult or expensive, an employer may choose to provide an easier or less costly accommodation as long as it is effective in meeting the employee's needs.

May an Employer Be Required to Provide More than One Accommodation for the Same Employee with Diabetes?

Yes. The duty to provide a reasonable accommodation is an ongoing one. Although some employees with diabetes may require only one reasonable accommodation, others may need more than one. For example, an employee with diabetes may require leave to attend a class on how to administer insulin injections and later may request a part-time or modified schedule to better control his glucose levels. An employer must consider each request for a reasonable accommodation and determine whether it would be effective and whether providing it would pose an undue hardship.

May an Employer Automatically Deny a Request for Leave from Someone with Diabetes Because the Employee Cannot Specify an Exact Date of Return?

No. Granting leave to an employee who is unable to provide a fixed date of return may be a reasonable accommodation. Although diabetes can be successfully treated, some individuals experience serious complications that may be unpredictable and do not permit exact timetables. An employee requesting leave because of diabetes or resulting complications (for example, a foot or toe amputation), therefore, may be able to provide only an approximate date of return (e.g., "in six to eight weeks," "in about three months"). In such situations, or in situations in which a return date must be postponed because of unforeseen medical developments, employees should stay in regular communication with their employers to inform them of their progress and discuss the need for continued leave beyond what originally was granted. The employer also has the right to require that the employee provide periodic updates on his condition and possible date of return. After receiving these updates, the employer may reevaluate whether continued leave constitutes an undue hardship.

Concerns about Safety

When it comes to safety concerns, an employer should be careful not to act on the basis of myths, fears, or stereotypes about diabetes. Instead, the employer should evaluate each individual on his/her skills, knowledge, experience, and how having diabetes affects him/her.

Questions on Safety Concerns

When May an Employer Refuse to Hire, Terminate, or Temporarily Restrict the Duties of a Person Who Has Diabetes Because of Safety Concerns?

An employer only may exclude an individual with diabetes from a job for safety reasons when the individual poses a direct threat. A "direct threat" is a significant risk of substantial harm to the individual or others that cannot be eliminated or reduced through reasonable accommodation. This determination must be based on objective, factual evidence, including the best recent medical evidence and advances in the treatment of diabetes.

In making a direct threat assessment, the employer must evaluate the individual's present ability to safely perform the job. The employer also must consider:

1. the duration of the risk;

2. the nature and severity of the potential harm;

3. the likelihood that the potential harm will occur; and

4. the imminence of the potential harm.

The harm must be serious and likely to occur, not remote or speculative. Finally, the employer must determine whether any reasonable accommodation (for example, temporarily limiting an employee's duties, temporarily reassigning an employee, or placing an employee on leave) would reduce or eliminate the risk.

May an Employer Require an Employee Who Has Had an Insulin Reaction at Work to Submit Periodic Notes from His/Her Doctor Indicating That His/Her Diabetes Is under Control?

Yes, but only if the employer has a reasonable belief that the employee will pose a direct threat if he/she does not regularly see his/her doctor. In determining whether to require periodic documentation, the employer should consider the safety risks associated with the position the employee holds, the consequences of the employee's inability or impaired ability to perform his/her job, how long the employee has had diabetes, and how many insulin reactions the employee has had on the job.

What Should an Employer Do When Another Federal Law Prohibits It from Hiring Anyone Who Uses Insulin?

If a federal law prohibits an employer from hiring a person who uses insulin, the employer is not liable under the ADA. The employer should be certain, however, that compliance with the law actually is required, not voluntary. The employer also should be sure that the law does not contain any exception or waivers. For example, the Department of Transportation's Federal Motor Carrier Safety Administration (FMCSA) issues exemptions to certain individuals with diabetes who wish to drive commercial motor vehicles (CMVs).

Harassment

The ADA prohibits harassment, or offensive conduct, based on disability just as other federal laws prohibit harassment based on race, sex, color, national origin, religion, age, and genetic information. Offensive conduct may include, but is not limited to, offensive jokes, slurs, epithets or name calling, physical assaults or threats, intimidation, ridicule or mockery, insults or put-downs, offensive objects or pictures, and interference with work performance. Although the law does not prohibit simple teasing, offhand comments, or isolated incidents that are not very serious, harassment is illegal when it is so frequent or severe that it creates a hostile or offensive work environment or when it results in an adverse employment decision (such as the victim being fired or demoted).

Questions on Harassment of People with Diabetes at Workplace

What Should Employers Do to Prevent and Correct Harassment?

Employers should make clear that they will not tolerate harassment based on disability or on any other basis. This can be done in a number of ways, such as through a written policy, employee handbooks, staff meetings, and periodic training. The employer should emphasize that harassment is prohibited and that employees should promptly report such conduct to a manager. Finally, the employer should immediately conduct a thorough investigation of any report of harassment and take swift and appropriate corrective action.

Retaliation

The ADA prohibits retaliation by an employer against someone who opposes discriminatory employment practices, files a charge of employment discrimination, or testifies or participates in any way in an investigation, proceeding, or litigation related to a charge of employment discrimination. It is also unlawful for an employer to retaliate against someone for requesting a reasonable accommodation. Persons who believe that they have experienced retaliation may file a charge of retaliation as described below.

How to File a Charge of Employment Discrimination

Against Private Employers and State/Local Governments

Any person who believes that his or her employment rights have been violated on the basis of disability and wants to make a claim against an employer must file a charge of discrimination with the EEOC. A third party may also file a charge on behalf of another person who believes he or she experienced discrimination. For example, a family member, social worker, or other representative can file a charge on behalf of someone who is incapacitated because of diabetes. The charge must be filed by mail or in person with the local EEOC office within 180 days from the date of the alleged violation. The 180-day filing deadline is extended to 300 days if a state or local antidiscrimination agency has the authority to grant or seek relief as to the challenged unlawful employment practice.

The EEOC will send the parties a copy of the charge and may ask for responses and supporting information. Before formal investigation, the EEOC may select the charge for EEOC's mediation program. Both parties have to agree to mediation, which may prevent a time-consuming investigation of the charge. Participation in mediation is free, voluntary, and confidential.

If mediation is unsuccessful, the EEOC investigates the charge to determine if there is "reasonable cause" to believe discrimination has occurred. If reasonable cause is found, the EEOC will then try to resolve the charge with the employer. In some cases, where the charge cannot be resolved, the EEOC will file a court action. If the EEOC finds no discrimination, or if an attempt to resolve the charge fails and the EEOC decides not to file suit, it will issue a notice of a "right to sue," which gives the charging party 90 days to file a court action. A charging party can also request a notice of a "right to sue" from the EEOC 180 days after the charge was first filed with the Commission, and may then bring suit within 90 days after receiving the notice.

Against the Federal Government

If you are a federal employee or job applicant and you believe that a federal agency has discriminated against you, you have a right to file a complaint. Each agency is required to post information about how to contact the agency's EEO Office. You can contact an EEO Counselor by calling the office responsible for the agency's EEO complaints program. Generally, you must contact the EEO Counselor within 45 days from the day the discrimination occurred. In most cases the EEO Counselor will give you the choice of participating either in EEO counseling or in an alternative dispute resolution (ADR) program, such as a mediation program.

If you do not settle the dispute during counseling or through ADR, you can file a formal discrimination complaint against the agency with the agency's EEO Office. You must file within 15 days from the day you receive notice from your EEO Counselor about how to file.

Once you have filed a formal complaint, the agency will review the complaint and decide whether or not the case should be dismissed for a procedural reason (for example, your claim was filed too late). If the agency doesn't dismiss the complaint, it will conduct an investigation. The agency has 180 days from the day you filed your complaint to finish the investigation. When the investigation is finished, the agency will issue a notice giving you two choices: either request a hearing before an EEOC Administrative Judge or ask the agency to issue a decision as to whether the discrimination occurred.

Chapter 34

Emergency Situations

Chapter Contents

Section 34.1

Insulin Storage and Switching between Products in an Emergency

This section includes text excerpted from "Information Regarding Insulin Storage and Switching between Products in an Emergency," U.S. Food and Drug Administration (FDA), September 19, 2017.

Insulin Storage and Effectiveness

Insulin for Injection

Insulin from various manufacturers is often made available to patients in an emergency and may be different from a patient's usual insulin. After a disaster, patients in the affected area may not have access to refrigeration. According to the product labels from all three U.S. insulin manufacturers, it is recommended that insulin be stored in a refrigerator at approximately 36–46°F. Unopened and stored in this manner, these products maintain potency until the expiration date on the package.

Insulin products contained in vials or cartridges supplied by the manufacturers (opened or unopened) may be left unrefrigerated at a temperature between 59–86°F for up to 28 days and continue to work. However, an insulin product that has been altered for the purpose of dilution or by removal from the manufacturer's original vial should be discarded within two weeks.

Note: Insulin loses some effectiveness when exposed to extreme temperatures. The longer the exposure to extreme temperatures, the less effective the insulin becomes. This can result in loss of blood glucose control over time. Under emergency conditions, you might still need to use insulin that has been stored above 86°F.

You should try to keep insulin as cool as possible. If you are using ice, avoid freezing the insulin. Do not use insulin that has been frozen. Keep insulin away from direct heat and out of direct sunlight.

When properly stored insulin becomes available again, the insulin vials that have been exposed to these extreme conditions should be discarded and replaced as soon as possible. If patients or healthcare providers have specific questions about the suitability of their insulin, they may call the respective manufacturer at the following numbers:

Lilly: 800-545-5979
Sanofi-Aventis: 800-633-1610
Novo Nordisk: 800-727-6500

Additional Storage Information for Insulin Pumps

Insulin contained in the infusion set of a pump device (e.g., reservoir, tubing, and catheters) should be discarded after 48 hours. Insulin contained in the infusion set of a pump device and exposed to temperature exceeding 98.6°F should be discarded.

Insulin Switching

Switching insulin should always be done in consultation with a physician and requires close medical supervision, and if possible, close monitoring of blood glucose. If medical supervision is not possible under emergency conditions, the following recommendations may be considered. Make sure to closely monitor your blood glucose and seek medical attention as soon as possible.

Short-Acting (Regular Insulin) and Rapid-Acting Insulins

One brand of regular insulin (e.g., Humulin R, Novolin R) may be substituted for another brand of regular insulin and for rapid-acting insulins (e.g., Humalog, NovoLog, Apidra), and vice-versa, on a unit-per-unit basis in emergency conditions.

Regular insulins are to be injected approximately 30 minutes before the start of each meal. Rapid-acting insulins begin working more rapidly than regular insulin and are to be injected no more than 15 minutes before the start of each meal to avoid dangerously low blood glucose levels.

Intermediate- and Long-Acting Insulins

One intermediate-acting insulin product (e.g., Humulin N, Novolin N) may be substituted for another intermediate-acting insulin product on a unit-per-unit basis in emergency conditions. Likewise, these intermediate insulins may also be substituted for long-acting insulins (e.g., Lantus, Levemir) on a total unit-per-day basis, or vice versa in emergency conditions.

- Importantly, when switching from a once-a-day, long-acting insulin (e.g., Lantus, Levemir) to an intermediate-acting insulin, the dose of the once-a-day, long-acting insulin should be cut in half and given as two injections of intermediate-acting insulin, one in the morning with breakfast and one in the evening with dinner to avoid dangerously low blood glucose levels.

- When switching from an intermediate-acting to a once-a-day, long-acting insulin, add up the total amount of intermediate-acting insulin units for one day, and give it as a single long-acting insulin dose once-a-day.

Close monitoring of blood glucose and adjustment in insulin dose may be needed in the transition period.

Insulin Mixes

Switching between types of insulin should be done in consultation with a physician and requires medical supervision, and if possible, close monitoring of blood glucose.

What Is an Insulin Mix?

Insulin mixes contain a ratio of intermediate- and short/rapid-acting insulin. The first number denotes the quantity of intermediate insulin and the second number denotes the quantity of short/rapid-acting insulin delivered with each dose administered. For example, each dose of a 70/30 mix contains 70 percent intermediate-acting insulin and 30 percent short/rapid-acting insulin.

Switching from Your Insulin Mix: Substitution or Replacement

Patients using premixed insulin products (e.g., Humulin 70/30, Humalog Mix 75/25, Novolin 70/30, NovoLog Mix 70/30) have the following options to consider:

- In emergency conditions, one insulin mix product may be substituted for another on a unit-per-unit basis.

- Insulin mixes containing a rapid-acting insulin analog (e.g., Humalog Mix, Novolog Mix) should be injected closer (within 15 minutes) to the start of the meal compared to mixes containing regular insulin (e.g., Humulin 70/30).

- If an insulin mix is not available, patients should follow this two-step process:

- **Step 1.** Substitute an intermediate-acting component of the mix (e.g., for most of the examples listed above this will be approximately 70 percent of the total units for each dose) with an intermediate-acting or a long-acting insulin on a unit-per-unit basis.

  - Substituting with an intermediate-acting insulin:

    - Give 70 percent of total units for each dose

  - Substituting with a long-acting insulin:

    - Add up the total insulin units given in one day

    - Give 70 percent as one daily dose

- **Step 2.** If regular or rapid-acting insulins are also available, they may be used before major meals in doses equivalent to approximately 30 percent of the total dose of premixed insulin and in combination with the intermediate- or long-acting insulin usually taken before that meal.

Note: Inject longer and shorter acting insulins separately unless directed otherwise by a physician.

Insulin Pumps

Switching between types of insulin should be done in consultation with a physician and requires medical supervision, and if possible, close monitoring of blood glucose.

Using a Different Insulin in Your Insulin Pump

- Patients administering insulin using a pump device may be able to substitute rapid-acting insulin (e.g., Humalog, Novolog, Apidra) for another on a unit-per-unit basis in emergency conditions. Patients should check the instructions for use of the pump device to see if available insulins are compatible with their devices.

Switching from an Insulin Pump to Injected Insulin

- Patients using insulin pumps who must switch to injected insulin may substitute intermediate or long-acting insulin for the total "basal" dose infused over 24-hours on a unit-per-unit basis in emergency conditions.

- For example, an individual using a pump with a basal rate of one unit per hour has a total 24-hour "basal" dose of 24 units.

- For an intermediate insulin, the 24 units should generally be administered as two injections of 12 units, and for a long-acting insulin, the 24 units should generally be administered as one injection daily.

- If regular or rapid-acting insulin is also available, patients should administer these insulins with each meal. The individual should substitute their meal-time "bolus" dose on a unit-per-unit basis to an injected dose.

  - For example, an individual using a "bolus" dose of five units on the pump to cover the breakfast meal should inject five units of regular or rapid-acting insulin to cover the breakfast meal.

Section 34.2

Managing Diabetes in the Heat

This section includes text excerpted from "Managing Diabetes in the Heat," Centers for Disease Control and Prevention (CDC), July 12, 2018.

Did you know that people who have diabetes—both type 1 and type 2—feel the heat more than people who don't have diabetes? Some reasons why:

- Certain diabetes complications, such as damage to blood vessels and nerves, can affect your sweat glands so your body can't cool as effectively. That can lead to heat exhaustion and heat stroke, which is a medical emergency.

- People with diabetes get dehydrated (lose too much water from their bodies) more quickly. Not drinking enough liquids can raise blood sugar, and high blood sugar can make you urinate more, causing dehydration. Some commonly used medicines like diuretics ("water pills" to treat high blood pressure) can dehydrate you, too.

- High temperatures can change how your body uses insulin. You may need to test your blood sugar more often and adjust your insulin dose and what you eat and drink.

It's the Heat and the Humidity

Even when it doesn't seem very hot outside, the combination of heat and humidity (moisture in the air) can be dangerous. When sweat evaporates (dries) on your skin, it removes heat and cools you. It's harder to stay cool in high humidity because sweat can't evaporate as well.

Whether you're working out or just hanging out, it's a good idea to check the heat index—a measurement that combines temperature and humidity. Take steps to stay cool when it reaches 80°F in the shade with 40 percent humidity or above.

Important to know: The heat index can be up to 15°F higher in full sunlight, so stick to the shade when the weather warms up.

Physical activity is key to managing diabetes, but don't get active outdoors during the hottest part of the day or when the heat index is high. Get out early in the morning or in the evening when temperatures are lower, or go to an air-conditioned mall or gym to get active.

Your Summer Checklist

- Drink plenty of water.

- Test your blood sugar often.

- Keep medicines, supplies, and equipment out of the heat.

- Stay inside in air-conditioning when it's hottest.

- Wear loose, light clothing.

- Get medical attention for heat-related illness.

- Make a plan in case you lose power.

- Have a go-bag ready for emergencies.

Your Blood Sugar Knows Best

Kids out of school, vacations, get-togethers, family reunions. The summer season can throw off your routine, and possibly your diabetes management plan. Check your blood sugar more often to make sure it's in your target range no matter what the summer brings. It's especially important to recognize what low blood sugar feels like and treat it as soon as possible.

Warm-weather wisdom:

- Drink plenty of water—even if you're not thirsty—so you don't get dehydrated.

- Avoid alcohol and drinks with caffeine, like coffee and energy or sports drinks. They can lead to water loss and spike your blood sugar levels.

- Check your blood sugar before, during, and after you're active. You may need to change how much insulin you use. Ask your doctor if you would like help in adjusting your dosage.

- Wear loose-fitting, lightweight, light-colored clothing.

- Wear sunscreen and a hat when you're outside. Sunburn can raise your blood sugar levels.

- Don't go barefoot, even on the beach or at the pool.

- Use your air conditioner or go to an air-conditioned building or mall to stay cool. In very high heat, a room fan won't cool you enough.

Too Hot to Handle

- Don't store insulin or oral diabetes medicine in direct sunlight or in a hot car. Check package information about how high temperatures can affect insulin and other medicines.

- If you're traveling, keep insulin and other medicines in a cooler. Don't put insulin directly on ice or on a gel pack.

- Heat can damage your blood sugar monitor, insulin pump, and other diabetes equipment. Don't leave them in a hot car, by a pool, in direct sunlight, or on the beach. The same goes for supplies such as test strips.

But don't let the summer heat stop you from taking your diabetes medicine and supplies with you when you're out and about. You'll need to be able to test your blood sugar and take steps if it's too high or too low. Just make sure to protect your diabetes gear from the heat.

Stormy Weather

Severe thunderstorms with hail, high winds, and tornadoes are more likely in warm weather, too. People with diabetes face extra challenges if a strong storm knocks out the power or they have to seek shelter away from home. Plan how you'll handle medicine that needs refrigeration, such as insulin. And be prepared by packing an emergency go-bag—a supply kit you can grab quickly if you need to leave your home.

Here's to staying cool, staying safe, and enjoying the long summer days!

Section 34.3

Importance of Wearing Medical Alert Bracelets and Necklaces

Medical alert bracelets and necklaces, also known as personal identification jewelry, are tags that people with certain illness, including diabetes, wear to save their lives in case of a medical emergency. The bracelets or necklaces are engraved with critical information such as the patient's personal details and medical conditions.

How the Medical Alert Jewelry Works

Patients with diabetes may sometimes face adverse conditions such as a sudden drop in blood glucose level, dizziness, and loss of consciousness, during which time the patients may not be able to express themselves clearly and seek medical help. In such situations, medical alert jewelry will be helpful in conveying the message that the wearer is suffering from a specific illness and may need immediate medical aid.

Information to Put on Medical Alert Jewelry

Medical information such as the person's medical condition ("diabetes"), allergies to any food or medicine, and life-saving medicines should be engraved boldly on one side of the jewelry for easy identification. The other side should contain other necessary information, such as:

- Patient's name

- Blood type

- Name of physician

- Emergency contact information

Information provided on the jewelry should be simple and precise and abbreviations of medical terms should be used to save room. When using abbreviations, however, make sure that they comply with international medical standards. Also, pay attention to the use of upper- and lower-case letters of the alphabet in the abbreviations.

Benefits of Medical Alert Jewelry

- Acts as a tool to convey the medical condition of the patient in case of emergencies

- Ensures quick recognition of ailments, allergies, and medications, and facilitates prompt diagnosis

- Ensures appropriate and timely medical care

- Reduces potentially harmful medical errors at the time of admission and discharge

How to Buy a Medical Alert Jewelry

Medical alert jewelry is available in most of surgical supply stores and many pharmacies. It is also available online on many websites. The jewelry is usually made of metals such as gold, silver, or stainless steel. However, nonmetallic jewelry made of leather, rubber, or nylon is also available. These nonmetallic bracelets are more popular among youth and are suitable for those who have skin sensitivity to metals. Although the bracelets come in different colors and designs, it is always preferable to choose the simpler ones because the simpler the design, the easier it is to read the message contained on it.

References

1. "The Basics of Medical Alert Bracelets," StickyJ Medical ID, October 25, 2017.

2. "Importance of Medical IDs," MedicAlert Foundation, October 10, 2014.

3. "The Benefits of Wearing a Medical ID Bracelet," MyIDShop, September 21, 2017.

4. "Importance of Wearing a Medical Alert Bracelet with Diabetes," Joslin Diabetes Center, October 17, 2008.

Part Five

Complications of Diabetes and Co-Occurring Disorders

Chapter 35

How to Prevent Diabetes Complications

Chapter Contents

Section 35.1

Preventing Complications: Overview

This section includes text excerpted from "Living with Diabetes—Prevent Complications," Centers for Disease Control and Prevention (CDC), April 16, 2018.

Diabetes can affect any part of your body. The good news is that you can prevent most of these problems by keeping your blood glucose (blood sugar) under control, eating healthy, being physically active, working with your healthcare provider to keep your blood pressure and cholesterol under control, and getting necessary screening tests.

Heart Disease (Cardiovascular Health)

How Can Diabetes Affect Your Heart?

Heart disease is the leading cause of early death among people with diabetes. Adults with diabetes are two to three times more likely than people without diabetes to die of heart disease or have a stroke. Also, about 74 percent of people with diabetes have high blood pressure, a risk factor for heart disease.

How Can You Be "Heart Healthy" and Avoid Heart Disease If You Have Diabetes?

To protect your heart and blood vessels:

- **Eat healthily.** Choose a healthy diet, low in salt. Work with a dietitian to plan healthy meals.

- **Get physically active.** If you're overweight, talk to your doctor about how to safely lose weight. Ask about a physical activity or exercise program that would be best for you.

- **Don't smoke.** Quit smoking, if you currently do.

- **Maintain healthy blood glucose, blood pressure, and cholesterol levels.** Get an A1C test at least twice a year to determine what your average blood glucose level was for the past three months. Get your blood pressure checked at every doctor's visit, and get your cholesterol checked at least once a year. Take medications if prescribed by your doctor.

How Are Cholesterol, Triglyceride, Weight, and Blood Pressure Problems Related to Diabetes?

People with type 2 diabetes have high cholesterol and triglyceride rates, obesity, and high blood pressure, all of which are major contributors to higher rates of heart disease. Many people with diabetes have several of these conditions at the same time. This combination is often called metabolic syndrome. The metabolic syndrome is often defined as the presence of any three of the following conditions:

- excess weight around the waist
- high levels of triglycerides
- low levels of high-level lipoprotein (HDL), or "good," cholesterol
- high blood pressure
- high fasting blood glucose levels.

If you have one or more of these conditions, you are at an increased risk of having one or more of the others. The more conditions that you have, the greater the risk to your health.

Kidney Disease

How Can Diabetes Affect the Kidneys?

In diabetic kidney disease (also called diabetic nephropathy), cells and blood vessels in the kidneys are damaged, affecting the organs' ability to filter out waste. Waste builds up in your blood instead of being excreted. In some cases, this can lead to kidney failure. When your kidneys fail, you will have to have your blood filtered through a machine (dialysis) several times a week, or you will need a kidney transplant.

How Can You Keep Your Kidneys Healthy If You Have Diabetes?

You can do a lot to prevent kidney problems. Controlling your blood glucose and keeping your blood pressure under control can prevent or delay the onset of kidney disease.

Diabetic kidney disease happens slowly and silently, so you might not feel that anything is wrong until severe problems develop. Therefore, it is important to get your blood and urine checked for kidney problems each year.

Your doctor will see how well your kidneys are working by testing every year for microalbumin (a protein) in the urine. Microalbumin in the urine is an early sign of diabetic kidney disease. Your doctor can also do a yearly blood test to measure your kidney function.

If you develop a bladder or kidney infection, visit your doctor. Symptoms include cloudy or bloody urine, pain or burning when you urinate, an urgent need to urinate often, back pain, chills, or fever.

Nerve Damage

How Can Diabetes Affect Nerve Endings?

Having high blood glucose for many years can damage blood vessels that bring oxygen to some nerve endings. Damaged nerves may stop, slow, or send messages at wrong times. Numbness, pain, and weakness in the hands, arms, feet, and legs may develop. Problems may also occur in various organs, including the digestive tract, heart, and sex organs. Diabetic neuropathy is the medical term for damage to the nervous system from diabetes. The most common type is peripheral neuropathy, which affects the arms and legs.

An estimated 50 percent of people with diabetes have some nerve problems, but not all have symptoms. Nerve problems can develop at any time, but the longer a person has diabetes, the greater the risk. The highest rates of nerve problems are among people who have had the disease for at least 25 years.

Diabetic nerve problems also are more common in people who have problems controlling their blood glucose levels, blood pressure, weight, and in people over the age of 40.

How Can You Prevent Nerve Damage If You Have Diabetes?

You can help keep your nervous system healthy by keeping your blood glucose as close to normal as possible, getting regular physical activity, not smoking, taking good care of your feet each day, having your healthcare provider examine your feet at least four times a year, and getting your feet tested for nerve damage at least once a year.

Digestive Problems

How Can Diabetes Affect the Digestion?

Gastroparesis (delayed gastric emptying) is a disorder where the stomach takes too long to empty itself due to nerve damage. It frequently occurs in people with either type 1 or type 2 diabetes.

Symptoms of gastroparesis include heartburn, nausea, vomiting of undigested food, an early feeling of fullness when eating, weight loss, abdominal bloating, erratic blood glucose levels, lack of appetite, gastroesophageal reflux, and spasms of the stomach wall.

Foot Problems

Why Is It Especially Important to Take Care of Your Feet If You Have Diabetes?

Sometimes nerve damage can deform or mis-shape your feet, causing pressure points that can turn into blisters, sores, or ulcers. Poor circulation can make these injuries slow to heal. Sometimes this can lead to amputation of a toe, foot, or leg.

What Should You Do on a Regular Basis to Take Care of Your Feet?

- Look for cuts, cracks, sores, red spots, swelling, infected toenails, splinters, blisters, and calluses on the feet each day. Call your doctor if such wounds do not heal after one day.
- If you have corns and calluses, ask your doctor or podiatrist about the best way to care for them.
- Wash your feet in warm—not hot—water, and dry them well.
- Cut your toenails once a week or when needed. Cut toenails when they are soft from washing. Cut them to the shape of the toe and not too short. File the edges with an emery board.
- Rub lotion on the tops and bottoms of feet—but not between the toes—to prevent cracking and drying.
- Wear stockings or socks to avoid blisters and sores.
- Wear clean, lightly padded socks that fit well. Seamless socks are best.
- Wear shoes that fit well. Break in new shoes slowly, by wearing them 1–2 hours each day for 1–2 weeks.
- Always wear shoes or slippers, because when you are barefoot it is easy to step on something and hurt your feet.
- Protect your feet from extreme heat and cold.
- When sitting, keep the blood flowing to your lower limbs by propping your feet up and moving your toes and ankles for a few minutes at a time.

- Avoid smoking, which reduces blood flow to the feet.

- Keep your blood sugar, blood pressure, and cholesterol under control by eating healthy foods, staying active, and taking your diabetes medicines.

Sexual Response

How Can Diabetes Affect Your Sexual Response?

Many people with diabetic nerve damage have trouble having sex. For example, men can have trouble maintaining an erection and ejaculating. Women can have trouble with sexual response and vaginal lubrication. Both men and women with diabetes can get urinary tract infections and bladder problems more often than average.

Oral Health

How Can Diabetes Affect Your Mouth, Teeth, and Gums?

People with diabetes are more likely to have problems with their teeth and gums due to high blood glucose. And like all infections, dental infections can make your blood glucose go up. Sore, swollen, and red gums that bleed when you brush your teeth are a sign of a dental problem called gingivitis. Another problem, called periodontitis, happens when your gums shrink or pull away from your teeth.

People with diabetes can have tooth and gum problems more often if their blood glucose stays high. Smoking also makes it more likely for you to have gum disease, especially if you have diabetes and are age 45 or older.

How Can You Keep Your Mouth, Gums, and Teeth Healthy If You Have Diabetes?

You can help maintain your oral health by:

- Keeping your blood glucose as close to normal as possible

- Brushing your teeth at least twice a day, and flossing once a day

- Keeping any dentures clean

- Getting a dental cleaning and exam twice a year, and telling your dentist that you have diabetes

Call your dentist with any problems, such as gums that are red, sore, bleeding, or pulling away from the teeth; any possible tooth infection; or soreness from dentures.

Vision

How Can Diabetes Affect the Eyes?

In diabetic eye disease, high blood glucose, and high blood pressure cause small blood vessels to swell and leak liquid into the retina of the eye, blurring the vision and sometimes leading to blindness. People with diabetes are also more likely to develop cataracts (a clouding of the eye's lens) and glaucoma (optic nerve damage). Laser surgery can in some cases help these conditions.

How Can You Keep Your Eyes Healthy If You Have Diabetes?

There's a lot you can do to prevent eye problems. Keeping your blood glucose level closer to normal can prevent or delay the onset of diabetic eye disease. Also, keeping your blood pressure under control is important. Finding and treating eye problems early can help save your sight.

Have an eye doctor give you a dilated eye exam at least once a year. The doctor will use eye drops to enlarge (dilate) your pupils to examine the backs of your eyes. Your eyes will be checked for signs of cataracts or glaucoma, problems that people with diabetes are more likely to get.

Because diabetic eye disease may develop without symptoms, regular eye exams are important for finding problems early. Some people may notice signs of vision changes. If you're having trouble reading, if your vision is blurred, or if you're seeing rings around lights, dark spots, or flashing lights, you may have eye problems. Be sure to tell your healthcare team or eye doctor about any eye problems you may have.

Section 35.2

Putting the Brakes on Diabetes Complications

This section includes text excerpted from "Putting the Brakes on Diabetes Complications," Centers for Disease Control and Prevention (CDC), December 21, 2017.

Encouraging news: People with diabetes are living longer, healthier lives with fewer complications. What's the driving force? Greater awareness and better control of risk factors are moving the needle.

In the last 20 years, rates of several major complications have decreased among U.S. adults with diabetes. The greatest declines were for two leading causes of death: heart attack and stroke. (People with diabetes are at higher risk for heart disease, and they may get it more severely and at a younger age than people who don't have diabetes.) This is meaningful progress.

It's important to note that during that same 20 years, the number of adults diagnosed with diabetes has more than tripled as the American population has aged. Diabetes complications still take a heavy toll on the health of millions of people and on our healthcare system.

Why Complications Are So...Complicated

Diabetes complications often share the same risk factors, and one complication can make other complications worse. For example, many people with diabetes also have high blood pressure, which in turn worsens eye and kidney diseases. Diabetes tends to lower HDL ("good") cholesterol and raise triglycerides and LDL ("bad") cholesterol, which increases the risk for heart disease and stroke. Smoking doubles the risk of heart disease in people with diabetes.

Take a closer look at these major diabetes complications:

- **Heart disease and stroke:** People with diabetes are twice as likely to have heart disease or a stroke as people without diabetes.

- **Blindness and other eye problems:** Diabetic retinopathy (damage to blood vessels in the retina), cataract (clouding of the lens), and glaucoma (increase in fluid pressure in the eye) can all result in vision loss. Diabetic retinopathy is also one of the most preventable causes of vision loss. Early detection and treatment can prevent or delay blindness in 90 percent of people with diabetes.

- **Nerve damage (neuropathy):** One of the most common diabetes complications, nerve damage can cause numbness and pain and can even be disabling. Nerve damage most often affects the feet and legs but can also affect your digestion, blood vessels, and heart.

- **Kidney disease:** High blood sugar levels can damage the kidneys and cause chronic kidney disease (CKD). If not treated, CKD usually gets worse and can lead to kidney failure. A person with kidney failure needs regular dialysis (a treatment that filters the blood) or a kidney transplant to survive. About 1 in 3 adults with diabetes has CKD. You won't know if you have CKD unless your doctor tests you for it. The earlier treatment is started, the better the outcome.

- **Amputations:** Diabetes-related damage to blood vessels and nerves, especially in the feet, can lead to serious, hard-to-treat infections. Amputation can be necessary to stop the spread of infection.

- And more:
  - Diabetes is associated with gum disease, which can lead to tooth loss and increased blood sugar, making diabetes harder to control. Gum disease itself can increase the risk of type 2 diabetes.

  - Diabetes increases the risk of depression, and that risk grows as more diabetes-related health problems develop.

  - Gestational diabetes, diagnosed during pregnancy, can cause serious complications for mothers or their babies, such as preeclampsia (pregnancy-induced high blood pressure), birth-related trauma, and birth defects.

Complications usually develop over a long time without any symptoms. That's why it's so important to make and keep doctor and dentist appointments even if you feel fine. Early treatment can help prevent or delay diabetes-related health conditions and improve overall health.

Your Prevention Toolkit

- A healthy lifestyle is your road map for managing diabetes, which is the key to preventing or delaying complications:
  - Follow a healthy eating plan.

- Be physically active for at least 150 minutes a week (just 30 minutes, 5 days a week).

- Manage your ABCs:

  - A: Get a regular A1C test to measure your average blood sugar over 2 to 3 months; aim to stay in your target range as much as possible.

  - B: Try to keep your blood pressure below 140/90 mm Hg (or the target your doctor sets).

  - C: Control your cholesterol levels.

  - s: Stop smoking or don't start.

For people with diabetes, controlling blood pressure has big benefits: it reduces the risk of heart disease by as much as 50 percent and the risk of kidney, eye, and nerve disease by about 33 percent.

- Lose weight if you're overweight—just a 5–7 percent weight loss lowers the risk for complications. That's 10–14 pounds for someone who weighs 200 pounds.

- Take medicines as prescribed, and talk to your doctor if you have questions about or problems with your medicine.

- Make and keep appointments with your healthcare team (primary care doctor, dentist, foot doctor, eye doctor, and dietitian).

In Charge, but Not Alone

- You're in the driver's seat when it comes to managing your diabetes—watching what you eat, making time for physical activity, taking meds, checking your blood sugar. Also be sure to stay in touch with your healthcare team to keep going in the right direction.

- Everyone's diabetes is different. Some people will still have complications even with good control. Maybe that's you—you've been trying hard but not seeing results. Or you've developed a health problem related to diabetes in spite of your best efforts.

- If you feel discouraged and frustrated, you may slip into unhealthy habits, stop monitoring your blood sugar, even skip doctors' appointments. That's when your team can help you get back on track, from setting goals and reminding you of your progress to offering new ideas and strategies.

Chapter 36

Diabetes-Related Eye Disease

What Is Diabetic Eye Disease?

Diabetic eye disease is a group of eye problems that can affect people with diabetes. These conditions include diabetic retinopathy, diabetic macular edema (DME), cataracts, and glaucoma.

Over time, diabetes can cause damage to your eyes that can lead to poor vision or even blindness. But you can take steps to prevent diabetic eye disease, or keep it from getting worse, by taking care of your diabetes.

The best ways to manage your diabetes and keep your eyes healthy are to:

- manage your blood glucose (A1C test), blood pressure, and cholesterol sometimes called the diabetes ABCs.

- If you smoke, get help to quit smoking.

- have a dilated eye exam once a year.

Often, there are no warning signs of diabetic eye disease or vision loss when damage first develops. A full, dilated eye exam helps your

This chapter includes text excerpted from "Diabetic Eye Disease," National Institute of Diabetes and Digestive and Kidney Diseases (NIDDK), May 2017.

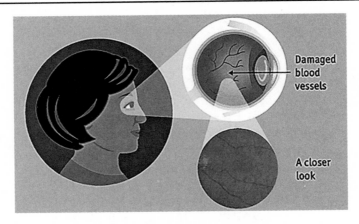

Figure 36.1. *How Diabetes Damages Your Eyes* (Source: "Diabetic Eye Disease: A Self-Guided Module," National Eye Institute (NEI).)

doctor find and treat eye problems early—often before much vision loss can occur.

How Does Diabetes Affect Your Eyes?

Diabetes affects your eyes when your blood glucose, also called blood sugar, is too high.

In the short term, you are not likely to have vision loss from high blood glucose. People sometimes have blurry vision for a few days or weeks when they're changing their diabetes care plan or medicines. High glucose can change fluid levels or cause swelling in the tissues of your eyes that help you to focus, causing blurred vision. This type of blurry vision is temporary and goes away when your glucose level gets closer to normal.

If your blood glucose stays high over time, it can damage the tiny blood vessels in the back of your eyes. This damage can begin during prediabetes, when blood glucose is higher than normal, but not high enough for you to be diagnosed with diabetes. Damaged blood vessels may leak fluid and cause swelling. New, weak blood vessels may also begin to grow. These blood vessels can bleed into the middle part of the eye, lead to scarring, or cause dangerously high pressure inside your eye.

Most serious diabetic eye diseases begin with blood vessel problems. The four eye diseases that can threaten your sight are:

Diabetic Retinopathy

The retina is the inner lining at the back of each eye. The retina senses light and turns it into signals that your brain decodes, so you can see the world around you. Damaged blood vessels can harm the retina, causing a disease called diabetic retinopathy.

In early diabetic retinopathy, blood vessels can weaken, bulge, or leak into the retina. This stage is called nonproliferative diabetic retinopathy (NPDR).

If the disease gets worse, some blood vessels close off, which causes new blood vessels to grow, or proliferate, on the surface of the retina. This stage is called proliferative diabetic retinopathy (PDR). These abnormal new blood vessels can lead to serious vision problems.

Diabetic Macular Edema (DME)

The part of your retina that you need for reading, driving, and seeing faces is called the macula. Diabetes can lead to swelling in the macula, which is called diabetic macular edema. Over time, this disease can destroy the sharp vision in this part of the eye, leading to partial vision loss or blindness. Macular edema usually develops in people who already have other signs of diabetic retinopathy.

Glaucoma

Glaucoma is a group of eye diseases that can damage the optic nerve—the bundle of nerves that connects the eye to the brain. Diabetes doubles the chances of having glaucoma, which can lead to vision loss and blindness if not treated early.

Cataracts

The lenses within our eyes are clear structures that help provide sharp vision—but they tend to become cloudy as we age. People with diabetes are more likely to develop cloudy lenses, called cataracts. People with diabetes can develop cataracts at an earlier age than people without diabetes. Researchers think that high glucose levels cause deposits to build up in the lenses of your eyes.

How Common Is Diabetic Eye Disease?

Diabetic Retinopathy

About one in three people with diabetes who are older than age 40 already have some signs of diabetic retinopathy. Diabetic retinopathy is the most common cause of vision loss in people with diabetes. Each person's outlook for the future, however, depends in large part on regular care. Finding and treating diabetic retinopathy early can reduce the risk of blindness by 95 percent.

Glaucoma and Cataracts

Your chances of developing glaucoma or cataracts are about twice that of someone without diabetes.

Who Is More Likely to Develop Diabetic Eye Disease?

Anyone with diabetes can develop diabetic eye disease. Your risk is greater with:

- high blood glucose that is not treated
- high blood pressure that is not treated

High blood cholesterol and smoking may also raise your risk for diabetic eye disease.

Some groups are affected more than others. African Americans, American Indians, and Alaska Natives, Hispanics/Latinos, Pacific Islanders, and older adults are at greater risk of losing vision or going blind from diabetes.

If you have diabetes and become pregnant, you can develop eye problems very quickly during your pregnancy. If you already have some diabetic retinopathy, it can get worse during pregnancy. Changes that help your body support a growing baby may put stress on the blood vessels in your eyes. Your healthcare team will suggest regular eye exams during pregnancy to catch and treat problems early and protect your vision.

Diabetes that occurs only during pregnancy, called gestational diabetes, does not usually cause eye problems. Researchers aren't sure why this is the case.

Your chances of developing diabetic eye disease increase the longer you have diabetes.

What Are the Symptoms of Diabetic Eye Disease?

Often there are no early symptoms of diabetic eye disease. You may have no pain and no change in your vision as damage begins to grow inside your eyes, particularly with diabetic retinopathy.

When symptoms do occur, they may include:

- blurry or wavy vision
- frequently changing vision—sometimes from day to day
- dark areas or vision loss
- poor color vision
- spots or dark strings (also called floaters)
- flashes of light

Talk with your eye doctor if you have any of these symptoms.

When Should You See a Doctor Right Away?

Call a doctor right away if you notice sudden changes to your vision, including flashes of light or many more spots (floaters) than usual. You also should see a doctor right away if it looks like a curtain is pulled over your eyes. These changes in your sight can be symptoms of a detached retina, which is a medical emergency.

How Do Doctors Diagnose Eye Problems from Diabetes?

Having a full, dilated eye exam is the best way to check for eye problems from diabetes. Your doctor will place drops in your eyes to widen your pupils. This allows the doctor to examine a larger area at the back of each eye, using a special magnifying lens. Your vision will be blurry for a few hours after a dilated exam.

Your doctor will also:

- test your vision
- measure the pressure in your eyes

Your doctor may suggest other tests, too, depending on your health history.

Most people with diabetes should see an eye-care professional once a year for a complete eye exam. Your own healthcare team may suggest a different plan, based on your type of diabetes and the time since you were first diagnosed.

How Do Doctors Treat Diabetic Eye Disease?

Your doctor may recommend having eye exams more often than once a year, along with management of your diabetes. This means managing your diabetes ABCs, which include your A1C, blood pressure, and cholesterol; and quitting smoking. Ask your healthcare team what you can do to reach your goals.

Doctors may treat advanced eye problems with medicine, laser treatments, surgery, or a combination of these options.

Medicine

Your doctor may treat your eyes with antivascular endothelial growth factor (VEGF) medicine, such as aflibercept, bevacizumab, or ranibizumab. These medicines block the growth of abnormal blood vessels in the eye. Anti-VEGF medicines can also stop fluid leaks, which can help treat diabetic macular edema (DME).

The doctor will inject an anti-VEGF medicine into your eyes during office visits. You'll have several treatments during the first few months, then fewer treatments after you finish the first round of therapy. Your doctor will use medicine to numb your eyes so you don't feel pain. The needle is about the thickness of a human hair.

Anti-VEGF treatments can stop further vision loss and may improve vision in some people.

Laser Treatment

Laser treatment, also called photocoagulation, creates tiny burns inside the eye with a beam of light. This method treats leaky blood vessels and extra fluid, called edema. Your doctor usually provides this treatment during several office visits, using medicine to numb your eyes. Laser treatment can keep eye disease from getting worse, which is important to prevent vision loss or blindness. But laser treatment is less likely to bring back vision you've already lost compared with anti-VEGF medicines.

There are two types of laser treatment:

1. **Focal/grid laser treatment** works on a small area of the retina to treat diabetic macular edema.

2. **Scatter laser treatment,** also called panretinal photocoagulation (PRP), covers a larger area of the retina. This method treats the growth of abnormal blood vessels, called proliferative diabetic retinopathy (PDR).

Vitrectomy

Vitrectomy is a surgery to remove the clear gel that fills the center of the eye, called the vitreous gel. The procedure treats problems with severe bleeding or scar tissue caused by proliferative diabetic reti-nopathy (PDR). Scar tissue can force the retina to peel away from the tissue beneath it, like wallpaper peeling away from a wall. A retina that comes completely loose, or detaches, can cause blindness.

During vitrectomy, a clear salt solution is gently pumped into the eye to maintain eye pressure during surgery and to replace the removed vitreous. Vitrectomy is done in a surgery center or hospital with pain medicine.

Cataract Lens Surgery

In a surgery center or hospital visit, your doctor can remove the cloudy lens in your eye, where the cataract has grown, and replace it with an artificial lens. People who have cataract surgery generally have better vision afterward. After your eye heals, you may need a new prescription for your glasses. Your vision following cataract surgery may also depend on treating any damage from diabetic retinopathy or macular edema.

What Can You Do to Protect Your Eyes?

To prevent diabetic eye disease, or to keep it from getting worse, manage your diabetes ABCs: your A1C, blood pressure, and choles-terol; and quit smoking if you smoke.

Also, have a dilated eye exam at least once a year—or more often if recommended by your eye-care professional. These actions are power-ful ways to protect the health of your eyes—and can prevent blindness.

The sooner you work to manage your diabetes and other health conditions, the better. And, even if you've struggled in the past to manage your health, taking better care of yourself now can protect your eyes for the future. It's never too late to begin.

What If You Already Have Some Vision Loss from Diabetes?

Ask your eye-care professional to help you find a low vision and rehabilitation clinic. Special eye-care professionals can help you man-age vision loss that cannot be corrected with glasses, contact lenses, medicine, or surgery. Special devices and training may help you make the most of your remaining vision so that you can continue to be active, enjoy hobbies, visit friends and family members, and live without help from others.

Chapter 37

Diabetes and Flu Complications

People with diabetes (type 1 or type 2), even when well-managed, are at high risk of serious flu complications, often resulting in hospitalization and sometimes even death. Pneumonia, bronchitis, sinus infections, and ear infections are examples of flu-related complications. The flu also can make chronic health problems, like diabetes, worse. This is because diabetes can make the immune system less able to fight infections. In addition, illness can make it harder to control your blood sugar. The illness might raise your sugar but sometimes people don't feel like eating when they are sick, and this can cause blood sugar levels to fall. So it is important to follow the sick day guidelines for people with diabetes.

Vaccination Is the Best Protection against Flu

The Centers for Diseases Control and Prevention (CDC) recommends that all people who are six months and older get a flu vaccine. It is especially important for people with diabetes to get a flu vaccine.

- Flu shots are approved for use in people with diabetes and other health conditions. The flu shot has a long, established safety record in people with diabetes.

This chapter includes text excerpted from "Flu and People with Diabetes," Centers for Disease Control and Prevention (CDC), August 25, 2016.

People with type 1 or type 2 diabetes are at increased risk of developing pneumococcal pneumonia because of the flu, so being up to date with pneumococcal vaccination is also recommended. Pneumococcal vaccination should be part of a diabetes management plan. Talk to your doctor to find out which pneumococcal vaccines are recommended for you.

Take Action to Stop Flu

Take everyday preventive actions to stop the spread of flu:

- Cover your nose and mouth with a tissue when coughing or sneezing and throw the tissue away after using it;

- Wash your hands often with soap and water, especially after coughing or sneezing;

- Avoid touching your eyes, nose, and mouth (germs are spread that way); and

- Stay home when you are sick, except to get medical care. If you are sick with flu-like symptoms you should stay home for 24 hours after your fever is gone (without the use of fever-reducing medicine).

Everyday preventive actions can protect you from getting sick and, if you are sick, can help protect others from catching your illness

Treating Influenza

- If you do get sick with flu symptoms, call your doctor early in illness because prompt treatment is recommended for people who are at high risk of serious flu complications and who have influenza infection or suspected influenza infection.

  - Treatment should begin as soon as possible because antiviral drugs work best when started early (within 48 hours after symptoms start).

  - Antiviral drugs can make your flu illness milder and make you feel better faster. They may also prevent serious health problems that can result from flu illness.

  - There are three U.S. Food and Drug Administration (FDA)-approved influenza antiviral drugs recommended by CDC this season that can be used to treat the flu. These medicines fight against the flu by keeping flu viruses from making more viruses in your body.

- For you to get an antiviral drug, a doctor needs to write a prescription. These medicines fight against the flu by keeping flu viruses from making more viruses in your body.

Other Preventive Actions

In addition to getting vaccinated yearly, people with diabetes should take everyday precaution for protecting against the flu.

Using Nasal Spray Vaccine

The flu shot has a long, established safety record in people with diabetes. Your doctor or other healthcare professional can advise you on which flu vaccine is best for you.

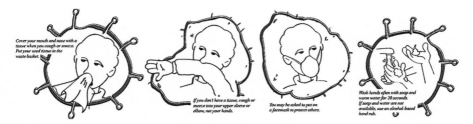

Figure 37.1. *Preventing the Flu: Good Health Habits Can Help Stop Germs* (Source: "Cover Your Cough," Centers for Disease Control and Prevention (CDC).)

Chapter 38

Diabetes-Related Foot Problems

Foot problems are common in people with diabetes. You might be afraid you'll lose a toe, foot, or leg to diabetes, or know someone who has, but you can lower your chances of having diabetes-related foot problems by taking care of your feet every day. Managing your blood glucose levels, also called blood sugar, can also help keep your feet healthy.

How Can Diabetes Affect Your Feet?

Over time, diabetes may cause nerve damage, also called diabetic neuropathy, that can cause tingling and pain, and can make you lose feeling in your feet. When you lose feeling in your feet, you may not feel a pebble inside your sock or a blister on your foot, which can lead to cuts and sores. Cuts and sores can become infected.

Diabetes also can lower the amount of blood flow in your feet. Not having enough blood flowing to your legs and feet can make it hard for a sore or an infection to heal. Sometimes, a bad infection never heals. The infection might lead to gangrene.

Gangrene and foot ulcers that do not get better with treatment can lead to an amputation of your toe, foot, or part of your leg. A surgeon

This chapter includes text excerpted from "Diabetes and Foot Problems," National Institute of Diabetes and Digestive and Kidney Diseases (NIDDK), January 2017.

may perform an amputation to prevent a bad infection from spreading to the rest of your body, and to save your life. Good foot care is very important to prevent serious infections and gangrene.

Although rare, nerve damage from diabetes can lead to changes in the shape of your feet, such as Charcot foot. Charcot foot may start with redness, warmth, and swelling. Later, bones in your feet and toes can shift or break, which can cause your feet to have an odd shape, such as a "rocker bottom."

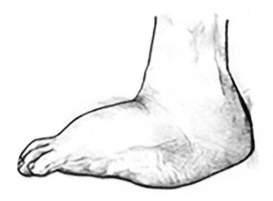

Figure 38.1. *Charcot Foot*

Charcot foot can cause your feet to have an odd shape, such as a "rocker bottom."

What Can You Do to Keep Your Feet Healthy?

Work with your healthcare team to make a diabetes self-care plan, which is an action plan for how you will manage your diabetes. Your plan should include foot care. A foot doctor, also called a podiatrist, and other specialists may be part of your healthcare team.

Check Your Feet Everyday

You may have foot problems, but feel no pain in your feet. Checking your feet each day will help you spot problems early before they get worse. A good way to remember is to check your feet each evening when you take off your shoes. Also, check between your toes. If you have trouble bending over to see your feet, try using a mirror to see them, or ask someone else to look at your feet.

Look for problems such as:

- Cuts, sores, or red spots

- Swelling or fluid-filled blisters
- Ingrown toenails, in which the edge of your nail grows into your skin
- Corns or calluses, which are spots of rough skin caused by too much rubbing or pressure on the same spot
- Plantar warts, which are flesh-colored growths on the bottom of the feet
- Athlete's foot
- Warm spots

If you have certain foot problems that make it more likely you will develop a sore on your foot, your doctor may recommend taking the temperature of the skin on different parts of your feet. A "hot spot" can be the first sign that a blister or an ulcer is starting.

Cover a blister, cut, or sore with a bandage. Smooth corns and calluses as explained below.

Wash Your Feet Every Day

Wash your feet with soap in warm, not hot, water. Test the water to make sure it is not too hot. You can use a thermometer (90–95°F is safe) or your elbow to test the warmth of the water. Do not soak your feet because your skin will get too dry.

After washing and drying your feet, put talcum powder or corn-starch between your toes. Skin between the toes tends to stay moist. Powder will keep the skin dry to help prevent an infection.

Smooth Corns and Calluses Gently

Thick patches of skin called corns or calluses can grow on the feet. If you have corns or calluses, talk with your foot doctor about the best way to care for these foot problems. If you have nerve damage, these patches can become ulcers.

If your doctor tells you to, use a pumice stone to smooth corns and calluses after bathing or showering. A pumice stone is a type of rock used to smooth the skin. Rub gently, only in one direction, to avoid tearing the skin.

Do not:

- cut corns and calluses
- use corn plasters, which are medicated pads

273

- use liquid corn and callus removers

Cutting and over-the-counter (OTC) corn removal products can damage your skin and cause an infection.

To keep your skin smooth and soft, rub a thin coat of lotion, cream, or petroleum jelly on the tops and bottoms of your feet. Do not put lotion or cream between your toes because moistness might cause an infection.

Trim Your Toenails Straight Across

Trim your toenails, when needed, after you wash and dry your feet. Using toenail clippers, trim your toenails straight across. Do not cut into the corners of your toenail. Gently smooth each nail with an emery board or nonsharp nail file. Trimming this way helps prevent cutting your skin and keeps the nails from growing into your skin.

Have a foot doctor trim your toenails if:

- you cannot see, feel, or reach your feet

- your toenails are thick or yellowed

- your nails curve and grow into the skin

If you want to get a pedicure at a salon, you should bring your own nail tools to prevent getting an infection. You can ask your health-care provider what other steps you can take at the salon to prevent infection.

Wear Shoes and Socks at All Times

Wear shoes and socks at all times. Do not walk barefoot or in just socks—even when you are indoors. You could step on something and hurt your feet. You may not feel any pain and may not know that you hurt yourself.

Check the inside of your shoes before putting them on, to make sure the lining is smooth and free of pebbles or other objects.

Make sure you wear socks, stockings, or nylons with your shoes to keep from getting blisters and sores. Choose clean, lightly padded socks that fit well. Socks with no seams are best.

Wear shoes that fit well and protect your feet. Here are some tips for finding the right type of shoes:

- Walking shoes and athletic shoes are good for daily wear. They support your feet and allow them to "breathe."

- Do not wear vinyl or plastic shoes, because they do not stretch or "breathe."

- When buying shoes, make sure they feel good and have enough room for your toes. Buy shoes at the end of the day, when your feet are the largest, so that you can find the best fit.

- If you have a bunion, or hammertoes, which are toes that curl under your feet, you may need extra-wide or deep shoes. Do not wear shoes with pointed toes or high heels, because they put too much pressure on your toes.

- If your feet have changed shape, such as from Charcot foot, you may need special shoes or shoe inserts, called orthotics. You also may need inserts if you have bunions, hammertoes, or other foot problems.

When breaking in new shoes, only wear them for a few hours at first and then check your feet for areas of soreness.

Medicare-Part B insurance and other health insurance programs may help pay for these special shoes or inserts. Ask your insurance plan if it covers your special shoes or inserts.

Protect Your Feet from Hot and Cold

If you have nerve damage from diabetes, you may burn your feet and not know you did. Take the following steps to protect your feet from heat:

- Wear shoes at the beach and on hot pavement.

- Put sunscreen on the tops of your feet to prevent sunburn.

- Keep your feet away from heaters and open fires.

- Do not put a hot water bottle or heating pad on your feet.

Wear socks in bed if your feet get cold. In the winter, wear lined, waterproof boots to keep your feet warm and dry.

Keep the Blood Flowing to Your Feet

Try the following tips to improve blood flow to your feet:

- Put your feet up when you are sitting.

- Wiggle your toes for a few minutes throughout the day. Move your ankles up and down and in and out to help blood flow in your feet and legs.

- Do not wear tight socks or elastic stockings. Do not try to hold up loose socks with rubber bands.

- Be more physically active. Choose activities that are easy on your feet, such as walking, dancing, yoga, or stretching, swimming, or bike riding.

- Stop smoking. Smoking can lower the amount of blood flow to your feet. If you smoke, ask for help to stop. You can get help by calling the national quitline at 800-QUIT-NOW or 800-784-8669.

Get a Foot Check at Every Healthcare Visit

Ask your healthcare team to check your feet at each visit. Take off your shoes and socks when you're in the exam room so they will remember to check your feet. At least once a year, get a thorough foot exam, including a check of the feeling and pulses in your feet.

Get a thorough foot exam at each healthcare visit if you have:

- changes in the shape of your feet

- loss of feeling in your feet

- peripheral artery disease

- had foot ulcers or an amputation in the past

Ask your healthcare team to show you how to care for your feet.

When Should You See Your Healthcare Provider about Foot Problems?

Call your healthcare provider right away if you have:

- a cut, blister, or bruise on your foot that does not start to heal after a few days

- skin on your foot that becomes red, warm, or painful—signs of a possible infection

- a callus with dried blood inside of it, which often can be the first sign of a wound under the callus

- a foot infection that becomes black and smelly—signs you might have gangrene

Ask your provider to refer you to a foot doctor, or podiatrist, if needed.

Chapter 39

Diabetes, Heart Disease, and Stroke

Having diabetes means that you are more likely to develop heart disease and have a greater chance of a heart attack or a stroke. People with diabetes are also more likely to have certain conditions, or risk factors, that increase the chances of having heart disease or stroke, such as high blood pressure or high cholesterol. If you have diabetes, you can protect your heart and health by managing your blood glucose, also called blood sugar, as well as your blood pressure and cholesterol. If you smoke, get help to stop.

What Is the Link between Diabetes, Heart Disease, and Stroke?

Over time, high blood glucose from diabetes can damage your blood vessels and the nerves that control your heart and blood vessels. The longer you have diabetes, the higher the chances that you will develop heart disease.

People with diabetes tend to develop heart disease at a younger age than people without diabetes. In adults with diabetes, the most common causes of death are heart disease and stroke. Adults with

---

This chapter includes text excerpted from "Diabetes, Heart Disease, and Stroke," National Institute of Diabetes and Digestive and Kidney Diseases (NIDDK), February 2017.

diabetes are nearly twice as likely to die from heart disease or stroke as people without diabetes.

The good news is that the steps you take to manage your diabetes also help to lower your chances of having heart disease or stroke.

What Else Increases Your Chances of Heart Disease or Stroke If You Have Diabetes?

If you have diabetes, other factors add to your chances of developing heart disease or having a stroke.

Smoking

Smoking raises your risk of developing heart disease. If you have diabetes, it is important to stop smoking because of both smoking and diabetes narrow blood vessels. Smoking also increases your chances of developing other long-term problems such as lung disease. Smoking also can damage the blood vessels in your legs and increase the risk of lower leg infections, ulcers, and amputation.

High Blood Pressure

If you have high blood pressure, your heart must work harder to pump blood. High blood pressure can strain your heart, damage blood vessels, and increase your risk of heart attack, stroke, eye problems, and kidney problems.

Abnormal Cholesterol Levels

Cholesterol is a type of fat produced by your liver and found in your blood. You have two kinds of cholesterol in your blood: low-density lipoprotein (LDL) and high-density lipoprotein (HDL).

LDL, often called "bad" cholesterol, can build up and clog your blood vessels. High levels of LDL cholesterol raise your risk of developing heart disease.

Another type of blood fat, triglycerides, also can raise your risk of heart disease when the levels are higher than recommended by your healthcare team.

Obesity and Belly Fat

Being overweight or obese can affect your ability to manage your diabetes and increase your risk for many health problems, including heart disease and high blood pressure. If you are overweight, a healthy eating plan with reduced calories often will lower your glucose levels and reduce your need for medications.

Excess belly fat around your waist, even if you are not overweight, can raise your chances of developing heart disease.

You have excess belly fat if your waist measures:

- more than 40 inches and you are a man

- more than 35 inches and you are a woman

Family History of Heart Disease

A family history of heart disease may also add to your chances of developing heart disease. If one or more of your family members had a heart attack before age 50, you may have an even higher chance of developing heart disease.

You can't change whether heart disease runs in your family, but if you have diabetes, it's even more important to take steps to protect yourself from heart disease and decrease your chances of having a stroke.

How Can You Lower Your Chances of a Heart Attack or Stroke If You Have Diabetes?

Taking care of your diabetes is important to help you take care of your heart. You can lower your chances of having a heart attack or stroke by taking the following steps to manage your diabetes to keep your heart and blood vessels healthy.

Manage Your Blood Glucose Level, Blood Pressure, and Cholesterol

Knowing your diabetes ABCs will help you manage your blood glucose, blood pressure, and cholesterol. Stopping smoking if you have diabetes is also important to lower your chances of heart disease.

A is for the A1C test. The A1C test shows your average blood glucose level over the past three months. This is different from the blood glucose checks that you do every day. The higher your A1C number, the higher your blood glucose levels have been during the past three months. High levels of blood glucose can harm your heart, blood vessels, kidneys, feet, and eyes.

The A1C goal for many people with diabetes is below seven percent. Some people may do better with a slightly higher A1C goal. Ask your healthcare team what your goal should be.

B is for blood pressure. Blood pressure is the force of your blood against the wall of your blood vessels. If your blood pressure gets too high, it makes your heart work too hard. High blood pressure can cause a heart attack or stroke and damage your kidneys and eyes.

The blood pressure goal for most people with diabetes is below 140/90 mm Hg. Ask what your goal should be.

C is for cholesterol. You have two kinds of cholesterol in your blood: LDL and HDL. LDL or "bad" cholesterol can build up and clog your blood vessels. Too much bad cholesterol can cause a heart attack or stroke. HDL or "good" cholesterol helps remove the "bad" cholesterol from your blood vessels.

Ask your healthcare team what your cholesterol numbers should be. If you are over 40 years of age, you may need to take medicine such as a statin to lower your cholesterol and protect your heart. Some people with very high LDL ("bad") cholesterol may need to take medicine at a younger age.

S is for stop smoking. Not smoking is especially important for people with diabetes because both smoking and diabetes narrow blood vessels, so your heart has to work harder.

If you quit smoking:

- you will lower your risk for heart attack, stroke, nerve disease, kidney disease, eye disease, and amputation

- your blood glucose, blood pressure, and cholesterol levels may improve

- your blood circulation will improve

- you may have an easier time being physically active

If you smoke or use other tobacco products, stop. Ask for help so you don't have to do it alone. You can start by calling the national quitline at 800-QUIT-NOW or 800-784-8669.

Ask your healthcare team about your goals for A1C, blood pressure, and cholesterol, and what you can do to reach these goals.

Develop or Maintain Healthy Lifestyle Habits

Developing or maintaining healthy lifestyle habits can help you manage your diabetes and prevent heart disease.

- Follow your healthy eating plan.

- Make physical activity part of your routine.

- Stay at or get to a healthy weight.

- Get enough sleep.

Learn to Manage Stress

Managing diabetes is not always easy. Feeling stressed, sad, or angry is common when you are living with diabetes. You may know what to do to stay healthy but may have trouble sticking with your plan over time. Long-term stress can raise your blood glucose and blood pressure, but you can learn ways to lower your stress. Try deep breathing, gardening, taking a walk, doing yoga*, meditating, doing a hobby, or listening to your favorite music.

* A mind and body practice with origins in ancient Indian philosophy.

Take Medicine to Protect Your Heart

Medicines may be an important part of your treatment plan. Your doctor will prescribe medicine based on your specific needs. Medicine may help you:

- meet your A1C (blood glucose), blood pressure, and cholesterol goals

- reduce your risk of blood clots, heart attack, or stroke

- treat angina or chest pain that is often a symptom of heart disease. (Angina can also be an early symptom of a heart attack.)

Ask your doctor whether you should take aspirin. Aspirin is not safe for everyone. Your doctor can tell you whether taking aspirin is right for you and exactly how much to take.

Statins can reduce the risk of having a heart attack or stroke in some people with diabetes. Statins are a type of medicine often used to help people meet their cholesterol goals. Talk with your doctor to find out whether taking a statin is right for you.

Talk to your doctor if you have questions about your medicines. Before you start a new medicine, ask your doctor about possible side effects and how you can avoid them. If the side effects of your medicine bother you, tell your doctor. Don't stop taking your medicines without checking with your doctor first.

How Do Doctors Diagnose Heart Disease in Diabetes?

Doctors diagnose heart disease in diabetes based on:

- your symptoms
- your medical and family history
- how likely you are to have heart disease
- a physical exam
- results from tests and procedures

Tests used to monitor your diabetes—A1C, blood pressure, and cholesterol—help your doctor decide whether it is important to do other tests to check your heart health.

What Are the Warning Signs of Heart Attack and Stroke?

Call 9-1-1 right away if you have any of the following warning signs of a heart attack:

- pain or pressure in your chest that lasts longer than a few minutes or goes away and comes back
- pain or discomfort in one or both of your arms or shoulders; or your back, neck, or jaw
- shortness of breath
- sweating or light-headedness
- indigestion or nausea (feeling sick to your stomach)
- feeling very tired

Treatment works best when it is given right away. Warning signs can be different in different people. You may not have all of these symptoms.

If you have angina, it's important to know how and when to seek medical treatment.

Women sometimes have nausea and vomiting, feel very tired (sometimes for days), and have pain in the back, shoulders, or jaw without any chest pain.

People with diabetes-related nerve damage may not notice any chest pain.

Call 9-1-1 right away if you have warning signs of a stroke, including sudden:

- weakness or numbness of your face, arm, or leg on one side of your body
- confusion, or trouble talking or understanding
- dizziness, loss of balance, or trouble walking
- trouble seeing out of one or both eyes
- sudden severe headache

If you have any one of these warning signs, call 9-1-1. You can help prevent permanent damage by getting to a hospital within an hour of a stroke.

Chapter 40

Diabetes-Related Kidney Disease

What Is Diabetic Kidney Disease?

Diabetic kidney disease is a type of kidney disease caused by diabetes.

Diabetes is the leading cause of kidney disease. About 1 out of 4 adults with diabetes have kidney disease.

The main job of the kidneys is to filter wastes and extra water out of your blood to make urine. Your kidneys also help control blood pressure and make hormones that your body needs to stay healthy.

When your kidneys are damaged, they can't filter blood like they should, which can cause wastes to build up in your body. Kidney damage can also cause other health problems.

Kidney damage caused by diabetes usually occurs slowly, over many years. You can take steps to protect your kidneys and to prevent or delay kidney damage.

Diabetic kidney disease is also called DKD, chronic kidney disease (CKD), kidney disease or diabetes, or diabetic nephropathy.

This chapter includes text excerpted from "Diabetic Kidney Disease," National Institute of Diabetes and Digestive and Kidney Diseases (NIDDK) February 2017.

How Does Diabetes Cause Kidney Disease?

High blood glucose, also called blood sugar, can damage the blood vessels in your kidneys. When the blood vessels are damaged, they don't work as well. Many people with diabetes also develop high blood pressure, which can also damage your kidneys.

What Increases Your Chances of Developing Diabetic Kidney Disease?

Having diabetes for a long time increases the chances that you will have kidney damage. If you have diabetes, you are more likely to develop kidney disease if your:

- blood glucose is too high

- blood pressure is too high

African Americans, American Indians, and Hispanics/Latinos develop diabetes, kidney disease, and kidney failure at a higher rate than Caucasians.

You are also more likely to develop kidney disease if you have diabetes and;

- smoke

- don't follow your diabetes eating plan

- eat foods high in salt

- are not active

- are overweight

- have heart disease

- have a family history of kidney failure

How Can You Tell If You Have Diabetic Kidney Disease?

Most people with diabetic kidney disease do not have symptoms. The only way to know if you have diabetic kidney disease is to get your kidneys checked.

Healthcare professionals use blood and urine tests to check for diabetic kidney disease. Your healthcare professional will check your urine for albumin and will also do a blood test to see how well your kidneys are filtering your blood.

You should get tested every year for kidney disease if you:

- have type 2 diabetes
- have had type 1 diabetes for more than five years

How Can You Keep Your Kidneys Healthy If You Have Diabetes?

The best way to slow or prevent diabetes-related kidney disease is to try to reach your blood glucose and blood pressure goals. Healthy lifestyle habits and taking your medicines as prescribed can help you achieve these goals and improve your health overall.

Reach Your Blood Glucose Goals

Your healthcare professional will test your A1C. The A1C is a blood test that shows your average blood glucose level over the past three months. This is different from the blood glucose checks that you may do yourself. The higher your A1C number, the higher your blood glucose levels have been during the past three months.

The A1C goal for many people with diabetes is below seven percent. Ask your healthcare team what your goal should be. Reaching your goal numbers will help you protect your kidneys.

To reach your A1C goal, your healthcare professional may ask you to check your blood glucose levels. Work with your healthcare team to use the results to guide decisions about food, physical activity, and medicines. Ask your healthcare team how often you should check your blood glucose level.

Control Your Blood Pressure

Blood pressure is the force of your blood against the wall of your blood vessels. High blood pressure makes your heart work too hard. It can cause heart attack, stroke, and kidney disease.

Your healthcare team will also work with you to help you set and reach your blood pressure goal. The blood pressure goal for most people with diabetes is below 140/90 mmHg. Ask your healthcare team what your goal should be.

Medicines that lower blood pressure can also help slow kidney damage. Two types of blood pressure medicines, angiotensin-converting enzyme (ACE) inhibitors and angiotensin-receptor blockers (ARBs), play a special role in protecting your kidneys. Each has been found to slow kidney damage in people with diabetes who have high blood pressure and DKD. The names of these medicines end in -pril or -sartan. ACE inhibitors and ARBs are not safe for women who are pregnant.

Develop or Maintain Healthy Lifestyle Habits

Healthy lifestyle habits can help you reach your blood glucose and blood pressure goals. Following the steps below will also help you keep your kidneys healthy:

- Stop smoking.

- Work with a dietitian to develop a diabetes meal plan and limit salt and sodium.

- Make physical activity part of your routine.

- Stay at or get to a healthy weight.

- Get enough sleep. Aim for 7–8 hours of sleep each night.

Take Medicines as Prescribed

Medicines may be an important part of your treatment plan. Your healthcare professional will prescribe medicine based on your specific needs. Medicine can help you meet your blood glucose and blood pressure goals. You may need to take more than one kind of medicine to control your blood pressure.

How Can You Cope with the Stress of Managing Your Diabetes?

Managing diabetes isn't always easy. Feeling stressed, sad, or angry is common when you are living with diabetes. You may know what to do to stay healthy but may have trouble sticking with your plan over time. Long-term stress can raise your blood glucose and blood pressure, but you can learn ways to lower your stress. Try deep breathing, gardening, taking a walk, doing yoga, meditating, doing a hobby, or listening to your favorite music.

Does Diabetic Kidney Disease Get Worse over Time?

Kidney damage from diabetes can get worse over time. However, you can take steps to keep your kidneys healthy and help slow kidney damage to prevent or delay kidney failure. Kidney failure means that your kidneys have lost most of their ability to function—less than 15 percent of normal kidney function. However, most people with diabetes and kidney disease don't end up with kidney failure.

Chapter 41

Diabetes and Kidney Failure

End-Stage Renal Disease (ESRD) or Kidney Failure[1]

Chronic kidney disease (CKD) is a public health problem that affects nearly 14 percent of the U.S. population and is disproportionately distributed among minority and disadvantaged groups. Most risk factors for CKD are modifiable; therefore, public health strategies targeting these factors may significantly reduce the disease burden.

Diabetes is the leading cause of CKD, and the increasing prevalence of diabetes together with improved availability of dialysis and transplants have sustained a continued rise in the proportion of CKD attributable to diabetes since the 1980s. In persons with type 1 diabetes, the incidence of CKD has declined in parallel with a significant trend for earlier initiation of antihypertensive treatment following the onset of diabetes, expansion of RAAS inhibitor (renin-angiotensin-aldosterone system) usage, and sustained improvements in glycemic control. On

This chapter includes text excerpted from documents published by three public domain sources. Text under the headings marked 1 are excerpted from "Kidney Disease in Diabetes," National Institute of Diabetes and Digestive and Kidney Diseases (NIDDK), July 10, 2017; Text under the heading marked 2 is excerpted from "Chronic Kidney Disease Tests and Diagnosis," National Institute of Diabetes and Digestive and Kidney Diseases (NIDDK), October 2016; Text under the heading marked 3 is excerpted from "Choosing a Treatment for Kidney Failure," National Institute of Diabetes and Digestive and Kidney Diseases (NIDDK), January 2018.

the other hand, in persons with type 2 diabetes, the incidence of CKD does not appear to be declining, possibly due to the higher number and prevalence of CKD risk factors associated with type 2 diabetes that outweigh current treatment options or their effectiveness. An ever-increasing number of persons with diabetes, 91 percent of whom have type 2 diabetes, are requiring renal replacement therapy, at an enormous cost to patients, their families, and to society.

Improved management of hyperglycemia, hypertension, hyperlipidemia, and albuminuria have dramatically slowed progression to end-stage renal disease (ESRD), as illustrated by a level incidence of ESRD attributed to diabetes since 2005. Trends in the incidence of ESRD due to diabetes, however, differ broadly by age and race/ethnicity. At the national level, the incidence of ESRD in persons with a primary diagnosis of diabetes remains higher in African Americans, Mexican Americans, Asians, and American Indians than in whites, with the highest rates being found in African Americans and American Indians.

Risk Factors for Diabetic Kidney Disease[1]

Numerous risk factors have been identified for the development and progression of diabetic kidney disease. Some of the more prominent factors are:

Duration of Diabetes

One of the most important risk factors for diabetic kidney disease is the duration of diabetes, its influence being far greater than that of age, sex, or type of diabetes. For a given duration of diabetes, the cumulative incidences of overt nephropathy and ESRD are similar in type 1 and type 2 diabetes.

Socioeconomic Factors

Socioeconomic factors are often taken into consideration when describing associations between risk factors and CKD in large populations with diabetes. A low socioeconomic status is associated with increased prevalence of diabetes, hypertension, and CKD. The mechanism of this association, however, is unclear and often difficult to separate from racial/ethnic predisposition or other environmental factors. Exposure to an adverse prenatal environment, such as that caused by poor maternal dietary habits, smoking, or poor health, may also introduce adverse health traits that persist in subsequent generations.

Hyperglycemia

Increased blood glucose concentration is a major risk factor for the development and progression of moderate albuminuria in both types of diabetes but may have a lesser influence on progression of more advanced kidney dysfunction, when hypertension, hypercholesterolemia, and genetic factors play a greater role in shaping the outcome.

Hypertension

High blood pressure is related to diabetic kidney disease in many cross-sectional and longitudinal studies of both type 1 and type 2 diabetes. In type 1 diabetes, this relationship frequently reflects elevation of blood pressure in response to kidney disease; whereas in type 2 diabetes, the onset of hypertension generally precedes diabetic kidney disease and is often associated with obesity.

Obesity

Obesity is a major risk factor for diabetes, hypertension, and CVD, all of which increase the risk for kidney disease. It increasingly affects young people, particularly Hispanics, African Americans, and American Indians, leading to an earlier onset of diabetes and its major complications, including kidney disease.

Lipids

Many of the abnormalities in plasma lipoproteins associated with kidney disease are sequelae of kidney dysfunction, yet dyslipidemia may also play a role in the pathogenesis of glomerular injury. Dyslipidemia might contribute to onset and progression of diabetic kidney disease through mechanisms similar to those responsible for arterial atherogenesis. The diabetic environment facilitates glomerular production of triglycerides and cholesterol, which appear to cause kidney injury.

Screening for Chronic Kidney Disease in Diabetes[2]

Blood Test for Glomerular Filtration Rate (GFR)

Your healthcare provider will use a blood test to check your kidney function. The results of the test mean the following:

- a GFR of 60 or more is in the normal range. Ask your healthcare provider when your GFR should be checked again.

- a GFR of less than 60 may mean you have kidney disease. Talk with your healthcare provider about how to keep your kidney health at this level.

- a GFR of 15 or less is called kidney failure. Most people below this level need dialysis or a kidney transplant. Talk with your healthcare provider about your treatment options.

You can't raise your GFR, but you can try to keep it from going lower.

Creatinine. Creatinine is a waste product from the normal breakdown of muscles in your body. Your kidneys remove creatinine from your blood. Providers use the amount of creatinine in your blood to estimate your GFR. As kidney disease gets worse, the level of creatinine goes up.

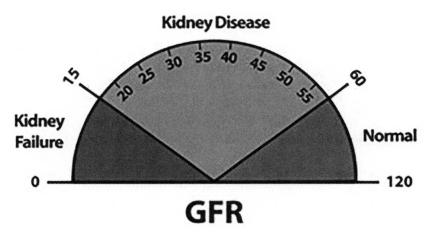

Figure 41.1. *Glomerular Filtration Rate (GFR)*

GFR results show whether your kidneys are filtering at a normal level.

Urine Test for Albumin

If you are at risk for kidney disease, your provider may check your urine for albumin.

Albumin is a protein found in your blood. A healthy kidney doesn't let albumin pass into the urine. A damaged kidney lets some albumin pass into the urine. The less albumin in your urine, the better. Having albumin in the urine is called albuminuria.

Inside a *healthy* kidney   **Inside a *damaged* kidney**

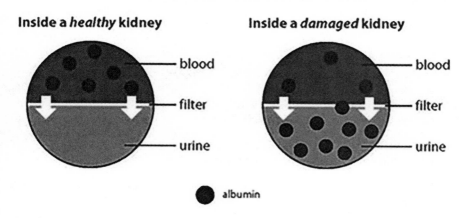

Figure 41.2. *Healthy versus Damaged Kidney*

A healthy kidney doesn't let albumin pass into the urine. A damaged kidney lets some albumin pass into the urine.

A healthcare provider can check for albumin in your urine in two ways:

Dipstick test for albumin. A provider uses a urine sample to look for albumin in your urine. You collect the urine sample in a container in a healthcare provider's office or lab. For the test, a provider places a strip of chemically treated paper, called a dipstick, into the urine. The dipstick changes color if albumin is present in the urine.

Urine albumin-to-creatinine ratio (UACR). This test measures and compares the amount of albumin with the amount of creatinine in your urine sample. Providers use your UACR to estimate how much albumin would pass into your urine over 24 hours. A urine albumin result of:

- 30 mg/g or less is normal
- more than 30 mg/g may be a sign of kidney disease

If you have albumin in your urine, your provider may want you to repeat the urine test one or two more times to confirm the results. Talk with your provider about what your specific numbers mean for you.

If you have kidney disease, measuring the albumin in your urine helps your provider know which treatment is best for you. A urine albumin level that stays the same or goes down may mean that treatments are working.

Managing ESRD[3]

You can choose one of three treatment options to filter your blood and take over a small part of the work your damaged kidneys can no longer do. A fourth option offers care without replacing the work of the kidneys. None of these treatments will help your kidneys get better. However, they all can help you feel better.

- **Hemodialysis** uses a machine to move your blood through a filter outside your body, removing wastes.

- **Peritoneal dialysis** uses the lining of your belly to filter your blood inside your body, removing wastes.

- **Kidney transplant** is surgery to place a healthy kidney from a person who has just died, or from a living person, into your body to filter your blood.

- **Conservative management** treats kidney failure without dialysis or a transplant. You'll work with your healthcare team to manage symptoms and preserve your kidney function and quality of life as long as possible.

Doing well with kidney failure is a challenge, and it works best if you:

- stick to your treatment schedule.

- review your medicines with your healthcare provider at every visit. You are the only one who knows how your body is responding to each of your medicines. It's really important that your provider knows which medicines you are taking.

- follow a special eating plan.

- are active most days of the week.

Prognosis for Persons with Diabetic ESRD[1]

Persons with diabetes make up the fastest growing group of kidney dialysis and transplant recipients in the United States. In 1985, 20,961 persons with diabetes were receiving renal replacement therapy, representing 29 percent of all new cases of end-stage renal disease (ESRD). By 2012, 239,837 persons with diabetes were on renal replacement therapy, accounting for 44 percent of all new ESRD cases. The increased count reflects growth in diabetes prevalence and increased access to dialysis and transplantation. Those with a primary diagnosis of diabetes have lower survival relative to other causes of ESRD, primarily because of the coexistent morbidity associated with diabetes, particularly cardiovascular diseases (CVD). While survival on dialysis has slowly improved across modalities since the 1990s, it remains reduced in persons with diabetes, half of whom die within 3 years of beginning dialysis in the United States. Similar to persons with ESRD in general, the leading causes of death among adults with diabetes who started dialysis before 2009 were CVD (58% of the deaths) and infections (13% of the deaths). Kidney transplant recipients with diabetes have much better survival than those on dialysis, indicating a significant impact of the type of renal replacement therapy (transplant versus dialysis) on long-term survival.

Chapter 42

Diabetes and Pregnancy-Related Complications

Chapter Contents

Section 42.1

Type 1 or Type 2 Diabetes and Pregnancy

This section includes text excerpted from "Pregnancy—
Type 1 or Type 2 Diabetes and Pregnancy," Centers for
Disease Control and Prevention (CDC), June 1, 2018.

Problems of Diabetes in Pregnancy

Blood sugar that is not well-controlled in a pregnant woman with Type
1 or Type 2 diabetes could lead to problems for the woman and the baby:

Birth Defects

The organs of the baby form during the first two months of pregnancy, often before a woman knows that she is pregnant. Blood sugar
that is not in control can affect those organs while they are being
formed and cause serious birth defects in the developing baby, such
as those of the brain, spine, and heart.

An Extra Large Baby

Diabetes that is not well-controlled causes the baby's blood sugar to
be high. The baby is "overfed" and grows extra large. Besides causing
discomfort to the woman during the last few months of pregnancy,
an extra large baby can lead to problems during delivery for both the
mother and the baby. The mother might need a cesarean section (C-section) to deliver the baby. The baby can be born with nerve damage due
to pressure on the shoulder during delivery.

C- Section (Cesarean Section)

A C-section is a surgery to deliver the baby through the mother's
belly. A woman who has diabetes that is not well-controlled has a
higher chance of needing a C-section to deliver the baby. When the
baby is delivered by a C-section, it takes longer for the woman to
recover from childbirth.

High Blood Pressure (Preeclampsia)

When a pregnant woman has high blood pressure, protein in her
urine, and often swelling in fingers and toes that doesn't go away,
she might have preeclampsia. It is a serious problem that needs to be

watched closely and managed by her doctor. High blood pressure can cause harm to both the woman and her unborn baby. It might lead to the baby being born early and also could cause seizures or a stroke (a blood clot or a bleed in the brain that can lead to brain damage) in the woman during labor and delivery. Women with type 1 or type 2 diabetes have high blood pressure more often than women without diabetes.

Early (Preterm) Birth

Being born too early can result in problems for the baby, such as breathing problems, heart problems, bleeding into the brain, intestinal problems, and vision problems. Women with type 1 or type 2 diabetes are more likely to deliver early than women without diabetes.

Low Blood Sugar (Hypoglycemia)

People with diabetes who take insulin or other diabetes medications can develop blood sugar that is too low. Low blood sugar can be very serious, and even fatal, if not treated quickly. Seriously low blood sugar can be avoided if women watch their blood sugar closely and treat low blood sugar early.

If a woman's diabetes was not well-controlled during pregnancy, her baby can very quickly develop low blood sugar after birth. The baby's blood sugar must be watched for several hours after delivery.

Miscarriage or Stillbirth

A miscarriage is a loss of the pregnancy before 20 weeks. Stillbirth means that after 20 weeks, the baby dies in the womb. Miscarriages and stillbirths can happen for many reasons. A woman who has diabetes that is not well-controlled has a higher chance of having a miscarriage or stillbirth.

Seven Tips for Women with Diabetes

If a woman with diabetes keeps her blood sugar well-controlled before and during pregnancy, she can increase her chances of having a healthy baby. Controlling blood sugar also reduces the chance that a woman will develop common problems of diabetes, or that the problems will get worse during pregnancy.

Steps women can take before and during pregnancy to help prevent problems includes:

1. **Plan for pregnancy.** Before getting pregnant, see your doctor. The doctor needs to look at the effects that diabetes has had on your body already, talk with you about getting and keeping control of your blood sugar, change medications if needed, and plan for frequent follow-up. If you are overweight, the doctor might recommend that you try to lose weight before getting pregnant as part of the plan to get your blood sugar under control.

2. **See your doctor early and often.** During pregnancy, a woman with diabetes needs to see the doctor more often than a pregnant woman without diabetes. Together, you and your doctor can work to prevent or catch problems early.

3. **Eat healthy foods.** Eat healthy foods from a meal plan made for a person with diabetes. A dietitian can help you create a healthy meal plan. A dietitian can also help you learn how to control your blood sugar while you are pregnant.

4. **Exercise regularly.** Exercise is another way to keep blood sugar under control. It helps to balance food intake. After checking with your doctor, you can exercise regularly before, during, and after pregnancy. Get at least 30 minutes of moderate-intensity physical activity at least five days a week. This could be brisk walking, swimming, or actively playing with children.

5. **Take pills and insulin as directed.** If diabetes pills or insulin are ordered by your doctor, take it as directed in order to help keep your blood sugar under control.

6. **Control and treat low blood sugar quickly.** Keeping blood sugar well-controlled can lead to a chance of low blood sugar at times. If you are taking diabetes pills or insulin, it's helpful to have a source of quick sugar, such as hard candy, glucose tablets or gel, on hand at all times. It's also good to teach family members and close co-workers or friends how to help in case of a severe low blood sugar reaction.

7. **Monitor blood sugar often.** Because pregnancy causes the body's need for energy to change, blood sugar levels can change very quickly. You need to check your blood sugar

often, as directed by your doctor. It is important to learn how to adjust food intake, exercise, and insulin, depending on the results of your blood sugar tests.

Section 42.2

Gestational Diabetes and Pregnancy

This section includes text excerpted from "Gestational Diabetes and Pregnancy," Centers for Disease Control and Prevention (CDC), June 1, 2018.

Gestational diabetes is a type of diabetes that is first seen in a pregnant woman who did not have diabetes before she was pregnant. Some women have more than one pregnancy affected by gestational diabetes. Gestational diabetes usually shows up in the middle of pregnancy. Doctors most often test for it between 24–28 weeks of pregnancy.

Often gestational diabetes can be controlled through eating healthy foods and regular exercise. Sometimes a woman with gestational diabetes must also take insulin.

Problems of Gestational Diabetes in Pregnancy

Blood sugar that is not well controlled in a woman with gestational diabetes can lead to problems for the pregnant woman and the baby. Some of them are described below:

An Extra Large Baby

Diabetes that is not well controlled causes the baby's blood sugar to be high. The baby is "overfed" and grows extra large. Besides causing discomfort to the woman during the last few months of pregnancy, an extra large baby can lead to problems during delivery for both the mother and the baby. The mother might need a Cesarean section (C-section) to deliver the baby. The baby can be born with nerve damage due to pressure on the shoulder during delivery.

Cesarean Section

A C-section is an operation to deliver the baby through the mother's belly. A woman who has diabetes that is not well controlled has a higher chance of needing a C-section to deliver the baby. When the baby is delivered by a C-section, it takes longer for the woman to recover from childbirth.

High Blood Pressure (Preeclampsia)

When a pregnant woman has high blood pressure, protein in her urine, and often swelling in fingers and toes that doesn't go away, she might have preeclampsia. It is a serious problem that needs to be watched closely and managed by her doctor. High blood pressure can cause harm to both the woman and her unborn baby. It might lead to the baby being born early and also could cause seizures or a stroke (a blood clot or a bleed in the brain that can lead to brain damage) in the woman during labor and delivery. Women with diabetes have high blood pressure more often than women without diabetes.

Low Blood Sugar (Hypoglycemia)

People with diabetes who take insulin or other diabetes medications can develop blood sugar that is too low. Low blood sugar can be very serious, and even fatal, if not treated quickly. Seriously low blood sugar can be avoided if women watch their blood sugar closely and treat low blood sugar early.

If a woman's diabetes was not well controlled during pregnancy, her baby can very quickly develop low blood sugar after birth. The baby's blood sugar must be watched for several hours after delivery.

Five Tips for Women with Gestational Diabetes

Tip 1. Eat Healthy Foods

Eat healthy foods from a meal plan made for a person with diabetes. A dietitian can help you create a healthy meal plan. A dietitian can also help you learn how to control your blood sugar while you are pregnant.

Tip 2. Exercise Regularly

Exercise is another way to keep blood sugar under control. It helps to balance food intake. After checking with your doctor, you can exercise regularly during and after pregnancy. Get at least 30 minutes of moderate-intensity physical activity at least five days a week. This could be brisk walking, swimming, or actively playing with children.

Tip 3. Monitor Blood Sugar Often

Because pregnancy causes the body's need for energy to change, blood sugar levels can change very quickly. Check your blood sugar often, as directed by your doctor.

Tip 4. Take Insulin, If Needed

Sometimes a woman with gestational diabetes must take insulin. If insulin is ordered by your doctor, take it as directed in order to help keep blood sugar under control.

Tip 5. Get Tested for Diabetes after Pregnancy

Get tested for diabetes 6–12 weeks after your baby is born, and then every 1–3 years. For most women with gestational diabetes, diabetes goes away soon after delivery. When it does not go away, the diabetes is called type 2 diabetes. Even if diabetes does go away after the baby is born, half of all women who had gestational diabetes develop type 2 diabetes later. It's important for a woman who has had gestational diabetes to continue to exercise and eat a healthy diet after pregnancy to prevent or delay getting type 2 diabetes. She should also remind her doctor to check her blood sugar every 1–3 years.

Chapter 43

Diabetes and Sexual and Bladder Problems

Sexual problems and bladder problems are common as people age, but diabetes can make these problems worse. You or your partner may have trouble having or enjoying sex. Or, you may leak urine or have trouble emptying your bladder normally.

Blood vessels and nerves can be damaged by the effects of high blood glucose, also called blood sugar. This damage can lead to sexual and bladder problems. Keeping your blood glucose levels in your target range is an important way to prevent damage to your blood vessels and nerves.

Work with your healthcare team to help prevent or treat sexual and bladder problems. These problems may be signs that you need to manage your diabetes in a different way. Remember, a healthy sex life and a healthy bladder can improve your quality of life, so take action now if you have concerns.

Can Sexual and Bladder Problems Be Symptoms of Diabetes?

Yes. Changes in sexual function or bladder habits may be a sign that you have diabetes. Nerve damage caused by diabetes, also called

This chapter includes text excerpted from "Diabetes, Sexual, and Bladder Problems," National Institute of Diabetes and Digestive and Kidney Diseases (NIDDK), June 2018.

diabetic neuropathy, can damage parts of your body—like your genitals or urinary tract. For example, men with diabetes may develop erectile dysfunction (ED) 10–15 years earlier than men without diabetes.

Talk with a healthcare professional if you have any symptoms of diabetes, including sexual and bladder problems.

When Should You See a Doctor about Your Sexual or Bladder Problems?

See a healthcare professional for problems with sex or your bladder. These problems could be a sign that you need to manage your diabetes differently. You may find it embarrassing and difficult to talk about these things. However, remember that healthcare professionals are trained to speak with people about every kind of health problem. Everyone deserves to have healthy relationships and enjoy the activities they love.

What Makes You More Likely to Develop Sexual or Bladder Problems?

You're more likely to develop sexual or bladder problems if you have diabetes and:

- have high blood glucose that is not well controlled, also called high blood sugar
- have nerve damage, also called neuropathy
- have high blood pressure that is not treated
- have high cholesterol that is not treated
- are overweight or have obesity
- are not physically active
- are taking certain medicines
- drink too many alcoholic drinks
- smoke

Research also suggests that certain genes may make people more likely to develop diabetic neuropathy.

What Sexual Problems Can Men with Diabetes Have?

Changes in your blood vessels, nerves, hormones, and emotional health during diabetes may make it more difficult for you to have

308

satisfactory sex. Diabetes and its related challenges also may make it harder for you to have a child.

Erectile Dysfunction

You have ED if you're unable to get or keep an erection firm enough for satisfactory sexual intercourse. More than half of men with diabetes will get ED. Men who have diabetes are more than three times more likely to develop ED than men who do not have diabetes. Good diabetes management may help prevent and treat ED caused by nerve damage and circulation problems. A doctor can help treat ED with medicine or a change in your diabetes care plan.

Retrograde Ejaculation

Rarely, diabetes can cause retrograde ejaculation, which is when part or all of your semen goes into your bladder instead of out of your penis during ejaculation. During retrograde ejaculation, semen enters your bladder, mixes with urine, and is safely urinated out. A urine sample after ejaculation can show if you have retrograde ejaculation. Some men with retrograde ejaculation may not ejaculate at all.

Penile Curvature

Men with diabetes are more likely to have Peyronie disease, also called penile curvature, than men who don't have diabetes. Men with Peyronie disease have scar tissue, called a plaque, in the penis, making it curve when erect. Curves in the penis can make sexual intercourse painful or difficult. Some men with Peyronie disease may have ED.

Low Testosterone

Men's testosterone levels naturally lower with age. However, lower-than-normal testosterone levels may be the cause of some men's ED or can explain why some men often feel tired, depressed, or have a low sex drive. Men with diabetes, especially those who are older and overweight, are more likely to have low testosterone, or "low T."

If your doctor thinks you might have low T, you will probably be asked to give a blood sample, and a healthcare professional will give you a physical exam. Your doctor may suggest treating your low testosterone with a prescription gel, injection, or patch.

Several studies show that, along with good diabetes management, testosterone therapy can lessen a man's sexual problems. However, testosterone therapy may have serious risks and may not be safe for all men. Talk with your doctor about testosterone therapies side effects and whether it's right for you.

Fertility Problems

Some studies show that men with diabetes can have problems with their sperm that make it harder to conceive. Your sperm could be slow or not move well, or your sperm may not be able to fertilize a woman's egg well. Working closely with your partner and a healthcare professional trained in fertility issues may help.

If you and your partner want to conceive a child, your doctor may treat retrograde ejaculation caused by diabetes with medicine or by changing your diabetes care plan. Or, talk with a urologist who is a fertility expert. He or she may be able to collect your sperm from your urine and then use it for artificial insemination.

What Sexual Problems Can Women with Diabetes Have?

Low sexual desire and response, vaginal dryness, and painful sex can be caused by nerve damage, reduced blood flow to the genitals, and hormonal changes. Other conditions can cause these problems, too, including menopause. If you notice a change in your sex life, talk with your healthcare team. A physical exam, which will include a pelvic exam, and blood and urine tests may help your doctor find the cause of your problems.

Low Sexual Desire and Response

Low sexual desire and sexual response can include:

- being unable to become or stay aroused
- not having enough vaginal lubrication
- having little to no feeling in your genitals
- being unable to have an orgasm or rarely having one

With diabetes, your body and mind will likely go through many changes. For example, both high and low blood glucose levels can affect how and if you become aroused. Or, you may find yourself more tired than usual or depressed and anxious, making you less interested in sex.

Your healthcare team can help you make changes to your diabetes care plan so that you're back on track. Women who keep blood glucose levels in their target range are less likely to have nerve damage, which can lead to low sexual desire and response.

Painful Sex

Some women with diabetes say they have uncomfortable or painful sexual intercourse. The nerves that tell your vagina to lubricate during stimulation can become damaged by diabetes. A prescription or over-the-counter (OTC) vaginal lubricant may help if you have vaginal dryness. Managing your blood glucose well over many weeks, months, and years can help prevent nerve damage.

Yeast and Bladder Infections

Women with diabetes are more likely to have yeast infections because yeast organisms can grow more easily when your blood glucose levels are higher. Yeast infections can be uncomfortable or painful and prevent you from enjoying activities, including having sex.

Although some yeast infections can be treated at home, talk with a healthcare professional first about your symptoms. Some symptoms of yeast infections are similar to other types of infections, including sexually transmitted diseases.

Pregnancy Concerns and Fertility Problems

If you have diabetes and plan to become pregnant, it's important to get your blood glucose levels close to your target range before you get pregnant. High blood glucose can harm your baby during the first weeks of pregnancy, even before you know you're pregnant.

If you have diabetes and are already pregnant, see your doctor as soon as possible to make a plan to manage your diabetes. Working with your healthcare team and following your diabetes management plan can help you have a healthy pregnancy and a healthy baby.

Conditions such as obesity and polycystic ovarian syndrome (PCOS) that are linked to diabetes can make it harder to conceive a child. Talk with a healthcare professional, such as a gynecologist or a fertility specialist, if you're having problems conceiving a child.

What Bladder Problems Can Men and Women with Diabetes Have?

Diabetes can cause nerve damage to your urinary tract, causing bladder problems. Overweight and obesity also can increase bladder problems, such as urinary incontinence (UI). Managing diabetes is an important part of preventing problems that can lead to excess urination.

Your healthcare team may be able to help you manage your blood glucose levels and help you lose weight if needed. Doctors use blood and urine tests to diagnose bladder problems or conditions with similar symptoms. Doctors also may use urodynamic testing to see what kind of bladder problem you have.

Frequent and Urgent Urination

Some people with diabetes who regularly have high blood glucose levels may have to urinate too often, also called urinary frequency. Even men and women with diabetes who manage their blood glucose levels within their target range sometimes feel the sudden urge to urinate, called urgency incontinence. This can happen at night, also. Medicines may help reduce the symptoms of bladder control problems.

Trouble "Going"

You may find that diabetes causes you to no longer feel when your bladder is full. Many people with diabetes report that they have trouble "going." Over time, having a too-full bladder can cause damage to your bladder muscles that push urine out. When these muscles don't work correctly, urine may stay in your bladder too long, also called urinary retention. Urinary retention can cause bladder infections, urine leaks, and the feeling that you always have to go.

Leaking Urine

People with diabetes are more likely to have other types of UI, such as stress incontinence. Nerve damage, obesity, and bladder infections, which are linked with diabetes, are often related to bladder control problems. Leaking urine can cause you to avoid activities you once enjoyed, including sex.

If you're overweight, losing weight can help you have fewer leaks. Avoiding weight gain may prevent UI. Studies suggest that, as your body mass index (BMI) increases, you're more likely to leak. If you're overweight or have obesity, talk with your doctor about how to lose weight.

Work with your healthcare team to help manage and prevent urine leaks. Bladder control problems are often treatable and are very common, even in people who don't have diabetes. You don't have to accept rushing to the bathroom all the time to avoid leaks.

Bladder Infections

People with diabetes are more likely to have urinary tract infections, also called bladder infections or cystitis. See a doctor right away if you have frequent, urgent urination that may be painful. Bladder infections can develop into kidney infections and can make bladder symptoms, such as leaks and urine retention, worse. Also, bladder infections can get in the way of your everyday life, including intimacy. Managing your blood glucose levels can help prevent bladder infections.

How Can You Prevent and Treat Your Sexual or Bladder Problems?

Managing your diabetes can help prevent nerve damage and other diabetes problems that can lead to sexual and bladder problems. With your healthcare team, you can help prevent and treat your sexual or bladder control problems by:

- keeping your blood glucose, blood pressure, and cholesterol levels close to your target numbers

- being physically active

- keeping a healthy weight

- quitting smoking if you smoke

- getting help for any emotional or psychological problems

Sex is a physical activity, so be sure to check your blood glucose level before and after sex, especially if you take insulin. Both high blood glucose levels and low blood glucose levels can cause problems during sex.

Counseling may also be helpful when you notice changes in your sexual function or desire. These types of changes are very common as people age or adjust to health problems.

If you have a partner, he or she also may be an important member of your healthcare team. You may find it helpful to share your concerns and have that person join you at the doctor's office or at counseling. Your friends and family may also be able to support you if you're having bladder problems.

Chapter 44

Diabetes-Related Tooth and Gum Disease

How Can Diabetes Affect Your Mouth?

Too much glucose, also called sugar, in your blood from diabetes can cause pain, infection, and other problems in your mouth. Your mouth includes:

- your teeth

- your gums

- your jaw

- tissues such as your tongue, the roof, and bottom of your mouth, and the inside of your cheeks

Glucose is present in your saliva—the fluid in your mouth that makes it wet. When diabetes is not controlled, high glucose levels in your saliva help harmful bacteria grow. These bacteria combine with food to form a soft, sticky film called plaque. Plaque also comes from eating foods that contain sugars or starches. Some types of plaque cause tooth decay or cavities. Other types of plaque cause gum disease and bad breath.

This chapter includes text excerpted from "Diabetes, Gum Disease, and Other Dental Problems," National Institute of Diabetes and Digestive and Kidney Diseases (NIDDK), September 2014. Reviewed September 2018.

315

High Glucose Levels = Increase in Plague

Gum disease can be more severe and take longer to heal if you have diabetes. In turn, having gum disease can make your blood glucose hard to control.

What Happens If You Have Plaque?

Plaque that is not removed hardens over time into tartar and collects above your gum line. Tartar makes it more difficult to brush and clean between your teeth. Your gums become red and swollen, and bleed easily—signs of unhealthy or inflamed gums, called gingivitis.

When gingivitis is not treated, it can advance to gum disease called periodontitis. In periodontitis, the gums pull away from the teeth and form spaces, called pockets, which slowly become infected. This infection can last a long time. Your body fights the bacteria as the plaque spreads and grows below the gum line. Both the bacteria and your body's response to this infection start to break down the bone and the tissue that hold the teeth in place. If periodontitis is not treated, the gums, bones, and tissue that support the teeth are destroyed. Teeth may become loose and might need to be removed. If you have periodontitis, your dentist may send you to a periodontist, an expert in treating gum disease.

What Are the Most Common Mouth Problems from Diabetes?

More symptoms of a problem in your mouth are:

- a sore, or an ulcer, that does not heal
- dark spots or holes in your teeth
- pain in your mouth, face, or jaw that doesn't go away
- loose teeth
- pain when chewing
- a changed sense of taste or a bad taste in your mouth
- bad breath that doesn't go away when you brush your teeth

How Will You Know If You Have Mouth Problems from Diabetes?

Check your mouth for signs of problems from diabetes. If you notice any problems, see your dentist right away. Some of the first signs of

Table 44.1. Common Mouth Problems Due to Diabetes

Problem	What It Is	Symptoms	Treatment
Gingivitis	Unhealthy or inflamed gums	Red, swollen, and bleeding gums	Daily brushing and flossing regular cleanings at the dentist
Periodontitis	Gum disease, which can change from mild to severe	Red, swollen, and bleeding gums Gums that have pulled away from the teeth Long-lasting infection between the teeth and gums Bad breath that won't go away Permanent teeth that are loose or moving away from one another Changes in the way your teeth fit together when you bite Sometimes pus between the teeth and gums Changes in the fit of dentures, which are teeth you can remove	Deep cleaning at your dentist Medicine that your dentist prescribes Gum surgery in severe cases
Thrush, called candidiasis	The growth of a naturally occurring fungus that the body is unable to control	Sore, white—or sometimes red—patches on your gums, tongue, cheeks, or the roof of your mouth Patches that have turned into open sores	Medicine that your doctor or dentist prescribes to kill the fungus Cleaning dentures Removing dentures for part of the day or night, and soaking them in medicine that your doctor or dentist prescribes

Table 44.1. Continued

Problem	What It Is	Symptoms	Treatment
Dry mouth, called xerostomia	A lack of saliva in your mouth, which raises your risk for tooth decay and gum disease	Dry feeling in your mouth, often or all of the time Dry, rough tongue Pain in the mouth Cracked lips Mouth sores or infection Problems chewing, eating, swallowing, or talking	Taking medicine to keep your mouth wet that your doctor or dentist prescribes Rinsing with a fluoride mouth rinse to prevent cavities Using sugarless gum or mints to increase saliva flow Taking frequent sips of water Avoiding tobacco, caffeine, and alcoholic beverages Using a humidifier, a device that raises the level of moisture in your home, at night Avoiding spicy or salty foods that may cause pain in a dry mouth
Oral burning	A burning sensation inside the mouth caused by uncontrolled blood glucose levels	Burning feeling in the mouth Dry mouth Bitter taste Symptoms may worsen throughout the day	Seeing your doctor, who may change your diabetes medicine Once your blood glucose is under control, the oral burning will go away

gum disease are swollen tender or bleeding gums. Sometimes you won't have any signs of gum disease. You may not know you have it until you have serious damage. Your best defense is to see your dentist twice a year for a cleaning and checkup.

How Can You Prepare for a Visit to Your Dentist?

Plan ahead. Talk to your doctor and dentist before the visit about the best way to take care of your blood glucose during dental work.

You may be taking a diabetes medicine that can cause low blood glucose, also called hypoglycemia. If you take insulin or other diabetes medicines, take them and eat as usual before visiting the dentist. You may need to bring your diabetes medicines and your snacks or meal with you to the dentist's office.

You may need to postpone any nonemergency dental work if your blood glucose is not under control.

If you feel nervous about visiting the dentist, tell your dentist and the staff about your feelings. Your dentist can adapt the treatment to your needs. Don't let your nerves stop you from having regular checkups. Waiting too long to take care of your mouth may make things worse.

What If Your Mouth Is Sore after Your Dental Work?

A sore mouth is common after dental work. If this happens, you might not be able to eat or chew the foods you normally eat for several hours or days. For guidance on how to adjust your usual routine while your mouth is healing, ask your doctor:

- what foods and drinks you should have
- if you should change the time when you take your diabetes medicines
- if you should change the dose of your diabetes medicines
- how often you should check your blood glucose

How Does Smoking Affect Your Mouth?

Smoking makes problems with your mouth worse. Smoking raises your chances of getting gum disease, oral and throat cancers, and oral fungal infections. Smoking also discolors your teeth and makes your breath smell bad.

Smoking and diabetes are a dangerous mix. Smoking raises your risk for many diabetes problems. If you quit smoking:

- you will lower your risk for heart attack, stroke, nerve disease, kidney disease, and amputation

- your cholesterol, and blood pressure levels might improve

- your blood circulation will improve

If you smoke, stop smoking. Ask for help so that you don't have to do it alone. You can start by calling 800–QUIT-NOW or 800–784–8669.

How Can You Keep Your Mouth Healthy?

You can keep your mouth healthy by taking these steps:

- Keep your blood glucose numbers as close to your target as possible. Your doctor will help you set your target blood glucose numbers and teach you what to do if your numbers are too high or too low.

- Eat healthy meals and follow the meal plan that you and your doctor or dietitian have worked out.

- Brush your teeth at least twice a day with fluoride toothpaste. Fluoride protects against tooth decay.

  - Aim for brushing first thing in the morning, before going to bed, and after each meal and sugary or starchy snack.

  - Use a soft toothbrush.

  - Gently brush your teeth with the toothbrush angled towards the gum line.

  - Use small, circular motions.

  - Brush the front, back, and top of each tooth. Brush your tongue, too.

  - Change your toothbrush every three months or sooner if the toothbrush looks worn or the bristles spread out. A new toothbrush removes more plaque.

- Drink water that contains added fluoride or ask your dentist about using a fluoride mouth rinse to prevent tooth decay.

- Ask your dentist about using an antiplaque or antigingivitis mouth rinse to control plaque or prevent gum disease.

- Use dental floss to clean between your teeth at least once a day. Flossing helps prevent plaque from building up on your teeth. When flossing,

  - Slide the floss up and down and then curve it around the base of each tooth under the gums.

  - Use clean sections of floss as you move from tooth to tooth.

- Another way of removing plaque between teeth is to use a dental pick or brush—thin tools designed to clean between the teeth. You can buy these picks at drug stores or grocery stores.

- If you wear dentures, keep them clean and take them out at night. Have them adjusted if they become loose or uncomfortable.

- Call your dentist right away if you have any symptoms of mouth problems.

- See your dentist twice a year for a cleaning and checkup. Your dentist may suggest more visits if you need them.

- Follow your dentist's advice.

  - If your dentist tells you about a problem, take care of it right away.

  - Follow any steps or treatments from your dentist to keep your mouth healthy.

- Tell your dentist that you have diabetes.

  - Tell your dentist about any changes in your health or medicines.

  - Share the results of some of your diabetes blood tests, such as the A1C test or the fasting blood glucose test.

  - Ask if you need antibiotics before and after dental treatment if your diabetes is uncontrolled.

- If you smoke, stop smoking.

Chapter 45

Diabetic Neuropathies

What Is Diabetic Neuropathy?

Diabetic neuropathy is nerve damage that is caused by diabetes.

Nerves are bundles of special tissues that carry signals between your brain and other parts of your body. The signals:

- send information about how things feel

- move your body parts

- control body functions such as digestion

What Are the Different Types of Diabetic Neuropathy?

Types of diabetic neuropathy include the following:

- peripheral neuropathy

- autonomic neuropathy

This chapter contains text excerpted from the following sources: Text beginning with the heading "What Is Diabetic Neuropathy?" is excerpted from "Diabetic Neuropathy," National Institute of Diabetes and Digestive and Kidney Diseases (NIDDK), February 2018; Text beginning with the heading "How Are Diabetic Neuropathies Diagnosed?" is excerpted from "Diabetic Neuropathies: The Nerve Damage of Diabetes," Department of Veterans Affairs (VA), July 2013. Reviewed September 2018; Text under the heading "Interventions" is excerpted from "Effectiveness of Treatments for Diabetic Peripheral Neuropathy, U.S. Department of Health and Human Services (HHS), May 9, 2016.

- focal neuropathies

- proximal neuropathy

Who Is Most Likely to Get Diabetic Neuropathy?

If you have diabetes, your chance of developing nerve damage caused by diabetes increases the older you get and the longer you have diabetes. Managing your diabetes is an important part of preventing health problems such as diabetic neuropathy.

You are also more likely to develop nerve damage if you have diabetes and,

- are overweight

- have high blood pressure

- have high cholesterol

- have advanced kidney disease

- drink too many alcoholic drinks

- smoke

Research also suggests that certain genes may make people more likely to develop diabetic neuropathy.

What Causes Diabetic Neuropathy?

Over time, high blood glucose levels, also called blood sugar, and high levels of fats, such as triglycerides, in the blood from diabetes can damage your nerves. High blood glucose levels can also damage the small blood vessels that nourish your nerves with oxygen and nutrients. Without enough oxygen and nutrients, your nerves cannot function well.

How Common Is Diabetic Neuropathy?

Although different types of diabetic neuropathy can affect people who have diabetes, research suggests that up to one-half of people with diabetes have peripheral neuropathy. More than 30 percent of people with diabetes have autonomic neuropathy.

The most common type of focal neuropathy is carpal tunnel syndrome (CTS), in which a nerve in your wrist is compressed. Although less than 10 percent of people with diabetes feel symptoms of CTS, about 25 percent of people with diabetes have some nerve compression at the wrist.

Other focal neuropathies and proximal neuropathy are less common.

What Are the Symptoms of Diabetic Neuropathy?

Your symptoms depend on which type of diabetic neuropathy you have. In peripheral neuropathy, some people may have a loss of sensation in their feet, while others may have burning or shooting pain in their lower legs. Most nerve damage develops over many years, and some people may not notice symptoms of mild nerve damage for a long time. In some people, severe pain begins suddenly.

What Problems Does Diabetic Neuropathy Cause?

Peripheral neuropathy can lead to foot complications, such as sores, ulcers, and infections, because nerve damage can make you lose feeling in your feet. As a result, you may not notice that your shoes are causing a sore or that you have injured your feet. Nerve damage can also cause problems with balance and coordination, leading to falls and fractures.

These problems may make it difficult for you to get around easily, causing you to lose some of your independence. In some people with diabetes, nerve damage causes chronic pain, which can lead to anxiety and depression.

Autonomic neuropathy can cause problems with how your organs work, including problems with your heart rate and blood pressure, digestion, urination, and ability to sense when you have low blood glucose.

How Can You Prevent Diabetic Neuropathy?

To prevent diabetic neuropathy, it is important to manage your diabetes by managing your blood glucose, blood pressure, and cholesterol levels.

You should also take the following steps to help prevent diabetes-related nerve damage:

- be physically active
- follow your diabetes meal plan
- get help to quit smoking
- limit alcoholic drinks to no more than one drink per day for women and no more than two drinks per day for men
- take any diabetes medicines and other medicines your doctor prescribes

How Can You Prevent Diabetic Neuropathy from Getting Worse?

If you have diabetic neuropathy, you should manage your diabetes, which means managing your blood glucose, blood pressure, cholesterol levels, and weight to keep nerve damage from getting worse.

Foot care is very important for all people with diabetes, and it's even more important if you have peripheral neuropathy. Check your feet for problems every day, and take good care of your feet. See your doctor for a neurological exam and a foot exam at least once a year—more often if you have foot problems.

What Is Peripheral Neuropathy?

Peripheral neuropathy is a type of nerve damage that typically affects the feet and legs and sometimes affects the hands and arms. This type of neuropathy is very common. Up to one-half of people with diabetes have peripheral neuropathy.

What Causes Peripheral Neuropathy?

Over time, high blood glucose also called blood sugar, and high levels of fats, such as triglycerides, in the blood from diabetes can damage your nerves and the small blood vessels that nourish your nerves, leading to peripheral neuropathy.

What Are the Symptoms of Peripheral Neuropathy?

If you have peripheral neuropathy, your feet, legs, hands, or arms may feel:

- burning
- tingling, like "pins and needles"
- numb
- painful
- weak

You may feel extreme pain in your feet, legs, hands, and arms, even when they are touched lightly. You may also have problems sensing pain or temperature in these parts of your body.

Symptoms are often worse at night. Most of the time, you will have symptoms on both sides of your body. However, you may have symptoms only on one side.

If you have peripheral neuropathy, you might experience:

- changes in the way you walk

- loss of balance, which could make you fall more often

- loss of muscle tone in your hands and feet

- pain when you walk

- problems sensing movement or position

- swollen feet

What Problems Does Peripheral Neuropathy Cause?

Peripheral neuropathy can cause foot problems that lead to blisters and sores. If peripheral neuropathy causes you to lose feeling in your feet, you may not notice pressure or injuries that lead to blisters and sores. Diabetes can make these wounds difficult to heal and increase the chance of infections. These sores and infections can lead to the loss of a toe, foot, or part of your leg. Finding and treating foot problems early can lower the chances that you will develop serious infections.

This type of diabetes-related nerve damage can also cause changes to the shape of your feet and toes. A rare condition that can occur in some people with diabetes is Charcot foot, a problem in which the bones and tissue in your foot are damaged.

Peripheral neuropathy can make you more likely to lose your balance and fall, which can increase your chance of fractures and other injuries. The chronic pain of peripheral neuropathy can also lead to grief, anxiety, and depression.

How Do Doctors Diagnose Peripheral Neuropathy?

Doctors diagnose peripheral neuropathy based on your symptoms, family and medical history, a physical exam, and tests. A physical exam will include a neurological exam and a foot exam.

Examination for Neuropathy

If you have diabetes, you should get a thorough exam to test how you feel in your feet and legs at least once a year. During this exam, your doctor will look at your feet for signs of problems and check the blood flow and feeling, or sensation, in your feet by:

- placing a tuning fork against your great toes and higher on your feet to check whether you can feel vibration

- touching each foot and some toes with a nylon strand to see if you can feel it—a procedure called a monofilament test

- reviewing your gait, or the patterns you make when you walk

- testing your balance

Your doctor may also check if you can feel temperature changes in your feet.

What Tests Do Doctors Use to Diagnose Peripheral Neuropathy?

Your doctor may perform tests to rule out other causes of nerve damage, such as a blood test to check for thyroid problems, kidney disease, or low vitamin B12 levels. If low B12 levels are found, your doctor will do additional tests to determine the cause. Metformin use is among several causes of low vitamin B12 levels. If B12 deficiency is due to metformin, metformin can be continued with B12 supplementation.

How Can You Prevent the Problems Caused by Peripheral Neuropathy?

You can prevent the problems caused by peripheral neuropathy by managing your diabetes, which means managing your blood glucose, blood pressure, and cholesterol. Staying close to your goal numbers can keep nerve damage from getting worse.

If you have diabetes, check your feet for problems every day and take good care of your feet. If you notice any foot problems, call or see your doctor right away.

Remove your socks and shoes in the exam room to remind your doctor to check your feet at every office visit. See your doctor for a foot exam at least once a year—more often if you have foot problems. Your doctor may send you to a podiatrist.

How Do Doctors Treat Peripheral Neuropathy?

Doctors may prescribe medicine and other treatments for pain.

Medicines for Nerve Pain

Your doctor may prescribe medicines to help with pain, such as certain types of:

- antidepressants, including:
  - tricyclic antidepressants, such as nortriptyline, desipramine, imipramine, and amitriptyline
  - other types of antidepressants, such as duloxetine, venlafaxine, paroxetine, and citalopram
- anticonvulsants—medicines designed to treat seizures—such as gabapentin and pregabalin
- skin creams, patches, or sprays, such as lidocaine

Although these medicines can help with the pain, they do not change the nerve damage. Therefore, if there is no improvement with a medicine to treat pain, there is no benefit to continuing to take it and another medication may be tried.

All medicines have side effects. Ask your doctor about the side effects of any medicines you take. Doctors don't recommend some medicines for older adults or for people with other health problems, such as heart disease.

Some doctors recommend avoiding over-the-counter (OTC) pain medicines, such as acetaminophen and ibuprofen. These medicines may not work well for treating most nerve pain and can have side effects.

Other Treatments for Nerve Pain

Your doctor may recommend other treatments for pain, including:

- physical therapy to improve your strength and balance
- a bed cradle, a device that keeps sheets and blankets off your legs and feet while you sleep

Diabetes experts have not made special recommendations about supplements for people with diabetes. For safety reasons, talk with your doctor before using supplements or any complementary or alternative medicines or medical practices.

What Is Autonomic Neuropathy?

Autonomic neuropathy is damage to nerves that control your internal organs.

Autonomic neuropathy can lead to problems with your:

- heart rate and blood pressure
- digestive system

- bladder
- sex organs
- sweat glands
- eyes

ability to sense hypoglycemia, also called low blood glucose or low blood sugar—a condition called hypoglycemia unawareness

What Causes Autonomic Neuropathy?

Over time, high blood glucose and high levels of fats, such as triglycerides, in the blood from diabetes can damage your nerves and the small blood vessels that nourish your nerves, leading to autonomic neuropathy.

What Are the Symptoms of Autonomic Neuropathy?

The symptoms of autonomic neuropathy depend on which of your body's functions are affected.

Heart Rate and Blood Pressure

Damage to the nerves that control your heart rate and blood pressure may make these nerves respond more slowly to a change in your body's position, stress, physical activity, sleep, and breathing patterns. You may feel light-headed or faint when you stand up from lying down or sitting, or when you do a physical activity. You may have a rapid heart rate, or your heart rate may suddenly speed up or slow down. Nerve damage can also prevent you from feeling chest pain when your heart is not getting enough oxygen or when you are having a heart attack.

Digestive System

Damage to the nerves of your digestive system can cause symptoms such as the following:

- bloating, fullness, and nausea
- constipation
- diarrhea, especially at night
- diarrhea alternating with constipation

- fecal incontinence
- problems swallowing
- vomiting

Autonomic neuropathy may also cause gastroparesis. Gastroparesis is a disorder that slows or stops the movement of food from your stomach to your small intestine. Gastroparesis can keep your body from absorbing glucose and using insulin properly. These problems can make it hard to manage your blood glucose.

Bladder

Damage to the nerves of your bladder may make it hard to know when you need to urinate and when your bladder is empty. This damage can cause you to hold urine for too long, which can lead to bladder infections. You may also leak drops of urine. Leaking urine or not being able to hold urine is called urinary incontinence (UI).

Sex Organs

In men, damage to nerves in the sex organs may prevent the penis from getting firm when a man wants to have sex. This condition is called erectile dysfunction (ED). Men also may have problems with ejaculation.

In women, damage to the nerves in the sex organs can prevent the vagina from getting wet when a woman wants to have sex. A woman might also have less feeling around her vagina and may have trouble having an orgasm.

Sweat Glands

Damage to the nerves that control your sweat glands may cause you to sweat a lot at night or while eating. Your sweat glands may not work at all, or certain parts of your body may sweat while other parts are dry. If your sweat glands do not work properly, your body may not be able to control its temperature.

Eyes

Damage to the nerves in your pupils may make them slow to respond to changes in light and darkness. Your eyes may take longer to adjust when you enter a dark room. You may have trouble seeing the lights of other cars when driving at night.

Ability to Feel Symptoms of Hypoglycemia

Autonomic neuropathy can cause hypoglycemia unawareness, meaning that you don't feel the symptoms of low blood glucose. Normally, early symptoms of low blood glucose can include feeling confused, dizzy, hungry, irritable, or nervous. If nerve damage keeps you from feeling these symptoms, you may not take steps to treat your low blood glucose. Without treatment, you may develop severe hypoglycemia, which can cause you to pass out. You will need help right away to deal with severe hypoglycemia.

How Do Doctors Diagnose Autonomic Neuropathy?

Doctors diagnose autonomic neuropathy based on your symptoms, family and medical history, a physical exam, and tests. Your doctor will check your heart rate and blood pressure and may perform additional tests to check for different types of autonomic nerve damage.

What Tests Do Doctors Use to Diagnose Autonomic Neuropathy?

To diagnose autonomic neuropathy, your doctor may use a few tests to assess changes in your heart rate in response to simple movements such as deep breathing or standing. Your doctor may also use tests to check your sweat function to know how your nerves and sweat glands are working.

Depending on your symptoms, your doctor may also use:

- tests to rule out other causes of digestive symptoms, such as constipation and diarrhea

- gastric emptying scintigraphy and gastric emptying breath tests to diagnose gastroparesis

- ultrasounds of your bladder and urinary tract to check how your bladder is working

- blood pressure checks while you are lying down and then after you stand up

How Can You Help Treat Autonomic Neuropathy?

You can help treat autonomic neuropathy by managing your diabetes, which means managing your blood glucose, blood pressure, and cholesterol. Staying close to your goal numbers can keep nerve damage from getting worse.

How Do Doctors Treat Autonomic Neuropathy?

Your doctor may treat the symptoms caused by autonomic nerve damage.

Heart Rate and Blood Pressure

Your doctor will treat the symptoms of nerve damage that affect your heart rate and blood pressure. Your doctor may recommend:

- getting more physical activity
- increasing salt in your diet if your blood pressure drops too low when you stand up
- increasing the amount of liquids you drink
- raising the head of your bed or wearing elastic stockings to improve blood flow
- sitting or standing slowly to prevent lightheadedness or fainting
- avoiding hypoglycemia

Your doctor may also prescribe medicines that help your body retain salt, medicines to help raise your blood pressure, or medicines that raise or lower your heart rate.

Digestive System

Your doctor may recommend changes to your diet and OTC or prescription medicines to treat digestive symptoms and problems such as:

- constipation
- diarrhea
- fecal incontinence
- gastroesophageal reflux
- gastroparesis

Talk with your doctor before taking any OTC medicines to treat problems with digestion. Your doctor may refer you to a gastroenterologist for treatment.

Bladder

Your doctor will treat your bladder problems by focusing on your symptoms. If you have incontinence, your doctor may recommend planning regular trips to the bathroom because you may not be able to tell when your bladder is full.

Your doctor may also prescribe medicines to help with incontinence or help if you have problems completely emptying your bladder.

If you have a bladder infection, your doctor may prescribe an antibiotic and suggest drinking plenty of liquids to help prevent future infections.

Sex Organs

Doctors may recommend medicines or devices to treat ED. Doctors may refer men to a urologist to treat sexual problems.

To treat sexual problems in women, doctors may refer women to a gynecologist. Doctors may recommend vaginal lubricants when neuropathy causes vaginal dryness.

Sweat Glands

If you have too much sweating, your doctor may suggest:

• Avoiding too much heat or humidity

• A prescription antiperspirant or medicine to decrease sweating

• Surgery to cut the nerves in the sweat glands or to remove sweat glands

Hypoglycemia Unawareness

• If diabetes-related nerve damage leads to hypoglycemia unawareness, you may need to check your blood glucose more often, so you know when you need to treat hypoglycemia or take steps to prevent it.

Your doctor may prescribe a continuous glucose monitor (CGM). A CGM checks your blood glucose levels at regular times throughout the day and night. CGMs can tell you if your blood glucose is falling quickly and sound an alarm if your blood glucose falls too low.

If you pass out due to severe hypoglycemia, someone will need to give you a glucagon injection and call 9-1-1. An injection of glucagon will quickly raise your blood glucose back to normal. Ask your doctor about when and how to use a glucagon emergency kit. Consider wearing a diabetes medical alert identity (ID) bracelet or pendant. If you pass out, this medical alert ID will tell other people that you have diabetes and need care right away.

What Are Focal Neuropathies?

Focal neuropathies are conditions in which you typically have damage to single nerves, most often in your hand, head, torso, or leg. This type of nerve damage is less common than peripheral or autonomic neuropathy.

Many different focal neuropathies can affect people who have diabetes.

Entrapments. Entrapments, or entrapment syndromes, are the most common type of focal neuropathy. Entrapments occur when nerves become compressed or trapped in areas where nerves pass through narrow passages between bones and tissues. People with diabetes are more likely to have entrapments than people without diabetes.

The most common entrapment is called CTS. Although less than 10 percent of people with diabetes feel symptoms of CTS, about 25 percent of people with diabetes have some nerve compression at the wrist.

Other focal neuropathies. Other focal neuropathies that do not involve trapped nerves are much less common. These focal neuropathies most often affect older adults. Examples include cranial neuropathies, which affect the nerves of the head. Cranial neuropathies can cause eye problems or problems with the muscles of the face. Symptoms depend on which nerve is affected.

What Causes Focal Neuropathies?

Over time, high blood glucose, also called blood sugar, and high levels of fats, such as triglycerides, in the blood from diabetes can damage your nerves and the small blood vessels that nourish your nerves, leading to focal neuropathies.

What Are the Symptoms of Focal Neuropathies?

Entrapments—focal neuropathies that involve trapped nerves—cause symptoms that begin gradually and get worse over time. Examples include:

- CTS, which causes pain, numbness, and tingling in your thumb, index finger, and middle finger, and sometimes weakness of your grip

- ulnar entrapment, which causes pain, numbness, and tingling in your little and ring fingers

- peroneal entrapment, which causes pain on the outside of your lower leg and weakness in your big toe

Focal neuropathies that do not involve trapped nerves cause symptoms that begin suddenly and improve after several weeks or months. Depending on which nerve is affected, you may have pain and other symptoms in your:

- hand
- leg
- foot
- torso

Cranial neuropathies—focal neuropathies that affect the nerves in the head—may cause symptoms such as:

- aching behind one eye
- double vision
- paralysis on one side of your face, called Bell palsy
- problems focusing your eyes

How Do Doctors Diagnose Focal Neuropathies?

Doctors diagnose focal neuropathies by asking about your symptoms and performing tests, such as nerve conduction studies and electromyography (EMG). Nerve conduction studies check how fast electrical signals move through your nerves in different parts of your body. EMG shows how your muscles respond to your nerves.

How Do Doctors Treat Focal Neuropathies?

Your doctor may treat focal neuropathy pain with the same medicines used to treat peripheral neuropathy pain.

To treat a focal neuropathy that involves a trapped nerve, your doctor may recommend:

- wearing a splint or brace to take pressure off the nerve
- medicines that reduce inflammation
- surgery, if other treatments don't work

For focal neuropathies that don't involve trapped nerves, most people recover within a few weeks or months, even without treatment.

What Is Proximal Neuropathy?

Proximal neuropathy is a rare and disabling type of nerve damage in your hip, buttock, or thigh. This type of nerve damage typically affects one side of your body and may rarely spread to the other side.

Proximal neuropathy is more common in men than in women and more common in people older than age 50. Most people with this condition have type 2 diabetes.

What Causes Proximal Neuropathy?

Over time, high blood glucose, also called blood sugar, and high levels of fats, such as triglycerides, in the blood from diabetes can damage your nerves and the small blood vessels that nourish your nerves, leading to proximal neuropathy.

What Are the Symptoms of Proximal Neuropathy?

Symptoms may include:

- sudden and sometimes severe pain in your hip, buttock, or thigh

- weakness in your legs that makes it difficult to stand from a sitting position

- loss of reflexes such as the knee-jerk reflex—the automatic movement of your lower leg when a doctor taps the area below your kneecap

- muscle wasting, or the loss of muscle tissue

- weight loss

After symptoms start, they typically get worse and then gradually improve over a period of months or years. In many cases, the symptoms do not go away completely.

How Do Doctors Diagnose Proximal Neuropathy?

Doctors diagnose proximal neuropathy by asking about your symptoms and performing tests, such as nerve conduction studies and EMG. Nerve conduction studies check how fast electrical signals move through your nerves in different parts of your body. EMG shows how your muscles respond to your nerves.

How Can You Help Treat Proximal Neuropathy?

You can help treat proximal neuropathy by managing your diabetes, which means managing your blood glucose, blood pressure, and cholesterol.

How Do Doctors Treat Proximal Neuropathy?

Your doctor may treat the pain of proximal neuropathy with the same medicines used to treat peripheral neuropathy pain.

Your doctor may also recommend physical therapy to help increase your strength, and occupational therapy to help you with daily activities.

Most people recover from proximal neuropathy within a few years, even without treatment.

How Are Diabetic Neuropathies Diagnosed?

Doctors diagnose neuropathy on the basis of symptoms and a physical exam. During the exam, your doctor may check blood pressure, heart rate, muscle strength, reflexes, and sensitivity to position changes, vibration, temperature, or light touch.

Foot Exams

Experts recommend that people with diabetes have a comprehensive foot exam each year to check for peripheral neuropathy. People diagnosed with peripheral neuropathy need more frequent foot exams. A comprehensive foot exam assesses the skin, muscles, bones, circulation, and sensation of the feet. Your doctor may assess protective sensation or feeling in your feet by touching your foot with a nylon monofilament—similar to a bristle on a hairbrush—attached to a wand or by pricking your foot with a pin. People who cannot sense pressure from a pinprick or monofilament have lost protective sensation and are at risk for developing foot sores that may not heal properly. The doctor may also check temperature perception or use a tuning fork, which is more sensitive than touch pressure, to assess vibration perception.

Other Tests

The doctor may perform other tests as part of your diagnosis.

- **Nerve conduction studies or electromyography** are sometimes used to help determine the type and extent of nerve damage. Nerve conduction studies check the transmission of electrical current through a nerve. Electromyography shows how well muscles respond to electrical signals transmitted by nearby nerves. These tests are rarely needed to diagnose neuropathy.

- **A check of heart rate variability** shows how the heart responds to deep breathing and to changes in blood pressure and posture.

- **Ultrasound** uses sound waves to produce an image of internal organs. An ultrasound of the bladder and other parts of the urinary tract, for example, can show how these organs preserve a normal structure and whether the bladder empties completely after urination.

How Are Diabetic Neuropathies Treated?

The first treatment step is to bring blood glucose levels within the normal range to help prevent further nerve damage. Blood glucose monitoring, meal planning, physical activity, and diabetes medicines or insulin will help control blood glucose levels. Symptoms may get worse when blood glucose is first brought under control, but over time, maintaining lower blood glucose levels helps lessen symptoms. Good blood glucose control may also help prevent or delay the onset of further problems. As scientists learn more about the underlying causes of neuropathy, new treatments may become available to help slow, prevent, or even reverse nerve damage.

As described in the following sections, additional treatment depends on the type of nerve problem and symptom. If you have problems with your feet, your doctor may refer you to a foot care specialist.

Pain Relief

Doctors usually treat painful diabetic neuropathy with oral medications, although other types of treatments may help some people. People with severe nerve pain may benefit from a combination of medications or treatments. Talk with your healthcare provider about options for treating your neuropathy.

Medications used to help relieve diabetic nerve pain include

- anticonvulsants, such as gabapentin (Neurontin®), carbamazepine (Tegretol®) and lamotrigine (Lamictal®), pregabalin (Lyrica®)

339

- other types of antidepressants, such as venlafaxine (Effexor®), bupropion (Wellbutrin®), fluoxetine (Prozac®) and citalopram (Celexa®), duloxetine (Cymbalta®)

- tricyclic antidepressants, such as amitriptyline (Elavil®), nortriptyline (Pamelor®), imipramine (Tofranil®), and desipramine (Norpramine®)

- opioids and opioid-like drugs, such as oxycodone, hydrocodone, codeine and morphine

- and tramadol (Ultram®), an opioid that also acts as an antidepressant

You do not have to be depressed for an antidepressant to help relieve your nerve pain. All medications have side effects, and some are not recommended for use in older adults or those with heart disease. Because over-the-counter (OTC) pain medicines such as acetaminophen and ibuprofen may not work well for treating most nerve pain and can have serious side effects, some experts recommend avoiding these medications.

Treatments that are applied to the skin—typically to the feet—include capsaicin cream and lidocaine patches. Studies suggest that nitrate sprays or patches for the feet may relieve pain. Studies of alpha-lipoic acid, an antioxidant, and evening primrose oil have shown that they can help relieve symptoms and may improve nerve function.

A device called a bed cradle can keep sheets and blankets from touching sensitive feet and legs.

Acupuncture, biofeedback, or physical therapy may help relieve pain in some people. Treatments that involve electrical nerve stimulation, magnetic therapy, and laser or light therapy may be helpful but need further study. Researchers are also studying several new therapies in clinical trials.

Gastrointestinal Problems

To relieve mild symptoms of gastroparesis—indigestion, belching, nausea, or vomiting—doctors suggest eating small, frequent meals; avoiding fats; and eating less fiber. When symptoms are severe, doctors may prescribe erythromycin to speed digestion, metoclopramide to speed digestion and help relieve nausea, or other medications to help regulate digestion or reduce stomach acid secretion.

To relieve diarrhea or other bowel problems, doctors may prescribe an antibiotic such as tetracycline, or other medications as appropriate.

Dizziness and Weakness

Sitting or standing slowly may help prevent the light-headedness, dizziness, or fainting associated with blood pressure and circulation problems. Raising the head of the bed or wearing elastic stockings may also help. Some people benefit from increased salt in the diet and treatment with salt-retaining hormones. Others benefit from high blood pressure medications. Physical therapy can help when muscle weakness or loss of coordination is a problem.

Urinary and Sexual Problems

To clear up a urinary tract infection, the doctor will probably prescribe an antibiotic. Drinking plenty of fluids will help prevent another infection. People who have incontinence should try to urinate at regular intervals—every 3 hours, for example—since they may not be able to tell when the bladder is full.

To treat erectile dysfunction in men, the doctor will first do tests to rule out a hormonal cause. Several methods are available to treat erectile dysfunction caused by neuropathy. Medicines are available to help men have and maintain erections by increasing blood flow to the penis. Some are oral medications and others are injected into the penis or inserted into the urethra at the tip of the penis. Mechanical vacuum devices can also increase blood flow to the penis. Another option is to surgically implant an inflatable or semirigid device in the penis.

Vaginal lubricants may be useful for women when neuropathy causes vaginal dryness. To treat problems with arousal and orgasm, the doctor may refer women to a gynecologist.

Foot Care

People with neuropathy need to take special care of their feet. The nerves to the feet are the longest in the body and are the ones most often affected by neuropathy. Loss of sensation in the feet means that sores or injuries may not be noticed and may become ulcerated or infected. Circulation problems also increase the risk of foot ulcers.

More than half of all lower-limb amputations in the United States occur in people with diabetes—86,000 amputations per year. Doctors estimate that nearly half of the amputations caused by neuropathy and poor circulation could have been prevented by careful foot care.

Interventions

Experimental pharmacologic interventions targeting diabetic peripheral neuropathy evaluated in recent clinical trials include aldose reductase inhibitors, such as ranirestat and epalrestat, the anti-nerve growth factor antibody fulranumab, the protein kinase C-beta inhibitor ruboxistaurin, gangliosides, and prostaglandin E1. These drugs focus on reducing the impact of oxidative stress on diabetes-induced microvascular complications. A 2007 Cochrane review evaluating the effectiveness of aldose reductase inhibitors on progression of diabetic neuropathies found no evidence for effectiveness.8 Ongoing Cochrane protocols are evaluating the effectiveness of several other classes of pharmacologic agents. However, all of these experimental interventions have not been FDA-approved, are not used in the United States, and thus are not within the scope of this review.

Pharmacologic Treatment Options to Prevent the Complications of Diabetic Peripheral Neuropathy

The cornerstone of pharmacologic interventions to prevent complications of diabetic peripheral neuropathy is medications and strategies that improve glucose control.

Key pharmacologic interventions that address comorbid conditions in patients with diabetes are statins and antihypertensives. These agents may also contribute to preventing DPN complications,13 since coexisting peripheral vascular disease can contribute to long-term diabetic complications such as foot ulcerations. Although DPN is not an outcome in studies addressing these comorbid conditions, they may be described as important comorbidities in studies of glucose control that report on diabetic neuropathy outcomes.

Nonpharmacologic Treatment Options to Prevent the Complications of Diabetic Peripheral Neuropathy

These interventions include nonpharmacologic glucose control interventions, such as diet and exercise, and interventions to prevent specific complications, such as foot care for prevention of foot ulcers, as well as exercise and balance training for the prevention of falls. Advances and technologies for foot care and balance management that have been proposed but not yet tested in trials (e.g., in-shoe micro compression pumps) will not be included in this review.

Pharmacologic Treatment Options to Improve the Symptoms of Diabetic Peripheral Neuropathy

For diabetic peripheral polyneuropathy (DPN), pain is the most commonly studied symptom in the literature, although other symptoms such as paresthesias that less commonly addressed in trials are also important to patients. A variety of pharmacological approaches have been evaluated to reduce pain and improve health-related quality of life through a variety of mechanisms. These include drugs with direct impact on neurotransmitters and inhibitory pathways or binding to opioid receptors. Several medications are FDA approved for DPN (e.g., pregabalin) or other types of neuropathy (e.g., gabapentin, lidocaine patches for herpes zoster), but most are approved for other indications (e.g., depression, seizure disorders) and evaluated and used off-label for painful diabetic peripheral neuropathy.

For pain outcomes, there are many studies on pharmacological agents, and recent systematic reviews have identified a number of different agents with supporting evidence. However, many studies include nondiabetic peripheral neuropathy or mixed populations.

Nonpharmacologic Treatment Options to Improve the Symptoms of Diabetic Peripheral Neuropathy

These interventions also focus mainly on treating pain. Although there is less evidence in this area, modalities that have been evaluated specifically for diabetic peripheral neuropathy and addressed in previous reviews include acupuncture, physical therapy and exercise, electrical stimulation,15 and surgical decompression.

Chapter 46

Gastroparesis

What Is Gastroparesis?

Gastroparesis, also called delayed gastric emptying, is a disorder that slows or stops the movement of food from your stomach to your small intestine. Normally, after you swallow food, the muscles in the wall of your stomach grind the food into smaller pieces and push them into your small intestine to continue digestion. When you have gastroparesis, your stomach muscles work poorly or not at all, and your stomach takes too long to empty its contents. Gastroparesis can delay digestion, which can lead to various symptoms and complications.

How Common Is Gastroparesis?

Gastroparesis is not common. Out of 100,000 people, about 10 men and about 40 women have gastroparesis. However, symptoms that are similar to those of gastroparesis occur in about 1 out of 4 adults in the United States.

Who Is More Likely to Get Gastroparesis?

You are more likely to get gastroparesis if you:

- have diabetes

This chapter includes text excerpted from "Gastroparesis," National Institute of Diabetes and Digestive and Kidney Diseases (NIDDK), January 2018.

- had surgery on your esophagus, stomach, or small intestine, which may injure the vagus nerve. The vagus nerve controls the muscles of the stomach and small intestine.

- had certain cancer treatments, such as radiation therapy on your chest or stomach area

What Other Health Problems Do People with Gastroparesis Have?

People with gastroparesis may have other health problems, such as

- Diabetes

- Scleroderma

- Hypothyroidism

- Nervous system disorders, such as migraine, Parkinson disease (PD), and multiple sclerosis (MS)

- Gastroesophageal reflux disease (GERD)

- Eating disorders

- Amyloidosis

What Are the Complications of Gastroparesis?

Complications of gastroparesis may include:

- Dehydration due to repeated vomiting

- Malnutrition due to poor absorption of nutrients

- Blood glucose, also called blood sugar, levels that are harder to control, which can worsen diabetes

- Low-calorie intake

- Bezoars

- Losing weight without trying

- Lower quality of life

What Are the Symptoms of Gastroparesis?

The symptoms of gastroparesis may include:

- feeling full soon after starting a meal

- feeling full long after eating a meal
- nausea
- vomiting
- too much bloating
- too much belching
- pain in your upper abdomen
- heartburn
- poor appetite

Certain medicines may delay gastric emptying or affect motility, resulting in symptoms that are similar to those of gastroparesis. If you have been diagnosed with gastroparesis, these medicines may make your symptoms worse. Medicines that may delay gastric emptying or make symptoms worse include the following:

- Narcotic pain medicines, such as codeine, hydrocodone, morphine, oxycodone, and tapentadol
- Some antidepressants, such as amitriptyline, nortriptyline, and venlafaxine
- Some anticholinergics—medicines that block certain nerve signals
- Some medicines used to treat overactive bladder
- Pramlintide

These medicines do not cause gastroparesis.

When Should You Seek a Doctor's Help?

You should seek a doctor's help right away if you have any of the following signs or symptoms:

- severe pain or cramping in your abdomen
- blood glucose levels that are too high or too low
- red blood in your vomit, or vomit that looks like coffee grounds
- sudden, sharp stomach pain that doesn't go away
- vomiting for more than an hour

- feeling extremely weak or fainting
- difficulty breathing
- fever

You should seek a doctor's help if you have any signs or symptoms of dehydration, which may include:

- extreme thirst and dry mouth
- urinating less than usual
- feeling tired
- dark-colored urine
- decreased skin turgor, meaning that when your skin is pinched and released, the skin does not flatten back to normal right away
- sunken eyes or cheeks
- lightheadedness or fainting

You should seek a doctor's help if you have any signs or symptoms of malnutrition, which may include:

- feeling tired or weak all the time
- losing weight without trying
- feeling dizzy
- loss of appetite
- abnormal paleness of the skin

What Causes Gastroparesis?

In most cases, doctors aren't able to find the underlying cause of gastroparesis, even with medical tests. Gastroparesis without a known cause is called idiopathic gastroparesis.

Diabetes is the most common known underlying cause of gastroparesis. Diabetes can damage nerves, such as the vagus nerve and nerves and special cells, called pacemaker cells, in the wall of the stomach. The vagus nerve controls the muscles of the stomach and small intestine. If the vagus nerve is damaged or stops working, the muscles of the stomach and small intestine do not work normally. The movement of food through the digestive tract is then slowed or stopped. Similarly, if nerves or pacemaker cells in the wall of the stomach are damaged or do not work normally, the stomach does not empty.

In addition to diabetes, other known causes of gastroparesis include:

- Injury to the vagus nerve due to surgery on your esophagus, stomach, or small intestine

- Hypothyroidism

- Certain autoimmune diseases, such as scleroderma

- Certain nervous system disorders, such as PD and MS

- Viral infections of your stomach

How Do Doctors Diagnose Gastroparesis?

Doctors diagnose gastroparesis based on your medical history, a physical exam, your symptoms, and medical tests. Your doctor may also perform medical tests to look for signs of gastroparesis complications and to rule out other health problems that may be causing your symptoms.

Medical History

Your doctor will ask about your medical history. He or she will ask for details about your current symptoms and medicines, and current and past health problems such as diabetes, scleroderma, nervous system disorders, and hypothyroidism.

Your doctor may also ask about:

- the types of medicines you are taking. Be sure to tell your doctor about all prescription medicines, over-the-counter (OTC) medicines, and dietary supplements you are taking.

- whether you've had surgery on your esophagus, stomach, or small intestine

- whether you've had radiation therapy on your chest or stomach area

Physical Exam

During a physical exam, your doctor will:

- check your blood pressure, temperature, and heart rate

- check for signs of dehydration and malnutrition

- check your abdomen for unusual sounds, tenderness, or pain

What Medical Tests Do Doctors Use to Diagnose Gastroparesis?

Doctors use lab tests, upper gastrointestinal (GI) endoscopy, imaging tests, and tests to measure how fast your stomach is emptying its contents to diagnose gastroparesis.

Lab Tests

Your doctor may use the following lab tests:

- Blood tests can show signs of dehydration, malnutrition, inflammation, and infection. Blood tests can also show whether your blood glucose levels are too high or too low.

- Urine tests can show signs of diabetes, dehydration, infection, and kidney problems.

Upper Gastrointestinal Endoscopy

Your doctor may perform an upper GI endoscopy to look for problems in your upper digestive tract that may be causing your symptoms.

Imaging Tests

Imaging tests can show problems, such as stomach blockage or intestinal obstruction, that may be causing your symptoms. Your doctor may perform the following imaging tests:

- Upper GI series

- Ultrasound of your abdomen

Tests to Measure Stomach Emptying

Your doctor may perform one of more of the following tests to see how fast your stomach is emptying its contents.

- **Gastric emptying scan, also called gastric emptying scintigraphy.** For this test, you eat a bland meal—such as eggs or an egg substitute—that contains a small amount of radioactive material. A camera outside your body scans your abdomen to show where the radioactive material is located. By tracking the radioactive material, a healthcare professional can measure how fast your stomach empties after the meal. The scan usually takes about four hours.

- **Gastric emptying breath test.** For this test, you eat a meal that contains a substance that is absorbed in your intestines and eventually passed into your breath. After you eat the meal, a healthcare professional collects samples of your breath over a period of a few hours—usually about four hours. The test can show how fast your stomach empties after the meal by measuring the amount of the substance in your breath.

- **Wireless motility capsule, also called a SmartPill.** The SmartPill is a small electronic device that you swallow. The capsule moves through your entire digestive tract and sends information to a recorder hung around your neck or clipped to your belt. A healthcare professional uses the information to find out how fast or slow your stomach empties, and how fast liquid and food move through your small intestine and large intestine. The capsule will pass naturally out of your body with a bowel movement.

How Do Doctors Treat Gastroparesis?

How doctors treat gastroparesis depends on the cause, how severe your symptoms and complications are, and how well you respond to different treatments. Sometimes, treating the cause may stop gastroparesis. If diabetes is causing your gastroparesis, your healthcare professional will work with you to help control your blood glucose levels. When the cause of your gastroparesis is not known, your doctor will provide treatments to help relieve your symptoms and treat complications.

Changing Eating Habits

Changing your eating habits can help control gastroparesis and make sure you get the right amount of nutrients, calories, and liquids. Getting the right amount of nutrients, calories, and liquids can also treat the disorders two main complications: malnutrition and dehydration.

Your doctor may recommend that you:

- eat foods low in fat and fiber

- eat five or six small, nutritious meals a day instead of two or three large meals

- chew your food thoroughly
- eat soft, well-cooked foods
- avoid carbonated, or fizzy, beverages
- avoid alcohol
- drink plenty of water or liquids that contain glucose and electrolytes, such as:
  - low-fat broths or clear soups
  - naturally sweetened, low-fiber fruit and vegetable juices
  - sports drinks
  - oral rehydration solutions
- do some gentle physical activity after a meal, such as taking a walk
- avoid lying down for two hours after a meal
- take a multivitamin each day.

If your symptoms are moderate to severe, your doctor may recommend drinking only liquids or eating well-cooked solid foods that have been processed into very small pieces or paste in a blender.

Controlling Blood Glucose Levels

If you have gastroparesis and diabetes, you will need to control your blood glucose levels, especially hyperglycemia. Hyperglycemia may further delay the emptying of food from your stomach. Your doctor will work with you to make sure your blood glucose levels are not too high or too low and don't keep going up or down. Your doctor may recommend:

- taking insulin more often, or changing the type of insulin you take
- taking insulin after, instead of before, meals
- checking your blood glucose levels often after you eat, and taking insulin when you need it

Your doctor will give you specific instructions for taking insulin based on your needs and the severity of your gastroparesis.

Medicines

Your doctor may prescribe medicines that help the muscles in the wall of your stomach work better. He or she may also prescribe medicines to control nausea and vomiting and reduce pain.

Your doctor may prescribe one or more of the following medicines:

- **Metoclopramide.** This medicine increases the tightening, or contraction, of the muscles in the wall of your stomach and may improve gastric emptying. Metoclopramide may also help relieve nausea and vomiting.

- **Domperidone.** This medicine also increases the contraction of the muscles in the wall of your stomach and may improve gastric emptying. However, this medicine is available for use only under a special program administered by the U.S. Food and Drug Administration (FDA).

- **Erythromycin.** This medicine also increases stomach muscle contraction and may improve gastric emptying.

- **Antiemetics.** Antiemetics are medicines that help relieve nausea and vomiting. Prescription antiemetics include ondansetron, prochlorperazine, and promethazine. Over-the-counter (OTC) antiemetics include bismuth subsalicylate and diphenhydramine. Antiemetics do not improve gastric emptying.

- **Antidepressants.** Certain antidepressants, such as mirtazapine, may help relieve nausea and vomiting. These medicines may not improve gastric emptying.

- **Pain medicines.** Pain medicines that are not narcotic pain medicines may reduce pain in your abdomen due to gastroparesis.

Oral or Nasal Tube Feeding

In some cases, your doctor may recommend oral or nasal tube feeding to make sure you're getting the right amount of nutrients and calories. A healthcare professional will put a tube either into your mouth or nose, through your esophagus and stomach, to your small intestine. Oral and nasal tube feeding bypass your stomach and deliver a special liquid food directly into your small intestine.

Jejunostomy Tube Feeding

If you aren't getting enough nutrients and calories from other treatments, your doctor may recommend jejunostomy tube feeding. Jejunostomy feedings are a longer-term method of feeding, compared to oral or nasal tube feeding.

Jejunostomy tube feeding is a way to feed you through a tube placed into part of your small intestine called the jejunum. To place the tube into the jejunum, a doctor creates an opening, called a jejunostomy, in your abdominal wall that goes into your jejunum. The feeding tube bypasses your stomach and delivers a liquid food directly into your jejunum.

Parenteral Nutrition

Your doctor may recommend parenteral, or intravenous (IV), nutrition if your gastroparesis is so severe that other treatments are not helping. Parenteral nutrition delivers liquid nutrients directly into your bloodstream. Parenteral nutrition may be short term, until you can eat again. Parenteral nutrition may also be used until a tube can be placed for oral, nasal, or jejunostomy tube feeding. In some cases, parenteral nutrition may be long term.

Venting Gastrostomy

Your doctor may recommend a venting gastrostomy to relieve pressure inside your stomach. A doctor creates an opening, called a gastrostomy, in your abdominal wall and into your stomach. The doctor then places a tube through the gastrostomy into your stomach. Stomach contents can then flow out of the tube and relieve pressure inside your stomach.

Gastric Electrical Stimulation

Gastric electrical stimulation (GES) uses a small, battery-powered device to send mild electrical pulses to the nerves and muscles in the lower stomach. A surgeon puts the device under the skin in your lower abdomen and attaches wires from the device to the muscles in the wall of your stomach. GES can help decrease long-term nausea and vomiting.

GES is used to treat people with gastroparesis due to diabetes or unknown causes only, and only in people whose symptoms can't be controlled with medicines.

How Can You Prevent Gastroparesis?

Gastroparesis without a known cause, called idiopathic gastroparesis, cannot be prevented.

If you have diabetes, you can prevent or delay nerve damage that can cause gastroparesis by keeping your blood glucose levels within the target range that your doctor thinks is best for you. Meal planning, physical activity, and medicines, if needed, can help you keep your blood glucose levels within your target range.

How Can Your Diet Help Prevent or Relieve Gastroparesis?

What you eat can help prevent or relieve your gastroparesis symptoms. If you have diabetes, following a healthy meal plan can help you manage your blood glucose levels. What you eat can also help make sure you get the right amount of nutrients, calories, and liquids if you are malnourished or dehydrated from gastroparesis.

What Should You Eat and Drink If You Have Gastroparesis?

If you have gastroparesis, your doctor may recommend that you eat or drink:

- foods and beverages that are low in fat
- foods and beverages that are low in fiber
- five or six small, nutritious meals a day instead of two or three large meals
- soft, well-cooked foods

If you are unable to eat solid foods, your doctor may recommend that you drink:

- liquid nutrition meals
- solid foods puréed in a blender

Your doctor may also recommend that you drink plenty of water or liquids that contain glucose and electrolytes, such as:

- low-fat broths and clear soups
- low-fiber fruit and vegetable juices
- sports drinks
- oral rehydration solutions

If your symptoms are moderate to severe, your doctor may recommend drinking only liquids or eating well-cooked solid foods that have been processed into very small pieces or paste in a blender.

What Should You Avoid Eating and Drinking If You Have Gastroparesis?

If you have gastroparesis, you should avoid:

- foods and beverages that are high in fat
- foods and beverages that are high in fiber
- foods that can't be chewed easily
- carbonated, or fizzy, beverages
- alcohol

Your doctor may refer you to a dietitian to help you plan healthy meals that are easy for you to digest and give you the right amount of nutrients, calories, and liquids.

Chapter 47

Hyperglycemic Hyperosmolar Syndrome

Hyperglycemic Hyperosmolar State (HHS) is defined as extreme elevation in blood glucose more than 600 mg/dL (>33.30 mmol/L) and serum osmolality more than 320 mOsm/kg in the absence of significant ketosis and acidosis. Small amounts of ketones may be present in blood and urine.

Pathogenesis

Decrease in the effective action of circulating insulin coupled with a concomitant elevation of counterregulatory hormones is the underlying mechanism for both HHS and diabetic ketoacidosis (DKA). These alterations lead to increased hepatic and renal glucose production and impaired glucose utilization in peripheral tissues, which result in hyperglycemia and parallel changes in osmolality of the extracellular space. HHS is associated with glycosuria, leading to osmotic diuresis, with loss of water, sodium, potassium, and other electrolytes. In HHS, insulin levels are inadequate for glucose utilization by insulin-sensitive tissues but sufficient to prevent lipolysis and ketogenesis.

This chapter includes text excerpted from "Acute Metabolic Complications in Diabetes," National Institute of Diabetes and Digestive and Kidney Diseases (NIDDK), March 12, 2016.

357

Incidence and Prevalence

The incidence of HHS is unknown because of the lack of population-based studies and multiple comorbidities often found in these patients. Estimated rates of hospital admissions for HHS are lower compared to DKA. HHS accounts for less than one percent of all admissions related to diabetes but may affect up to four percent of new type 2 diabetes patients. The prevalence of isolated HHS in adult patients with acute, significant hyperglycemia varies from 15 percent to 45 percent. HHS occurs at any age, but it is more prevalent in elderly patients who have additional comorbidities. Presence of other conditions, such as infection, cardiovascular disease, and cancer, seems to be responsible for the higher mortality associated with HHS compared to DKA.

The incidence of HHS is most likely underestimated in children, as the presenting clinical picture in many patients has elements of both HHS and DKA.

Several studies of pediatric and adolescent diabetic patients, mostly case series or single-institution reviews, have described more than 50 cases of HHS. Most patients were adolescents with newly diagnosed type 2 diabetes, and many were of African American descent. A study based on data from the Kids' Inpatient Database provided the first national estimate of hospitalizations due to HHS among U.S. children between 1997 and 2009. The estimated population rate for HHS diagnoses for children age 0–18 years was 2.1 per 1,000,000 children in 1997, rising to 3.2 in 2009. The majority (70.5%) of HHS hospitalizations occurred among children with type 1 diabetes.

Risk Factors

The majority of HHS episodes are precipitated by an infectious process; other precipitants include cerebrovascular accident, alcohol abuse, pancreatitis, myocardial infarction, trauma, and drugs. In a case series of 119 patients with HHS, nearly 60 percent of the patients had an infection, and 42 percent had a stroke. Medications affecting carbohydrate metabolism, such as corticosteroids, thiazides, and sympathomimetic agents (e.g., dobutamine and terbutaline), may also precipitate the development of HHS. Elderly individuals, particularly those with new-onset diabetes are at risk for HHS.

Prevention and Treatment

Appropriate diabetes education, adequate treatment, and frequent self-monitoring of blood glucose help to prevent HHS in patients with known diabetes. HHS can be precipitated by dehydration and medications, such as corticosteroids, thiazides, and sympathomimetic agents. Careful use of these medications is indicated in vulnerable patients, e.g., elderly cared for in nursing homes at risk of dehydration and unable to promptly communicate their medical problems. Patients with HHS require hospitalization, which can be prolonged due to underlying conditions. In cases not complicated by underlying conditions, treatment modalities are similar to DKA. Intravenous rehydration and insulin to correct hyperglycemia lead to prompt resolution of HHS.

Chapter 48

Hypoglycemia

What Is Hypoglycemia?

Hypoglycemia, also called low blood glucose or low blood sugar, occurs when the level of glucose in your blood drops below normal. For many people with diabetes, that means a level of 70 milligrams per deciliter (mg/dL) or less. Your numbers might be different, so check with your healthcare provider to find out what level is too low for you.

What Are the Symptoms of Hypoglycemia?

Symptoms of hypoglycemia tend to come on quickly and can vary from person to person. You may have one or more mild-to-moderate symptoms listed in the table below. Sometimes people don't feel any symptoms.

Severe hypoglycemia is when your blood glucose level becomes so low that you're unable to treat yourself and need help from another person. Severe hypoglycemia is dangerous and needs to be treated right away. This condition is more common in people with type 1 diabetes.

Some symptoms of hypoglycemia during sleep are:

- crying out or having nightmares

This chapter includes text excerpted from "Low Blood Glucose (Hypoglycemia)," National Institute of Diabetes and Digestive and Kidney Diseases (NIDDK), August 2016.

- sweating enough to make your pajamas or sheets damp
- feeling tired, irritable, or confused after waking up

Table 48.1. Hypoglycemia Symptoms

Mild-to-Moderate		Severe
Shaky or jittery	Uncoordinated	Unable to eat or drink
Sweaty	Irritable or nervous	Seizures or convulsions
Hungry	Argumentative or	(jerky movements)
Headache	combative	Unconsciousness
Blurred vision	Changed behavior or	
Sleepy or tired	personality	
Dizzy or lightheaded	Trouble concentrating	
Confused or disoriented	Weak	
Pale	Fast or irregular heartbeat	

What Causes Hypoglycemia in Diabetes?

Hypoglycemia can be a side effect of insulin or other types of diabetes medicines that help your body make more insulin. Two types of diabetes pills can cause hypoglycemia: sulfonylureas and meglitinides. Ask your healthcare team if your diabetes medicine can cause hypoglycemia.

Although other diabetes medicines don't cause hypoglycemia by themselves, they can increase the chances of hypoglycemia if you also take insulin, a sulfonylurea, or a meglitinide.

What Other Factors Contribute to Hypoglycemia in Diabetes?

If you take insulin or diabetes medicines that increase the amount of insulin your body makes—but don't match your medications with your food or physical activity—you could develop hypoglycemia. The following factors can make hypoglycemia more likely:

Not Eating Enough Carbohydrates (Carbs)

When you eat foods containing carbohydrates, your digestive system breaks down the sugars and starches into glucose. Glucose then enters your bloodstream and raises your blood glucose level. If you don't eat enough carbohydrates to match your medication, your blood glucose could drop too low.

Skipping or Delaying a Meal

If you skip or delay a meal, your blood glucose could drop too low. Hypoglycemia also can occur when you are asleep and haven't eaten for several hours.

Increasing Physical Activity

Increasing your physical activity level beyond your normal routine can lower your blood glucose level for up to 24 hours after the activity.

Drinking Too Much Alcohol without Enough Food

Alcohol makes it harder for your body to keep your blood glucose level steady, especially if you haven't eaten in a while. The effects of alcohol can also keep you from feeling the symptoms of hypoglycemia, which may lead to severe hypoglycemia.

Being Sick

When you're sick, you may not be able to eat as much or keep food down, which can cause low blood glucose.

How Can You Prevent Hypoglycemia If You Have Diabetes?

If you are taking insulin, a sulfonylurea, or a meglitinide, using your diabetes management plan and working with your healthcare team to adjust your plan as needed can help you prevent hypoglycemia. The following actions can also help prevent hypoglycemia:

Check Blood Glucose Levels

Knowing your blood glucose level can help you decide how much medicine to take, what food to eat, and how physically active to be. To find out your blood glucose level, check yourself with a blood glucose meter as often as your doctor advises.

Hypoglycemia unawareness. Sometimes people with diabetes don't feel or recognize the symptoms of hypoglycemia, a problem called hypoglycemia unawareness. If you have had hypoglycemia without feeling any symptoms, you may need to check your blood glucose more often so you know when you need to treat your hypoglycemia or take steps to prevent it. Be sure to check your blood glucose before you drive.

If you have hypoglycemia unawareness or have hypoglycemia often, ask your healthcare provider about a continuous glucose monitor (CGM). A CGM checks your blood glucose level at regular times throughout the day and night. CGMs can tell you if your blood glucose is falling quickly and sound an alarm if your blood glucose falls too low. CGM alarms can wake you up if you have hypoglycemia during sleep.

Eat Regular Meals and Snacks

Your meal plan is key to preventing hypoglycemia. Eat regular meals and snacks with the correct amount of carbohydrates to help keep your blood glucose level from going too low. Also, if you drink alcoholic beverages, it's best to eat some food at the same time.

Be Physically Active Safely

Physical activity can lower your blood glucose during the activity and for hours afterward. To help prevent hypoglycemia, you may need to check your blood glucose before, during, and after physical activity and adjust your medicine or carbohydrate intake. For example, you might eat a snack before being physically active or decrease your insulin dose as directed by your healthcare provider to keep your blood glucose from dropping too low.

Work with Your Healthcare Team

Tell your healthcare team if you have had hypoglycemia. Your healthcare team may adjust your diabetes medicines or other aspects of your management plan. Learn about balancing your medicines, eating plan, and physical activity to prevent hypoglycemia. Ask if you should have a glucagon emergency kit to carry with you at all times.

How Do You Treat Hypoglycemia?

If you begin to feel one or more hypoglycemia symptoms, check your blood glucose. If your blood glucose level is below your target or less than 70, eat or drink 15 grams of carbohydrates right away. Examples include:

- four glucose tablets or one tube of glucose gel

- half cup (four ounces) of fruit juice—not low-calorie or reduced sugar*

- half can (4–6 ounces) of soda—not low-calorie or reduced sugar

- one tablespoon of sugar, honey, or corn syrup

- two tablespoons of raisins

Wait 15 minutes and check your blood glucose again. If your glucose level is still low, eat or drink another 15 grams of glucose or carbohydrates. Check your blood glucose again after another 15 minutes. Repeat these steps until your glucose level is back to normal.

If your next meal is more than one hour away, have a snack to keep your blood glucose level in your target range. Try crackers or a piece of fruit.

People who have kidney disease shouldn't drink orange juice for their 15 grams of carbohydrates because it contains a lot of potassium. Apple, grape, or cranberry juice are good options.

Treating Hypoglycemia If You Take Acarbose or Miglitol

If you take acarbose or miglitol along with diabetes medicines that can cause hypoglycemia, you will need to take glucose tablets or glucose gel if your blood glucose level is too low. Eating or drinking other sources of carbohydrates won't raise your blood glucose level quickly enough.

What If You Have Severe Hypoglycemia and Can't Treat Yourself?

Someone will need to give you a glucagon injection if you have severe hypoglycemia. An injection of glucagon will quickly raise your blood glucose level. Talk with your healthcare provider about when and how to use a glucagon emergency kit. If you have an emergency kit, check the date on the package to make sure it hasn't expired.

If you are likely to have severe hypoglycemia, teach your family, friends, and coworkers when and how to give you a glucagon injection. Also, tell your family, friends, and coworkers to call 911 right away after giving you a glucagon injection or if you don't have a glucagon emergency kit with you.

If you have hypoglycemia often or have had severe hypoglycemia, you should wear a medical alert bracelet or pendant. A medical alert identity (ID) tells other people that you have diabetes and need care right away. Getting prompt care can help prevent the serious problems that hypoglycemia can cause.

Chapter 49

Ketoacidosis

What Is Ketoacidosis?

Ketoacidosis is a serious condition where the body produces high levels of blood acids called ketones. It may require hospitalization.

The U.S. Food and Drug Administration (FDA) is warning that the type 2 diabetes medicines canagliflozin, dapagliflozin, and empagliflozin may lead to ketoacidosis.

What Is Diabetic Ketoacidosis?

Diabetic ketoacidosis (DKA), a subset of ketoacidosis or ketosis in diabetic patients, is a type of acidosis that usually develops when insulin levels are too low or during prolonged fasting. DKA most commonly occurs in patients with type 1 diabetes and is usually accompanied by high blood sugar levels.

Potential DKA triggering factors identified in some cases included acute illness (e.g., urinary tract infection (UTI), urosepsis, gastroenteritis, influenza, or trauma), reduced caloric or fluid intake, and reduced insulin dose.

This chapter includes text excerpted from "Acute Metabolic Complications in Diabetes," National Institute of Diabetes and Digestive and Kidney Diseases (NIDDK), March 12, 2016.

What Are the Symptoms of Ketoacidosis?

Patients should pay close attention for any signs of ketoacidosis and seek medical attention immediately if they experience symptoms such as difficulty breathing, nausea, vomiting, abdominal pain, confusion, and unusual fatigue or sleepiness. Do not stop or change your diabetes medicines without first talking to your prescriber. Healthcare professionals should evaluate for the presence of acidosis, including ketoacidosis, in patients experiencing these signs or symptoms; discontinue sodium-glucose cotransporter-2 (SGLT2) inhibitors if acidosis is confirmed; and take appropriate measures to correct the acidosis and monitor sugar levels.

What Are the Basics of DKA Treatment?

The goal of therapy is to correct dehydration by restoring extracellular and intracellular fluid volume and correcting electrolytes imbalances, hyperglycemia, and acidosis. The recommended therapy differs between adults and children given the higher risk of development of cerebral edema in children. Pediatric DKA should be treated in a facility with appropriate pediatric expertise.

How to Prevent DKA

Prevention of DKA should be one of the main goals of diabetes education. Knowledge of the signs and symptoms of diabetes, such as the classic triad of polydipsia, polyuria, and polyphagia with weight loss, is the best strategy for early detection of type 1 diabetes and prevention of DKA at the time of diagnosis. Both public and health professional education should make people aware of those symptoms, as patients admitted with severe DKA are often seen hours or days earlier by healthcare providers who missed the diagnosis, particularly in the youngest children. The Diabetes Autoimmunity Study in the Young, an observational study following children at genetically high risk for type 1 diabetes by periodic testing for diabetes autoantibodies, glycosylated hemoglobin (A1c), and random blood glucose, demonstrated that prevention of DKA in newly diagnosed children is possible. The prevalence of DKA at the time of diagnosis among children enrolled in this study was significantly lower compared to the community level.

Chapter 50

Osteoporosis and Diabetes

What Is Osteoporosis?

Osteoporosis is a condition in which the bones become less dense and more likely to fracture. Fractures from osteoporosis can result in pain and disability. In the United States (U.S), more than 53 million people either already have osteoporosis or are at high risk due to low bone mass.

Risk factors for developing osteoporosis include:

- being thin or having a small frame

- having a family history of the disease

- for women, being postmenopausal, having an early menopause, or not having menstrual periods (amenorrhea)

- using certain medications, such as glucocorticoids

- not getting enough calcium

- not getting enough physical activity

- smoking

- drinking too much alcohol

This chapter includes text excerpted from "What People with Diabetes Need to Know about Osteoporosis," National Institutes of Health-Osteoporosis and Related Bone Diseases~National Resource Center (NIH ORBD~NRC), April 2016.

Osteoporosis is a disease that often can be prevented. If undetected, it can progress for many years without symptoms until a fracture occurs.

The Diabetes–Osteoporosis Link

Type 1 diabetes is linked to low bone density, although researchers don't know exactly why. Insulin, which is deficient in type 1 diabetes, may promote bone growth and strength. The onset of type 1 diabetes typically occurs at a young age when bone mass is still increasing. It is possible that people with type 1 diabetes achieve lower peak bone mass, the maximum strength, and density that bones reach. People usually reach their peak bone mass by age 30. Low peak bone mass can increase one's risk of developing osteoporosis later in life. Some people with type 1 diabetes also have celiac disease, which is associated with reduced bone mass. It is also possible that cytokines, substances produced by various cells in the body, play a role in the development of both type 1 diabetes and osteoporosis.

Research also suggests that women with type 1 diabetes may have an increased fracture risk, since vision problems and nerve damage associated with the disease have been linked to an increased risk of falls and related fractures. Hypoglycemia, or low blood sugar reactions, may also contribute to falls.

Increased body weight can reduce one's risk of developing osteoporosis. Since excessive weight is common in people with type 2 diabetes, affected people were long believed to be protected against osteoporosis. However, although bone density is increased in people with type 2 diabetes, fractures are increased. As with type 1 diabetes, this may be due to increased falls because of vision problems and nerve damage. Moreover, the sedentary lifestyle common in many people with type 2 diabetes also interferes with bone health; and the disease disproportionately affects older individuals. As well, researchers suspect that the increased fracture risk in people with type 2 diabetes may be due to the negative impact of the disease on bone structure and quality.

Osteoporosis Management Strategies

Strategies to prevent and treat osteoporosis in people with diabetes are the same as for those without diabetes.

Nutrition

A diet rich in calcium and vitamin D is important for healthy bones. Good sources of calcium include low-fat dairy products; dark green, leafy vegetables; and calcium-fortified foods and beverages. Many low-fat and low-sugar sources of calcium are available. Also, supplements can help you meet the daily requirements of calcium and other important nutrients.

Vitamin D plays an important role in calcium absorption and bone health. It is synthesized in the skin through exposure to sunlight. Although many people are able to obtain enough vitamin D naturally, older individuals are often deficient in this vitamin due, in part, to limited time spent outdoors. They may require vitamin D supplements to ensure an adequate daily intake.

Exercise

Like muscle, bone is living tissue that responds to exercise by becoming stronger. The best exercise for your bones is weight-bearing exercise that forces you to work against gravity. Some examples include walking, stair climbing, and dancing. Regular exercise can help prevent bone loss and, by enhancing balance and flexibility, reduce the likelihood of falling and breaking a bone. Exercise is especially important for people with diabetes since exercise helps insulin lower blood glucose levels.

Healthy Lifestyle

Smoking is bad for bones as well as for the heart and lungs. Women who smoke tend to go through menopause earlier, triggering an earlier bone loss. In addition, smokers may absorb less calcium from their diets. Alcohol can also negatively affect bone health. Heavy drinkers are more prone to bone loss and fracture because of poor nutrition as well as an increased risk of falling. Avoiding smoking and alcohol can also help with managing diabetes.

Bone Density Test

Specialized tests known as bone mineral density (BMD) tests measure bone density in various parts of the body. These tests can detect osteoporosis before a bone fracture occurs and predict one's chances of fracturing in the future. It can measure bone density at your hip and spine. People with diabetes should talk to their doctors about whether they might be candidates for a bone density test.

Medication

Like diabetes, there is no cure for osteoporosis. However, several medications are approved by the U.S. Food and Drug Administration

(FDA) for the prevention and treatment of osteoporosis in postmenopausal women and men. Medications are also approved for use in both women and men with glucocorticoid-induced osteoporosis.

Chapter 51

Polycystic Ovary Syndrome and Diabetes

Ever heard of polycystic ovary syndrome (PCOS)? If you're a woman who has had trouble getting pregnant, you might have. Just about everyone else? Probably not.

PCOS is one of the most common causes of female infertility, affecting 6–12 percent (as many as 5 million) of U.S. women of reproductive age. But it's a lot more than that. PCOS is a lifelong health condition that continues far beyond the childbearing years.

Women with PCOS are often insulin resistant; their bodies can make insulin but can't use it effectively, increasing their risk for type 2 diabetes. Women with PCOS have higher levels of androgens (male hormones that females also have), which can stop eggs from being released (ovulation) and cause irregular periods, acne, thinning scalp hair, and excess hair growth on the face and body.

Women with PCOS can develop serious health problems, especially if they are overweight:

- **Diabetes.** More than half of women with PCOS develop type 2 diabetes by age 40.

- **Gestational diabetes** (diabetes when pregnant)—which puts the pregnancy and baby at risk and can lead to type 2 diabetes later in life for both mother and child

This chapter includes text excerpted from "PCOS, and Diabetes, Heart Disease, Stroke," Centers for Disease Control and Prevention (CDC), March 14, 2018.

- **Heart disease.** Women with PCOS are at higher risk, and risk increases with age.

- **High blood pressure**—which can damage the heart, brain, and kidneys

- **High low-density lipoprotein (LDL) ("bad") cholesterol** and **low high-density lipoprotein (HDL) ("good")** cholesterol—increasing the risk for heart disease

- **Sleep apnea**—a disorder that causes breathing to stop during sleep and raises the risk for heart disease and type 2 diabetes

- **Stroke**—plaque (cholesterol and white blood cells) clogging blood vessels can lead to blood clots that in turn can cause a stroke

PCOS is also linked to depression and anxiety, though the connection is not fully understood.

What Causes Polycystic Ovary Syndrome?

The exact causes of PCOS aren't known at this time, but androgen levels that are higher than normal play an important part. Excess weight and family history—which are in turn related to insulin resistance—can also contribute to PCOS.

Weight

Does being overweight cause PCOS? Does PCOS make you overweight? The relationship is complicated and not well understood. Being overweight is associated with PCOS, but many women of normal weight have PCOS, and many overweight women don't.

Family History

PCOS tends to run in families. Women whose mother or sister has PCOS or type 2 diabetes are more likely to develop PCOS.

Insulin Resistance

Lifestyle can have a big impact on insulin resistance, especially if a woman is overweight because of an unhealthy diet and lack of physical activity. Insulin resistance also runs in families. Losing weight will often help improve symptoms no matter what caused the insulin resistance.

Finding out If You Have Polycystic Ovary Syndrome

Sometimes PCOS symptoms are clear, and sometimes they're less obvious. You may visit a dermatologist (skin doctor) for acne, hair growth, or darkening of the skin in body creases and folds such as the back of the neck (acanthosis nigricans), a gynecologist (doctor who treats medical conditions that affect women and female reproductive organs) for irregular monthly periods, and your family doctor for weight gain, not realizing these symptoms are all part of PCOS. Some women with PCOS will have just one symptom; others will have them all. Women of every race and ethnicity can have PCOS.

It's common for women to find out they have PCOS when they have trouble getting pregnant, but it often begins soon after the first menstrual period, as young as age 11 or 12. It can also develop in the 20s or 30s.

To determine if you have PCOS, your doctor will check that you have at least 2 of these 3 symptoms:

1. Irregular periods or no periods, caused from lack of ovulation

2. Higher than normal levels of male hormones that may result in excess hair on the face and body, acne, or thinning scalp hair

3. Multiple small cysts on the ovaries

Just having ovarian cysts isn't enough for a PCOS diagnosis. Lots of women without PCOS have cysts on their ovaries and lots of women with PCOS don't have cysts.

Ways to Manage Polycystic Ovary Syndrome

See your healthcare provider if you have irregular monthly periods, are having trouble getting pregnant, or have excess acne or hair growth. If you're told you have PCOS, ask about getting tested for type 2 diabetes and how to manage the condition if you have it. Making healthy changes such as losing weight if you're overweight and increasing physical activity can lower your risk for type 2 diabetes, help you better manage diabetes, and prevent or delay other health problems.

There are also medicines that can help you ovulate, as well as reduce acne and hair growth. Make sure to talk with your healthcare provider about all your treatment options.

Part Six

Diabetes in Specific Populations

Chapter 52

Diabetes in Children

Chapter Contents

Section 52.1

Type 1 and Type 2 Diabetes on the Rise among Children

This section includes text excerpted from "Rates of New Diagnosed Cases of Type 1 and Type 2 Diabetes on the Rise among Children, Teens," National Institutes of Health (NIH), April 13, 2017.

Rates of new diagnosed cases of type 1 and type 2 diabetes are increasing among youth in the United States, according to a report, Incidence Trends of Type 1 and Type 2 Diabetes among Youths, 2002–2012, published in the *New England Journal of Medicine.*

In the United States, 29.1 million people are living with diagnosed or undiagnosed diabetes, and about 208,000 people younger than 20 years are living with diagnosed diabetes.

This study is the first ever to estimate trends in new diagnosed cases of type 1 and type 2 diabetes in youth (those under the age of 20), from the five major racial/ethnic groups in the United States: non-Hispanic whites, non-Hispanic blacks, Hispanics, Asian Americans/Pacific Islanders, and Native Americans. However, the Native American youth who participated in the SEARCH study are not representative of all Native American youth in the United States. Thus, these rates cannot be generalized to all Native American youth nationwide.

The SEARCH for Diabetes in Youth study, funded by the Centers for Disease Control and Prevention (CDC) and the National Institutes of Health (NIH), found that from 2002 to 2012, incidence, or the rate of new diagnosed cases of type 1 diabetes in youth increased by about 1.8 percent each year. During the same period, the rate of new diagnosed cases of type 2 diabetes increased even more quickly, at 4.8 percent. The study included 11,244 youth ages 0–19 with type 1 diabetes and 2,846 youth ages 10–19 with type 2.

"Because of the early age of onset and longer diabetes duration, youth are at risk for developing diabetes-related complications at a younger age. This profoundly lessens their quality of life, shortens their life expectancy, and increases healthcare costs," said Giuseppina Imperatore, M.D., Ph.D., epidemiologist in CDC's Division of Diabetes Translation, National Center for Chronic Disease Prevention and Health Promotion.

The study results reflect the nation's first and only ongoing assessment of trends in type 1 and type 2 diabetes among youth and help identify how the epidemic is changing over time in Americans under the age of 20 years.

Key Diabetes Findings from the Report

- Across all racial/ethnic groups, the rate of new diagnosed cases of type 1 diabetes increased more annually from 2003-2012 in males (2.2 percent) than in females (1.4 percent) ages 0–19.

- Among youth ages 0–19, the rate of new diagnosed cases of type 1 diabetes increased most sharply in Hispanic youth, a 4.2 percent annual increase. In non-Hispanic blacks, the rate of new diagnosed cases of type 1 diabetes increased by 2.2 percent and in non-Hispanic whites by 1.2 percent per year.

- Among youth ages 10–19, the rate of new diagnosed cases of type 2 diabetes rose most sharply in Native Americans (8.9 percent), Asian Americans/Pacific Islanders (8.5 percent) and non-Hispanic blacks (6.3 percent).

Note: The rates for Native Americans cannot be generalized to all Native American youth nationwide.

- Among youth ages 10–19, the rate of new diagnosed cases of type 2 diabetes increased 3.1 percent among Hispanics. The smallest increase was seen in whites (0.6 percent).

- The rate of new diagnosed cases of type 2 diabetes rose much more sharply in females (6.2 percent) than in males (3.7 percent) ages 10–19.

Cause of Rising Diabetes Incidence Unclear

"These findings lead to many more questions," said Barbara Linder, M.D., Ph.D., senior advisor for childhood diabetes research at NIH's National Institute of Diabetes and Digestive and Kidney Diseases (NIDDK). "The differences among racial and ethnic groups and between genders raise many questions. We need to understand why the increase in rates of diabetes development varies so greatly and is so concentrated in specific racial and ethnic groups."

- Type 1 diabetes, the most common form of diabetes in young people, is a condition in which the body fails to make insulin. Causes of type 1 diabetes are still unknown. However, disease development is suspected to follow exposure of genetically predisposed people to an "environmental trigger," stimulating an immune attack against the insulin-producing beta cells of the pancreas.

- In type 2 diabetes, the body does not make or use insulin well. In the past, type 2 diabetes was extremely rare in youth, but it has become more common in recent years. Several NIH-funded studies are directly examining how to delay, prevent, and treat diabetes.

- Type 1 Diabetes TrialNet screens thousands of relatives of people with type 1 diabetes annually and conducts prevention studies with those at highest risk for the disease.

- The Environmental Determinants of Diabetes in the Young (TEDDY) study seeks to uncover factors that may increase development of type 1 diabetes.

- For youth with type 2 diabetes, the ongoing Treatment Options for Type 2 Diabetes in Adolescents and Youth (TODAY) study is examining methods to treat the disease and prevent complications.

Additionally, CDC's NEXT-D study aims to understand how population-targeted policies affect preventive behaviors and diabetes outcomes and answer questions about quantity and quality of care used, costs, and unintended consequences.

Section 52.2

Managing Diabetes at School

This section includes text excerpted from "Managing Diabetes at School Playbook," Centers for Disease Control and Prevention (CDC), August 3, 2016.

Getting back into the routine of school takes a little more preparation for kids with diabetes, but it pays off over and over as the weeks and months go by. And since kids spend nearly half their waking hours in school, reliable diabetes care during the school day really matters.

Some older students will be comfortable testing their blood sugar, injecting insulin, and adjusting levels if they use an insulin pump. Younger students and those who just found out they have diabetes will need help with everyday diabetes care.

In a perfect world, all teachers and other school staff would understand how to manage diabetes so they could support your child as needed. But here in the real world, you'll want to provide information to the school and work with staff to keep your son or daughter safe and healthy, no matter what the school day brings.

Put It in Writing

No two kids handle their diabetes exactly the same way. Before the year begins, meet with your child's healthcare team to develop a personalized Diabetes Medical Management Plan (DMMP). Then visit the school and review the DMMP with the principal, office secretary, school nurse, nutrition service manager, teachers, and other staff who may have responsibility for your son or daughter during the day and after school.

The DMMP explains everything about diabetes management and treatment, including:

- Target blood sugar range and whether your child needs help checking his or her blood sugar

- Your child's specific hypoglycemia (low blood sugar, or "low") symptoms and how to treat hypoglycemia

- Insulin or other medication used

- Meal and snack plans, including for special events

- How to manage physical activity/sports

The DMMP works with your child's daily needs and routine. Make sure to update it every year or more often if treatment changes.

You may want to work with the school to set up a 504 plan that explains what the school will do to make sure your son or daughter is safe and has the same education opportunities as other students. The 504 plan makes the school's responsibilities clear and helps avoid misunderstandings. A new plan should be set up each school year.

Making the Team

Team up with school staff to make sure all the bases are covered for a safe and successful year.

The school nurse is usually the main staff member in charge of your student's diabetes care, but may not always be available when needed. One or more backup school employees should be trained in diabetes care tasks and should be on site at all times during the day, including after-school activities.

Make sure to visit the classroom(s). Some teachers may have had kids with diabetes in class before, but there's still a learning curve because every student is unique—and so is every teacher.

This is a great time to talk about class rules. Are students allowed to leave the room without asking? Should they raise their hand? The more your child and teacher understand each other's needs, the less disruptive and awkward self-care activities will be. You may want to ask if the teacher could talk to the class about diabetes—what it is and isn't, what happens, and what needs to be done every day—without pointing out that your child has diabetes.

Also let the teacher know specific signs to look for if your son or daughter's blood sugar is too low. Does he or she get irritable or nervous? Hungry or dizzy? The teacher may notice the signs before your child does and can alert him or her to eat an appropriate snack or get help.

Check in with nutrition services (school cafeteria) to get menus and nutritional information to help your child plan insulin use. Some students bring lunch from home because it's easier to stick to their meal plan.

Kids with diabetes need to be physically active just like other kids. In fact, physical activity can help them use less insulin because it lowers blood sugar. Talk with the physical education instructor about what your kid needs to participate fully and safely.

And as the school year gets into full swing, get familiar with the daily school schedule, including any after-school activities. You'll want to know where and when you can find your child if needed. Some parents use a smartphone app (several free ones are available) to help them stay informed and in touch with their child.

The First Day and Beyond

Create a backpack checklist you and/or your child can use every day to be sure all necessary supplies are packed:

- Blood sugar meter, and extra batteries, testing strips, lancets
- Ketone testing supplies
- Insulin and syringes/pens (include for backup even if an insulin pump is used)
- Antiseptic wipes
- Water
- Glucose tablets or other fast-acting carbs like fruit juice or hard candy (about 10–15 grams) that will raise blood sugar levels quickly

Put together a "hypo" box with your child's name on it for the school office in case of hypoglycemia.

Also make sure your child:

- Wears a medical identity (ID) necklace or bracelet every day. Many options are available.
- Tests blood sugar according to schedule; older students can set phone reminders
- Knows where and when to go for blood sugar testing if help is needed
- Knows who to go to for help with hypoglycemia

Important—Treating Hypoglycemia

Hypoglycemia can happen quickly and needs to be treated immediately. It's most often caused by too much insulin, waiting too long for a meal or snack, not eating enough, or getting extra physical activity. Hypoglycemia symptoms vary, so school staff should be familiar with your child's specific symptoms, which could include:

- Shakiness
- Nervousness or anxiety
- Sweating, chills, or clamminess
- Irritability or impatience
- Dizziness and difficulty concentrating
- Hunger or nausea
- Blurred vision

- Weakness or fatigue

- Anger, stubbornness, or sadness

If your child has hypoglycemia several times a week, visit his or her healthcare provider to see if the treatment plan needs to be adjusted.

Staying Well Basics

- Make sure your child has had all recommended shots, including the flu shot. Kids with diabetes can get sicker from the flu and stay sick longer. Being sick can make blood sugar monitoring harder.

- Regular hand washing, especially before eating and after using the bathroom, is one of the best ways to avoid getting sick and spreading germs to others.

Section 52.3

How Diabetes Is Treated in Children

This section includes text excerpted from "How Is Diabetes Treated in Children?" U.S. Food and Drug Administration (FDA), January 3, 2018.

Is your child packing on the pounds? Becoming a couch potato? Then he or she may be at risk for getting type 2 diabetes.

Type 2 diabetes once occurred mainly in adults who are overweight and over 40, according to the National Institute of Diabetes and Digestive and Kidney Diseases (NIDDK). It is increasingly diagnosed in youths age 10–19.

Why Is This Happening?

Because just like adults, kids are heavier now. An estimated 1 in 6 children and teens is obese, according to the Centers for Disease Control and Prevention (CDC).

Along with a family history of diabetes, being overweight and inactive are the main risk factors for type 2 diabetes, says Ilan Irony, M.D., an endocrinologist at the U.S. Food and Drug Administration (FDA).

The two main types of diabetes—type 1 and type 2—are treatable, says Irony. "In addition to changes in diet and a healthier lifestyle, treatments can help control blood sugar and prevent or delay long-term complications of diabetes."

The FDA-approved treatments for both type 1 and type 2 diabetes are all about keeping the blood sugar (glucose) levels in a normal range.

But there is no one treatment that works for everybody, says Irony. And treatments may need to be changed if side effects of a particular medication are not tolerated. Also, additional medications may need to be added as diabetes gets worse over time.

Type 2 Diabetes

Type 2 diabetes is most often diagnosed in children starting at age 12 or 13, says Irony. "In children, the disease tends to get worse in puberty when the body produces hormones that make insulin less effective," he says. Insulin is the hormone that controls blood sugar levels.

"The first line of treatment is a healthy diet and other lifestyle changes," says Irony. "If a child is overweight or obese, losing weight and increasing physical activity can help lower blood sugar."

Ask the pediatrician if your child is a healthy weight or needs to lose weight. And children and adolescents should do at least one hour of physical activity each day, according to the federal government's 2008 Physical Activity Guidelines for Americans (PAGA).

Type 2 diabetes may be controlled with diet and exercise for a while—sometimes years—says Irony. "But the disease is progressive and medication will be needed later in the majority of patients."

The FDA has approved one glucose-lowering medication—metformin—in pill and liquid form for children. Metformin, used daily, increases the body's sensitivity to its own insulin so it becomes more active and pushes glucose into the cells. The most common side effects of metformin—upset stomach, nausea, and diarrhea—generally go away within a few weeks.

In rare cases, metformin can cause a serious and sometimes fatal side effect called lactic acidosis—a buildup of lactic acid in the blood. This rare condition has occurred mostly in people whose kidneys were not working normally.

The FDA has approved a number of different drugs for diabetes in adults that are currently being studied for use in children, Irony says.

Injectable insulins—which move glucose from the blood to the body's cells—are approved for children with diabetes. If the drug metformin alone doesn't bring the blood sugar down to normal, insulin can be injected and help achieve better control.

Type 1 Diabetes

Type 1 diabetes accounts for almost all diabetes in children younger than 10, and it is also on the rise in U.S. children and adolescents. Formerly called juvenile diabetes, type 1 occurs when the body's immune system destroys the insulin-making cells in the pancreas. Researchers are still investigating the causes of diabetes.

For children with type 1 diabetes, multiple injections of insulin are needed every day to keep the blood sugar in check.

"Treatment is individualized to the child and the spikes of high or low blood sugar need to be minimized," says Irony. It's a balancing act to lower the blood sugar but not get it too low, which could make the child feel shaky or pass out, he adds.

Diabetes Devices

Children with type 1 or type 2 diabetes, like adults, must test their blood sugar multiple times a day. The FDA regulates medical devices, including portable meters and monitors, used to check blood sugar levels. The agency also regulates devices such as syringes, pens, and pumps used to inject insulin.

Syringes and pens are used manually to inject insulin. Pumps are computerized devices programmed to deliver a continuous flow of insulin, even while you sleep. The FDA has approved more than 55 different insulin pumps. A pump system generally consists of:

- a pumping mechanism that holds batteries and a cartridge filled with insulin. The pump, which is similar in size to a pager, is worn outside the body on a belt or in a pocket.

- a tube (catheter) that carries insulin from the pump to another tube (cannula) implanted just under the skin, typically in the belly or back

Pump technology continues to evolve, says Alan Stevens, a mechanical engineer and FDA's infusion pump team leader. A newer type is the "patch" pump, he says, in which the tubing is contained within a pump directly attached to the body with adhesive. A small, hand-held computer similar to a Parenteral Drug Association (PDA), which directs the pump, can be carried in a purse or pocket.

Section 52.4

Weight and Diabetes in Children

This section includes text excerpted from "Helping Your Child Who Is Overweight," National Institute of Diabetes and Digestive and Kidney Diseases (NIDDK), September 2016.

As a parent or other caregiver, you can do a lot to help your child reach and maintain a healthy weight. Staying active and consuming healthy foods and beverages are important for your child's well-being. You can take an active role in helping your child—and your whole family—learn habits that may improve health.

How Can You Tell If Your Child Is Overweight?

Being able to tell whether a child is overweight is not always easy. Children grow at different rates and at different times. Also, the amount of a child's body fat changes with age and differs between girls and boys.

One way to tell if your child is overweight is to calculate his or her body mass index (BMI). BMI is a measure of body weight relative to height. The BMI calculator uses a formula that produces a score often used to tell whether a person is underweight, a normal weight, overweight, or obese. The BMI of children is age- and sex-specific and known as the "BMI-for-age."

BMI-for-age uses growth charts created by the Centers for Disease Control and Prevention (CDC). Doctors use these charts to track a child's growth. The charts use a number called a percentile to show how your child's BMI compares with the BMI of other children. The main BMI categories for children and teens are

- **Healthy weight:** 5th–84th percentile

- **Overweight:** 85th–94th percentile

- **Obese:** 95th percentile or higher

Why Should You Be Concerned?

You should be concerned if your child has extra weight because weighing too much may increase the chances that your child will develop health problems now or later in life.

In the short run, for example, he or she may have breathing problems or joint pain, making it hard to keep up with friends. Some children may develop health problems, such as type 2 diabetes, high blood pressure (BP), and high cholesterol. Some children also may experience teasing, bullying, depression, or low self-esteem.

Children who are overweight are at higher risk of entering adulthood with too much weight. The chances of developing health problems such as heart disease and certain types of cancer are higher among adults with too much weight.

BMI is a screening tool and does not directly measure body fat or an individual child's risk of health problems. If you are concerned about your child's weight, talk with your child's doctor or other healthcare professional. He or she can check your child's overall health and growth over time and tell you if weight management may be helpful. Many children who are still growing in length don't need to lose weight; they may need to decrease the amount of weight they gain while they grow taller. Don't put your child on a weight-loss diet unless your child's doctor tells you to.

How Can You Help Your Child Develop Healthy Habits?

You can play an important role in helping your child build healthy eating, drinking, physical activity, and sleep habits. For instance, teach your child about balancing the amount of food and beverages he or she eats and drinks with his or her amount of daily physical activity. Take your child grocery shopping and let him or her choose healthy foods and drinks, and help plan and prepare healthy meals and snacks. The *2015 U.S. Dietary Guidelines* explain the types of foods and beverages to include in a healthy eating plan.

Here are some other ways to help your child develop healthy habits:

- Be a good role model. Consume healthy foods and drinks, and choose active pastimes. Children are good learners, and they often copy what they see.

- Talk with your child about what it means to be healthy and how to make healthy decisions.

  - Discuss how physical activities and certain foods and drinks may help their bodies get strong and stay healthy.

    - Children should get at least an hour of physical activity daily and should limit their screen time (computers, television, and mobile devices) outside of school work to no more than 2 hours each day.

  - Chat about how to make healthy choices about food, drinks, and activities at school, at friends' houses, and at other places outside your home.

- Involve the whole family in building healthy eating, drinking, and physical activity habits. Everyone benefits, and your child who is overweight won't feel singled out.

- Make sure your child gets enough sleep. While research about the relationship between sleep and weight is ongoing, some studies link excess weight to not enough sleep in children and adults.

What Can You Do to Improve Your Child's Eating Habits?

Besides consuming fewer foods, drinks, and snacks that are high in calories, fat, sugar, and salt, you may get your child to eat healthier by offering these options more often:

- Fruits, vegetables, and whole grains such as brown rice

- Lean meats, poultry, seafood, beans, and peas, soy products, and eggs, instead of meat high in fat

- Fat-free or low-fat milk, and milk products, or milk substitutes, such as soy beverages with added calcium, and vitamin D, instead of whole milk or cream

- Fruit and vegetable smoothies made with fat-free or low-fat yogurt, instead of milkshakes or ice cream

- Water, fat-free, or low-fat milk, instead of soda and other drinks with added sugars

You also may help your child eat better by trying to:

- Avoid serving large portions, or the amount of food or drinks your child chooses for a meal or snack. Start with smaller amounts of food and let your child ask for more if he or she is still hungry. If your child chooses food or drinks from a package, container, or can, read the Nutrition Facts Label to see what amount is equal to one serving. Match your child's portion to the serving size listed on the label to avoid extra calories, fat, and sugar.

- Put healthy foods and drinks where they are easy to see and keep high-calorie foods and drinks out of sight—or don't buy them at all.

- Eat fast food less often. If you do visit a fast-food restaurant, encourage your child to choose healthier options, such as sliced fruit instead of fries. Also, introduce your child to different foods, such as hummus with veggies.

- Try to sit down to family meals as often as possible, and have fewer meals "on the run."

- Discourage eating in front of the television, computer, or other electronic device.

To help your child develop a healthy attitude toward food and eating:

- Don't make your child clean his or her plate.

- Offer rewards other than food or drinks when encouraging your child to practice healthy habits. Promising dessert for eating vegetables sends a message that vegetables are less valuable than dessert.

Healthy Snack Ideas

To help your child eat less candy, cookies, and other unhealthy snacks, try these healthier snack options instead:

- Air-popped popcorn without butter

- Fresh, frozen, or fruit canned in natural juices, plain or with fat-free, or low-fat yogurt

- Fresh vegetables, such as baby carrots, cucumbers, zucchini, or cherry tomatoes

- Low-sugar, whole-grain cereal with fat-free or low-fat milk, or a milk substitute with added calcium and vitamin D

How Can You Help Your Child Be More Active?

Try to make physical activity fun for your child. Children need about 60 minutes of physical activity a day, although the activity doesn't have to be all at once. Several short 10- or even 5-minute spurts of activity throughout the day are just as good. If your child is not used to being active, encourage him or her to start out slowly and build up to 60 minutes a day.

To encourage daily physical activity:

- Let your child choose a favorite activity to do regularly, such as climbing a jungle gym at the playground or joining a sports team or dance class.

- Help your child find simple, fun activities to do at home or on his or her own, such as playing tag, jumping rope, playing catch, shooting baskets, or riding a bike (wear a helmet).

- Limit time with the computer, television, cell phone, and other devices to two hours a day.

- Let your child and other family members plan active outings, such as a walk or hike to a favorite spot.

Where Can You Go for Help?

If you have tried to change your family's eating, drinking, physical activity, and sleep habits and your child has not reached a healthy weight, ask your child's healthcare professional about other options. He or she may be able to recommend a plan for healthy eating and physical activity, or refer you to a weight-management specialist, registered dietitian, or program. Your local hospital, a community health clinic, or health department also may offer weight-management programs for children and teens or information about where you can enroll in one.

What Should You Look for in a Weight-Management Program?

When choosing a weight-management program for your child, look for a program that:

- includes a variety of healthcare providers on staff, such as doctors, psychologists, and registered dietitians

- evaluates your child's weight, growth, and health before enrollment and throughout the program

- adapts to your child's specific age and abilities. Programs for elementary school-aged children should be different from those for teens.

- helps your family keep healthy eating, drinking, and physical activity habits after the program ends

How Else Can You Help Your Child?

You can help your child by being positive and supportive throughout any process or program you choose to help him or her achieve a healthy weight. Help your child set specific goals and track progress. Reward successes with praise and hugs.

Tell your child that he or she is loved, special, and important. Children's feelings about themselves are often based on how they think their parents and other caregivers feel about them.

Listen to your child's concerns about his or her weight. He or she needs support, understanding, and encouragement from caring adults.

Section 52.5

Prevent Type 2 Diabetes in Kids

This section includes text excerpted from "Prevent Type 2 Diabetes in Kids," Centers for Disease Control and Prevention (CDC), June 29, 2017.

There's a growing type 2 diabetes problem in our young people. But parents can help turn the tide with healthy changes that are good for the whole family.

Earlier, young children and teens almost never got type 2 diabetes, which is why it used to be called adult-onset diabetes. Now, about one-third of American youth are overweight, a problem closely related to the increase in kids with type 2 diabetes, some as young as 10 years old.

Weight Matters

People who are overweight—especially if they have excess belly fat—are more likely to have insulin resistance, kids included. Insulin resistance is a major risk factor for type 2 diabetes.

Insulin is a hormone made by the pancreas that acts like a key to let blood sugar into cells for use as energy. Because of heredity (traits inherited from family members) or lifestyle (eating too much and moving too little), cells can stop responding normally to insulin. That causes the pancreas to make more insulin to try to get cells to respond and take in blood sugar.

As long as enough insulin is produced, blood sugar levels remain normal. This can go on for several years, but eventually the pancreas can't keep up. Blood sugar starts to rise, first after meals and then all the time. Now the stage is set for type 2 diabetes.

Insulin resistance usually doesn't have any symptoms, though some kids develop patches of thickened, dark, velvety skin called acanthosis nigricans, usually in body creases and folds such as the back of the neck or armpits. They may also have other conditions related to insulin resistance, including:

- High blood pressure
- High cholesterol
- Polycystic ovary syndrome (PCOS)

Activity Matters

Being physically active lowers the risk for type 2 diabetes because it helps the body use insulin better, decreasing insulin resistance. Physical activity improves health in lots of other ways, too, from controlling blood pressure to boosting mental health.

Age Matters

Kids who get type 2 diabetes are usually diagnosed in their early teens. One reason is that hormones present during puberty make it harder for the body use insulin, especially for girls, who are more likely than boys to develop type 2 diabetes. That's an important reason to help your kids take charge of their health while they're young.

More Risk Factors

These factors also increase kids' risk for type 2 diabetes:

- Having a family member with type 2 diabetes

- Being born to a mom with gestational diabetes (diabetes while pregnant)

- Being African American, Hispanic/Latino, Native American/ Alaska Native, Asian American, or Pacific Islander

- Having one or more conditions related to insulin resistance

If your child is overweight and has any two of the risk factors listed above, talk to your doctor about getting his or her blood sugar tested. Testing typically begins at 10 years old or when puberty starts, whichever is first, and is repeated every three years.

Take Charge, Family Style

Parents can do a lot to help their kids prevent type 2 diabetes. Set a new normal as a family—healthy changes become habits more easily when everyone does them together. Here are some tips to get started:

Mealtime Makeover

- Drink more water and fewer sugary drinks.

- Eat more fruits and vegetables.

- Make favorite foods healthier.

- Get kids involved in making healthier meals.

- Eat slowly—it takes at least 20 minutes to start feeling full.

- Eat at the dinner table only, not in front of the TV or computer.

- Shop for food together.

- Shop on a full stomach so you're not tempted to buy unhealthy food.

- Teach your kids to read food labels to understand which foods are healthiest.

- Have meals together as a family as often as you can.

- Don't insist kids clean their plates.

- Don't put serving dishes on the table.
- Serve small portions; let kids ask for seconds.
- Reward kids with praise instead of food.

Getting Physical

- Aim for your child to get 60 minutes of physical activity a day, in several 10- or 15-minute sessions or all at once.
- Start slow and build up.
- Keep it positive—focus on progress.
- Take parent and kid fitness classes together.
- Make physical activity more fun; try new things.
- Ask kids what activities they like best—everyone is different.
- Encourage kids to join a sports team.
- Have a "fit kit" available—a jump rope, hand weights, resistance bands.
- Limit screen time to two hours a day.
- Plan active outings, like hiking or biking.
- Take walks together.
- Move more in and out of the house—vacuuming, raking leaves, gardening.
- Turn chores into games, like racing to see how fast you can clean the house.

Young kids and teens are still growing, so if they're overweight the goal is to slow down weight gain while allowing normal growth and development. Don't put them on a weight loss diet without talking to their doctor.

Chapter 53

Diabetes and Pregnancy

If you have diabetes and plan to have a baby, you should try to get your blood glucose levels close to your target range *before* you get pregnant.

Staying in your target range during pregnancy, which may be different than when you aren't pregnant, is also important. High blood glucose, also called blood sugar, can harm your baby during the first weeks of pregnancy, even before you know you are pregnant. If you have diabetes and are already pregnant, see your doctor as soon as possible to make a plan to manage your diabetes. Working with your healthcare team and following your diabetes management plan can help you have a healthy pregnancy and a healthy baby.

If you develop diabetes for the first time while you are pregnant, you have gestational diabetes.

How Can Diabetes Affect My Baby?

A baby's organs, such as the brain, heart, kidneys, and lungs, start forming during the first 8 weeks of pregnancy. High blood glucose levels can be harmful during this early stage and can increase the chance that your baby will have birth defects, such as heart defects or defects of the brain or spine.

This chapter includes text excerpted from "Pregnancy If You Have Diabetes," National Institute of Diabetes and Digestive and Kidney Diseases (NIDDK), January 2017.

High blood glucose levels during pregnancy can also increase the chance that your baby will be born too early, weigh too much, or have breathing problems or low blood glucose right after birth.

High blood glucose also can increase the chance that you will have a miscarriage or a stillborn baby. Stillborn means the baby dies in the womb during the second half of pregnancy.

How Can My Diabetes Affect Me during Pregnancy?

Hormonal and other changes in your body during pregnancy affect your blood glucose levels, so you might need to change how you manage your diabetes. Even if you've had diabetes for years, you may need to change your meal plan, physical activity routine, and medicines. If you have been taking an oral diabetes medicine, you may need to switch to insulin. As you get closer to your due date, your management plan might change again.

What Health Problems Could I Develop during Pregnancy because of My Diabetes?

Pregnancy can worsen certain long-term diabetes problems, such as eye problems and kidney disease, especially if your blood glucose levels are too high.

You also have a greater chance of developing preeclampsia, sometimes called toxemia, which is when you develop high blood pressure (BP) and too much protein in your urine during the second half of pregnancy. Preeclampsia can cause serious or life-threatening problems for you and your baby. The only cure for preeclampsia is to give birth. If you have preeclampsia and have reached 37 weeks of pregnancy, your doctor may want to deliver your baby early. Before 37 weeks, you and your doctor may consider other options to help your baby develop as much as possible before he or she is born.

How Can I Prepare for Pregnancy If I Have Diabetes?

If you have diabetes, keeping your blood glucose as close to normal as possible before and during your pregnancy is important to stay healthy and have a healthy baby. Getting check-ups before and during pregnancy, following your diabetes meal plan, being physically active as your healthcare team advises, and taking diabetes medicines if you need to will help you manage your diabetes. Stopping smoking and taking vitamins as your doctor advises also can help you and your baby stay healthy.

Work with Your Healthcare Team

Regular visits with members of a healthcare team who are experts in diabetes and pregnancy will ensure that you and your baby get the best care. Your healthcare team may include:

- A medical doctor who specializes in diabetes care, such as an endocrinologist or a diabetologist
- An obstetrician with experience treating women with diabetes
- A diabetes educator who can help you manage your diabetes
- A nurse practitioner who provides prenatal care during your pregnancy
- A registered dietitian to help with meal planning
- Specialists who diagnose and treat diabetes-related problems, such as vision problems, kidney disease, and heart disease
- A social worker or psychologist to help you cope with stress, worry, and the extra demands of pregnancy

You are the most important member of the team. Your healthcare team can give you expert advice, but you are the one who must manage your diabetes every day.

Get a Checkup

Have a complete checkup before you get pregnant or as soon as you know you are pregnant. Your doctor should check for:

- High blood pressure
- Eye disease
- Heart and blood vessel disease
- Nerve damage
- Kidney disease
- Thyroid disease

Pregnancy can make some diabetes health problems worse. To help prevent this, your healthcare team may recommend adjusting your treatment before you get pregnant.

Don't Smoke

Smoking can increase your chance of having a stillborn baby or a baby born too early. Smoking is especially harmful to people with diabetes. Smoking can increase diabetes-related health problems such as eye disease, heart disease, and kidney disease.

If you smoke or use other tobacco products, stop. Ask for help so you don't have to do it alone. You can start by calling the national quitline at 800-QUIT-NOW or 800-784-8669.

See a Registered Dietitian Nutritionist

If you don't already see a dietitian, you should start seeing one before you get pregnant. Your dietitian can help you learn what to eat, how much to eat, and when to eat to reach or stay at a healthy weight before you get pregnant. Together, you and your dietitian will create a meal plan to fit your needs, schedule, food preferences, medical conditions, medicines, and physical activity routine.

During pregnancy, some women need to make changes to their meal plans, such as adding extra calories, protein, and other nutrients. You will need to see your dietitian every few months during pregnancy as your dietary needs change.

Be Physically Active

Physical activity can help you reach your target blood glucose numbers. Being physically active can also help keep your blood pressure and cholesterol levels in a healthy range, relieve stress, strengthen your heart and bones, improve muscle strength, and keep your joints flexible.

Before getting pregnant, make physical activity a regular part of your life. Aim for 30 minutes of activity 5 days of the week.

Talk with your healthcare team about what activities are best for you during your pregnancy.

Avoid Alcohol

You should avoid drinking alcoholic beverages while you're trying to get pregnant and throughout pregnancy. When you drink, the alcohol also affects your baby. Alcohol can lead to serious, lifelong health problems for your baby.

Adjust Your Medicines

Some medicines are not safe during pregnancy and you should stop taking them before you get pregnant. Tell your doctor about all the medicines you take, such as those for high cholesterol and high blood pressure. Your doctor can tell you which medicines to stop taking and may prescribe a different medicine that is safe to use during pregnancy.

Doctors most often prescribe insulin for both type 1 and type 2 diabetes during pregnancy. If you're already taking insulin, you might need to change the kind, the amount, or how and when you take it. You may need less insulin during your first trimester but probably will need more as you go through pregnancy. Your insulin needs may double or even triple as you get closer to your due date. Your healthcare team will work with you to create an insulin routine to meet your changing needs.

Take Vitamin and Mineral Supplements

Folic acid is an important vitamin for you to take before and during pregnancy to protect your baby's health. You'll need to start taking folic acid at least one month before you get pregnant. You should take a multivitamin or supplement that contains at least 400 micrograms (mcg) of folic acid. Once you become pregnant, you should take 600 mcg daily. Ask your doctor if you should take other vitamins or minerals, such as iron or calcium supplements, or a multivitamin.

What Do I Need to Know about Blood Glucose Testing before and during Pregnancy?

How often you check your blood glucose levels may change during pregnancy. You may need to check them more often than you do now. If you didn't need to check your blood glucose before pregnancy, you will probably need to start. Ask your healthcare team how often and at what times you should check your blood glucose levels. Your blood glucose targets will change during pregnancy. Your healthcare team also may want you to check your ketone levels if your blood glucose is too high.

Target Blood Glucose Levels before Pregnancy

When you're planning to become pregnant, your daily blood glucose targets may be different than your previous targets. Ask your healthcare team which targets are right for you.

You can keep track of your blood glucose levels using My Daily Blood Glucose Record (niddk.nih.gov/-/media/Files/Diabetes/BloodGlucose_508.pdf?la=en). You can also use an electronic blood glucose tracking system on your computer or mobile device. Record the results every time you check your blood glucose. Your blood glucose records can help you and your healthcare team decide whether your diabetes care plan is working. You also can make notes about your insulin and ketones. Take your tracker with you when you visit your healthcare team.

Target Blood Glucose Levels during Pregnancy

Recommended daily target blood glucose numbers for most pregnant women with diabetes are:

- Before meals, at bedtime, and overnight: 90 or less
- 1 hour after eating: 130 to 140 or less
- 2 hours after eating: 120 or less

Ask your doctor what targets are right for you. If you have type 1 diabetes, your targets may be higher so you don't develop low blood glucose, also called hypoglycemia.

A1C Numbers

Another way to see whether you're meeting your targets is to have an A1C blood test. Results of the A1C test reflect your average blood glucose levels during the past three months. Most women with diabetes should aim for an A1C as close to normal as possible—ideally below 6.5 percent—before getting pregnant. After the first three months of pregnancy, your target may be as low as six percent. These targets may be different than A1C goals you've had in the past. Your doctor can help you set A1C targets that are best for you.

Ketone Levels

When your blood glucose is too high or if you're not eating enough, your body might make ketones. Ketones in your urine or blood mean your body is using fat for energy instead of glucose. Burning large amounts of fat instead of glucose can be harmful to your health and your baby's health.

You can prevent serious health problems by checking for ketones. Your doctor might recommend you test your urine or blood daily for ketones or when your blood glucose is above a certain level, such as 200. If you use an insulin pump, your doctor might advise you to test for ketones when your blood glucose level is higher than expected. Your healthcare team can teach you how and when to test your urine or blood for ketones.

Talk to your doctor about what to do if you have ketones. Your doctor might suggest making changes in the amount of insulin you take or when you take it. Your doctor also may recommend a change in meals or snacks if you need to consume more carbohydrates.

What Tests Will Check My Baby's Health during Pregnancy?

You will have tests throughout your pregnancy, such as blood tests and ultrasounds, to check your baby's health. Talk with your healthcare team about what prenatal tests you'll have and when you might have them.

Chapter 54

Diabetes in Older People

Diabetes is a serious disease. People get diabetes when their blood glucose level, sometimes called blood sugar, is too high. The good news is that there are things you can do to take control of diabetes and prevent its problems. And, if you are worried about getting diabetes, there are things you can do to lower your risk.

What Is Diabetes?

Our bodies turn the food we eat into glucose. Insulin helps glucose get into our cells, where it can be used to make energy. If you have diabetes, your body may not make enough insulin, may not use insulin in the right way, or both. That can cause too much glucose in the blood. Your family doctor may refer you to a doctor who specializes in taking care of people with diabetes, called an endocrinologist.

Types of Diabetes

There are two main kinds of diabetes.

- **Type 1 diabetes.** In type 1 diabetes, the body makes little or no insulin. Although adults can develop this type of diabetes, it occurs most often in children and young adults.

- **Type 2 diabetes.** In type 2 diabetes, the body makes insulin but doesn't use it the right way. It is the most common kind of

This chapter includes text excerpted from "Diabetes in Older People," National Institute on Aging (NIA), January 31, 2017.

diabetes. It occurs most often in middle-aged and older adults, but it can also affect children. Your chance of getting type 2 diabetes is higher if you are overweight, inactive, or have a family history of diabetes.

Diabetes can affect many parts of your body. It's important to keep diabetes under control. Over time, it can cause serious health problems like heart disease, stroke, kidney disease, blindness, nerve damage, and circulation problems that may lead to amputation. People with type 2 diabetes also have a greater risk for Alzheimer's disease.

What Is Prediabetes?

Many people have "prediabetes." This means their glucose levels are higher than normal but not high enough to be called diabetes. Prediabetes is a serious problem because people who have it are at high risk for developing type 2 diabetes.

There are things you can do to prevent or delay getting type 2 diabetes. Losing weight may help. Healthy eating and being physically active can make a big difference. Work with your doctor to set up a plan for good nutrition and regular exercise. Make sure to ask how often you should have your glucose levels checked.

Symptoms of Diabetes

Some people with type 2 diabetes may not know they have it. But, they may feel tired, hungry, or thirsty. They may lose weight without trying, urinate often, or have trouble with blurred vision. They may also get skin infections or heal slowly from cuts and bruises. See your doctor right away if you have one or more of these symptoms.

Tests for Diabetes

Doctors use several blood tests to help diagnose diabetes:

- **Random plasma glucose (RPG) test**—given at any time during the day

- **A1C test**—given at any time during the day; shows your glucose level for the past 3 months

- **Fasting plasma glucose (FPG) test**—taken after you have gone without food for at least 8 hours

- **Oral glucose tolerance test (OGTT)**—taken after fasting overnight and then again 2 hours after having a sugary drink

Your doctor may want you to be tested for diabetes twice before making a diagnosis.
(OGTT)

Managing Diabetes

Once you've been told you have diabetes, your doctor will choose the best treatment based on the type of diabetes you have, your everyday routine, and any other health problems you have. Many people with type 2 diabetes can control their blood glucose levels with diet and exercise alone. Others need diabetes medicines or insulin injections. Over time, people with diabetes may need both lifestyle changes and medication.

You can keep control of your diabetes by:

- **Tracking your glucose levels.** Very high glucose levels or very low glucose levels (called hypoglycemia) can be risky to your health. Talk to your doctor about how to check your glucose levels at home.

- **Making healthy food choices.** Learn how different foods affect glucose levels. For weight loss, check out foods that are low in fat and sugar. Let your doctor know if you want help with meal planning.

- **Getting exercise.** Daily exercise can help improve glucose levels in older people with diabetes. Ask your doctor to help you plan an exercise program.

- **Taking your diabetes medicines even when you feel good.** Tell your doctor if you have any side effects or cannot afford your medicines.

Your doctor may want you to see other healthcare providers who can help manage some of the extra problems caused by diabetes. He or she can also give you a schedule for other tests that may be needed. Talk to your doctor about how to stay healthy.

Here are some ways to stay healthy with diabetes:

- **Find out your average blood glucose level.** At least twice a year, get the A1C blood test. The result will show your average glucose level for the past 3 months.

- **Watch your blood pressure.** Get your blood pressure checked often.

- **Check your cholesterol.** At least once a year, get a blood test to check your cholesterol and triglyceride levels. High levels may increase your risk for heart problems.

- **Stop smoking.** Smoking raises your risk for many health problems, including heart attack and stroke.

- **Have yearly eye exams.** Finding and treating eye problems early may keep your eyes healthy.

- **Check your kidneys yearly.** Diabetes can affect your kidneys. A urine and blood test will show if your kidneys are okay.

- **Get flu shots every year and the pneumonia vaccine.** A yearly flu shot will help keep you healthy. If you're over 65, make sure you have had the pneumonia vaccine. If you were younger than 65 when you had the pneumonia vaccine, you may need another one. Ask your doctor.

- **Care for your teeth and gums.** Brush your teeth and floss daily. Have your teeth and gums checked twice a year by a dentist to avoid serious problems.

- **Protect your skin.** Keep your skin clean and use skin softeners for dryness. Take care of minor cuts and bruises to prevent infections.

- **Examine your feet.** Take time to examine your feet every day for any red patches. Ask someone else to check your feet if you can't. If you have sores, blisters, breaks in the skin, infections, or buildup of calluses, see a foot doctor, called a podiatrist.

- **Be Prepared.** Make sure you always have at least 3 days' worth of supplies on hand for testing and treating your diabetes in case of an emergency.

Medicare Can Help

Medicare may pay to help you learn how to care for your diabetes. It may also help pay for diabetes tests, supplies, flu and pneumonia shots, special shoes, foot exams, eye tests, and meal planning.

For more information about what Medicare covers, call 800-MEDI-CARE (800-633-4227) or visit the Medicare website (www.medicare.gov).

Part Seven

Research in Diabetes Care

Chapter 55

Blood Test May Identify Gestational Diabetes Risk in First Trimester

A blood test conducted as early as the tenth week of pregnancy may help identify women at risk for gestational diabetes, a pregnancy-related condition that poses potentially serious health risks for mothers and infants, according to researchers at the National Institutes of Health (NIH) and other institutions. The study appears in *Scientific Reports*.

Gestational diabetes occurs only in pregnancy and results when the level of blood sugar, or glucose, rises too high. Gestational diabetes increases the mother's chances for high blood pressure disorders of pregnancy and the need for cesarean delivery, and the risk for cardiovascular disease and type 2 diabetes later in life. For infants, gestational diabetes increases the risk for large birth size. Unless they have a known risk factor, such as obesity, women typically are screened for gestational diabetes between 24–28 weeks of pregnancy.

In the study, researchers evaluated whether the HbA1c test (also called the A1C test), commonly used to diagnose type 2 diabetes, could identify signs of gestational diabetes in the first trimester of pregnancy. The test approximates the average blood glucose levels over

This chapter includes text excerpted from "Blood Test May Identify Gestational Diabetes Risk in First Trimester," National Institutes of Health (NIH), August 16, 2018.

the previous two or three months, based on the amount of glucose that has accumulated on the surface of red blood cells. According to the authors, comparatively few studies have examined whether the HbA1c test could help identify the risk for gestational diabetes, and these studies have been limited to women already at high risk for the condition. The test is not recommended to diagnose gestational diabetes at any point in pregnancy.

The researchers analyzed records from the *Eunice Kennedy Shriver* National Institute of Child Health and Human Development (NICHD) Fetal Growth Study (www.nichd.nih.gov/about/org/diphr/officebranch/eb/fetal-growth-stud), a large observational study that recruited more than 2,000 low-risk pregnant women from 12 U.S. clinical sites between 2009–2013. The researchers compared HbA1c test results from 107 women who later developed gestational diabetes to test results from 214 women who did not develop the condition. Most of the women had tests at four intervals during pregnancy: early (weeks 8–13), middle (weeks 16–22 and 24–29) and late (weeks 34–37).

Women who went on to develop gestational diabetes had higher HbA1c levels (an average of 5.3 percent), compared to those without gestational diabetes (an average HbA1c level of 5.1 percent). Each 0.1 percent increase in HbA1c above 5.1 percent in early pregnancy was associated with a 22-percent higher risk for gestational diabetes.

In middle pregnancy, HbA1c levels declined for both groups. However, HbA1c levels increased in the final third of pregnancy, which is consistent with the decrease in sensitivity to insulin that often occurs during this time period.

"Our results suggest that the HbA1C test potentially could help identify women at risk for gestational diabetes early in pregnancy, when lifestyle changes may be more effective in reducing their risk," said the study's senior author, Cuilin Zhang, Ph.D., of the Epidemiology Branch at NIH's NICHD.

Exercise and a healthy diet may lower blood glucose levels during pregnancy. If these measures are not successful, physicians may prescribe insulin to bring blood glucose under control.

The authors noted that further studies are needed to confirm whether measuring HbA1c levels in early pregnancy could determine a woman's later risk for gestational diabetes. Similarly, research is needed to determine whether lowering HbA1c with lifestyle changes, either in early pregnancy or before pregnancy, could reduce the risk for the condition.

Chapter 56

Are Proteins in Infant Formula Linked to Type 1 Diabetes?

For decades, researchers have puzzled over why type 1 diabetes is becoming more common. Type 1 diabetes is a serious disease in which the body destroys the cells that make insulin. Insulin tells cells to take up sugar from your blood. People with type 1 diabetes need to take insulin every day to stay alive.

Researchers have wondered whether infant formula made from cow's milk might cause children to develop type 1 diabetes. Studies suggested that early exposure to the complex proteins in cow's milk might lead the body to mistakenly attack the cells that make insulin.

To test this idea, researchers used two formulas. One group of infants received a formula made from cow's milk. The other received a formula made from cow's milk that was processed to break complex proteins into small pieces. All the infants enrolled in the study had a genetic makeup that put them at higher risk of developing type 1 diabetes.

The mothers were encouraged to use the assigned formula whenever they didn't breastfeed. The analysis included infants who were fed formula at least 60 days.

This chapter includes text excerpted from "Are Proteins in Formula Linked to Type 1 Diabetes?" *NIH News in Health*, National Institutes of Health (NIH), March 2018.

The results showed that the chance of developing type 1 diabetes by age 10 was the same for children in both groups. The complex proteins in cow's milk did not raise the risk of developing type 1 diabetes.

"This once more shows us that there is no easy way to prevent type 1 diabetes," says researcher Dr. Dorothy Becker at the University of Pittsburgh.

Chapter 57

Breastfeeding May Help Health after Gestational Diabetes

A study suggests that breastfeeding may help women with a history of gestational diabetes from later developing type 2 diabetes.

About 5–9 percent of pregnant women nationwide develop high blood sugar levels even though they didn't have diabetes before pregnancy. This condition, called gestational diabetes, raises a woman's risk for type 2 diabetes later in life. Left untreated, type 2 diabetes can cause health problems such as heart disease, stroke, kidney disease, blindness, and amputation.

Past studies found that breastfeeding causes certain changes in the mother's body that may help protect against type 2 diabetes. However, the connection hadn't been proven, especially among women who'd had gestational diabetes. The National Institute of Health (NIH)-funded research team at the Kaiser Permanente Division of Research (KPDR) set out to address the question.

The team enrolled more than 1,000 ethnically diverse women who were diagnosed with gestational diabetes. Their lactation intensity and duration were assessed by feeding diaries, in-person exams, phone calls, and questionnaires. Researchers tested blood sugar 6–9 weeks after delivery and then annually for two years.

This chapter includes text excerpted from "Breastfeeding May Help Health after Gestational Diabetes," *NIH News in Health*, National Institutes of Health (NIH), January 2016.

During the two-year follow-up, nearly 12 percent of the women developed type 2 diabetes. After accounting for differences in age and other risk factors, the researchers estimated that women who exclusively breastfed or mostly breastfed were about half as likely to develop type 2 diabetes as those who didn't breastfeed.

How long women breastfeed also affected their chance of developing type 2 diabetes. Breastfeeding for longer than two months lowered the risk of type 2 diabetes by almost half. Breastfeeding beyond five months lowered the risk by more than half.

"These findings highlight the importance of prioritizing breastfeeding education and support for women with gestational diabetes as part of early diabetes prevention efforts," says study lead Dr. Erica P. Gunderson of the Kaiser Permanente Division of Research.

Chapter 58

Cone Snail Venom Reveals Insulin Insights

The marine cone snail has an unusual survival mechanism that offers new insights for managing diabetes. The snail releases an insulin-containing venom that acts within seconds to stun nearby fish, so they're easier to capture and eat. Scientists have been fascinated by how rapidly this insulin works compared to human insulin.

Insulin is important for people because it helps maintain blood sugar (glucose) levels. When glucose levels rise, such as after a meal, insulin is released into the bloodstream and travels throughout the body. When insulin binds to special cell-surface structures called receptors, it triggers cells to take in the glucose needed for energy. Diabetes arises when this process doesn't work correctly. Many people rely on injections of synthetic insulin to manage their diabetes, and rapid action can be crucial.

Human insulin is stored in the body in clusters of six. To work, the six parts must first separate, which might take up to an hour. In contrast, the insulin in cone snails is small and fast acting. It lacks the portion that would hold insulin clusters together.

The National Institute of Health (NIH)-supported research team, based partly at the University of Utah, analyzed the 3D structure of cone snail insulin. Despite its smaller structure, the snail insulin could bind and turn on the human insulin receptor.

This chapter includes text excerpted from "Cone Snail Venom Reveals Insulin Insights," *NIH News in Health*, National Institutes of Health (NIH), November 2016.

"We found that cone snail venom insulins work faster than human insulins by avoiding the structural changes that human insulins undergo in order to function—they are essentially primed and ready to bind to their receptors," says study co-author Dr. Michael Lawrence of the Walter and Eliza Hall Institute (WEHI) of Medical Research in Australia.

These findings provide insights that could help scientists design rapid-acting insulins that might help to manage diabetes.

Chapter 59

Diabetes Control and Prevention Studies

Chapter Contents

Section 59.1

Blood Glucose Control Studies for Type 1 Diabetes: DCCT and EDIC

This section includes text excerpted from "Blood Glucose
Control Studies for Type 1 Diabetes: DCCT and EDIC,"
National Institute of Diabetes and Digestive and
Kidney Diseases (NIDDK), March 27, 2018.

The National Institute of Diabetes and Digestive and Kidney
Diseases (NIDDK) funded the landmark Diabetes Control and Complications Trial (DCCT) to see if people with type 1 diabetes who
kept their blood glucose levels as close to normal as safely possible
with intensive diabetes treatment (three or more shots of insulin
per day or an insulin pump with self-monitoring of blood glucose at
least four times per day) could slow the development of eye, kidney,
and nerve disease, compared to people who used the conventional
treatment at the time of the study (one or two shots of insulin per
day with daily self-monitoring of urine or blood glucose). The DCCT
ended after 10 years in 1993—a year earlier than planned—when the
study proved that participants who kept their blood glucose levels
close to normal greatly lowered their chances of having eye, kidney,
and nerve disease.

A follow-up to the DCCT, the ongoing Epidemiology of Diabetes
Interventions and Complications (EDIC) study, has continued to follow
DCCT participants for the last 20-plus years. EDIC has shown that
there are long-term benefits of early and intensive blood glucose control on the future development of diabetes-related complications such
as heart, eye, kidney, and nerve disease, and that early and intensive
blood glucose control also lengthens life. EDIC has also shown that an
individualized eye exam schedule results in fewer eye exams, resulting in lower costs, and quicker diagnosis and treatment of advanced
diabetic eye disease.

Findings from DCCT/EDIC have changed the way diabetes is
treated worldwide. As a result of DCCT/EDIC, early and intensive
blood glucose control is now the standard treatment for people with
type 1 and even type 2 diabetes, and helps people with diabetes live
longer and healthier lives.

Diabetes Control and Complications Trial (DCCT)

DCCT Results

The DCCT showed that people with type 1 diabetes who kept their blood glucose levels as close to normal as safely possible with intensive diabetes treatment as early as possible in their disease had fewer diabetes-related health problems after 6.5 years, compared to people who used the conventional treatment.

DCCT showed that people who used intensive treatment lowered their risk of:

- **diabetic eye disease** by 76 percent; and advancement of eye disease by about half (54%), in people with some eye disease at the beginning of the study.

- **diabetic kidney disease** by 50 percent

- **diabetic nerve disease** by 60 percent

Researchers were not able to show whether people who used intensive treatment lowered their risk of heart disease during the DCCT, since only a few people had heart disease during the study.

Participants who used intensive treatment had an average A1C of seven percent, while participants who used the conventional treatment had an average A1C of nine percent. The A1C blood test shows a person's average blood glucose levels over the previous 2–3 months. A normal A1C value is six percent or less.

In the DCCT, the major side effect of intensive treatment was a higher risk for hypoglycemia, also called low blood glucose, which can be deadly if not treated immediately. Participants knew how to treat hypoglycemia.

DCCT Study Size, Participant Demographics, and Study Design

The DCCT took place from 1983–1993. The study involved 1,441 volunteers ages 13–39, and took place in 29 medical centers in the United States and Canada. At the start of the DCCT, participants had type 1 diabetes for at least an year but no longer than 15 years, and had no or only early signs of diabetic eye or kidney diseases.

DCCT participants were randomly assigned to one of the following groups:

- **Intensive diabetes treatment group.** Participants took insulin three or more times per day by injection or an insulin pump and self-monitored their blood glucose levels four or more times a day. The treatment goal was to keep A1C levels as close to normal as safely possible. Participants met with their healthcare team monthly.

- **Conventional diabetes treatment group.** Participants used what was conventional diabetes treatment at the time (in the early 1980s): one or two shots of insulin a day with daily urine or blood glucose testing. Participants met with their healthcare team every three months.

Researchers followed participants for an average of 6.5 years and compared the study groups to see if there was more eye, kidney, and nerve disease in one group or the other.

After DCCT ended participants who used conventional treatment were taught about intensive treatment. Participants who continued into the EDIC follow-up study were transferred to their own healthcare team for medical care and were able to choose between conventional treatment or intensive treatment.

Epidemiology of Diabetes Interventions and Complications (EDIC) Study

EDIC Results

EDIC researchers are trying to understand how diabetes affects the body over time, and the long-term benefits of a period of early and intensive blood glucose control in the development of later complications from diabetes. EDIC has shown that early and intensive blood glucose control during the DCCT lowers the risk of:

- **cardiovascular diseases (CVD), such as heart attack and stroke, and cardiovascular-related deaths** by 57 percent, 11 years after the DCCT ended and 32 percent, 20 years after the DCCT ended

- **eye surgery for diabetic eye disease** by 48 percent, 17 years after the DCCT ended

- **kidney disease and failure** by 50 percent, 18 years after the DCCT ended

- **nerve problems** by about 30 percent, 14 years after the DCCT ended

DCCT participants who had tight control of their blood glucose levels also lived longer. Historically, people with type 1 diabetes tended to die earlier than the general population. DCCT/EDIC researchers have found that this earlier death can be reduced or eliminated through careful management of blood glucose.

EDIC has shown that adjusting the frequency of eye screenings for people with type 1 diabetes based on their risk of severe eye problems and A1C level would result in:

- **fewer eye exams by 50 percent,** lowering the overall cost of care by one billion dollars over 20 years

- **quicker diagnosis and treatment of advanced diabetic eye disease,** a condition which can lead to vision loss

These long-term benefits occurred even though all participants had an average A1C of eight percent during the 20-plus years of the EDIC study. Participants from the DCCT intensive treatment and conventional treatment groups had similar blood glucose levels starting about five years after EDIC began.

EDIC Study Size, Participant Demographics, and Study Design

The EDIC follow-up study started in 1994, enrolling 96 percent of the living DCCT participants at the beginning of the study. When EDIC began, participants who used conventional treatment were taught about intensive treatment, and received follow-up care from their own healthcare team. The EDIC study is ongoing and includes the majority of the original surviving DCCT participants. These people continue to take part in studies of a variety of diabetes-related health problems, including hypoglycemia, irregular heartbeats, hearing loss, weakened bones, trouble thinking clearly, and problems with the eyes, kidneys, nerves, feet, bladder, and sexual function. Another study is looking at the small amount of insulin that some people with type 1 diabetes continue to make and whether this improves health.

Section 59.2

Diabetes Prevention Program

This section includes text excerpted from "Diabetes Prevention
Program (DPP)," National Institute of Diabetes and Digestive and
Kidney Diseases (NIDDK), March 29, 2018.

The National Institute of Diabetes and Digestive and Kidney Diseases (NIDDK)-sponsored Diabetes Prevention Program (DPP) and ongoing Diabetes Prevention Program Outcomes Study (DPPOS) are major studies that changed the way people approach type 2 diabetes prevention worldwide. The DPP showed that people who are at high risk for type 2 diabetes can prevent or delay the disease by losing a modest amount of weight through lifestyle changes (dietary changes and increased physical activity). Taking metformin, a safe and effective generic medicine to treat diabetes, was also found to prevent the disease, though to a lesser degree.

The DPPOS has continued to follow most DPP participants since 2002. To date, the DPPOS has shown that participants who took part in the DPP Lifestyle Change Program or are taking metformin continue to prevent or delay type 2 diabetes for at least 15 years. The DPPOS has also shown that the DPP Lifestyle Change Program is cost effective (costs are justified by the benefits of diabetes prevention, improved health, and fewer healthcare costs), and metformin is cost saving (leads to small savings in healthcare costs) after 10 years. DPPOS researchers are also continuing to follow other health problems in participants such as cancer, cardiovascular diseases (heart and blood vessel disease), nerve damage, kidney disease, and eye disease. As participants age, researchers are following age-related health problems such as trouble with physical function and difficulties with thinking or memory.

The NIDDK built on the success of the DPP by funding additional research to make modified versions of the DPP Lifestyle Change Program that are more cost effective and more easily available to the tens of millions of Americans at risk for type 2 diabetes. Several modified group versions of the DPP Lifestyle Change Program have shown great promise. One version tested in Young Men's Christian Association's (YMCA) is now widely available in the United States through a partnership with the Centers for Disease Control and Prevention's (CDC) National Diabetes Prevention Program (NDPP).

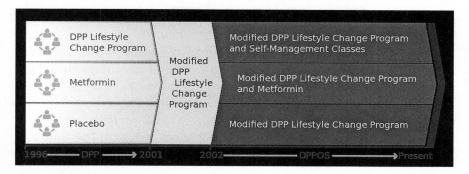

Figure 59.1. *DPP and DPPOS Timeline*

Diabetes Prevention Program (DPP)

DPP Goal

The DPP looked at whether the DPP Lifestyle Change Program or taking metformin would delay or prevent type 2 diabetes.

DPP Results

After about three years, the DPP showed that participants in the DPP Lifestyle Change Program lowered their chances of developing type 2 diabetes by 58 percent compared with participants who took a placebo (a pill without medicine). The DPP Lifestyle Change Program was effective for all participating racial and ethnic groups and both men and women. The program worked particularly well for participants ages 60 and older, lowering their chances of developing type 2 diabetes by 71 percent. About five percent of participants in the DPP Lifestyle Change Program developed diabetes each year during the study compared with 11 percent of participants who took a placebo.

Participants who took metformin lowered their chances of developing type 2 diabetes by 31 percent compared with participants who took a placebo. Metformin was effective for all participating racial and ethnic groups and both men and women. Metformin was most effective in women with a history of gestational diabetes, in people between the ages of 25–44, and in people with obesity who had a body mass index of 35 or higher.

DPP Study Design

The DPP was a randomized, controlled clinical trial conducted at 27 clinical centers around the United States from 1996–2001. The trial enrolled 3,234 participants; 55 percent were Caucasian, and 45 percent were from minority groups at high risk for the disease, including African American, Alaska Native, American Indian, Asian American, Hispanic/Latino, or Pacific Islander. The trial also recruited other groups at high risk for type 2 diabetes, including people ages 60 and older, women with a history of gestational diabetes, and people with a parent, brother, sister, or child who had type 2 diabetes.

DPP participants were randomly assigned to one of the following groups:

- **Lifestyle change group.** Group participants joined a DPP Lifestyle Change Program that provided intensive training. Participants tried to lose seven percent of their body weight and maintain that weight loss by eating less fat and fewer calories and exercising 150 minutes per week. Researchers met with participants individually at least 16 times in the first 24 weeks, and then every two months with at least one phone call between visits.

- **Metformin group.** Group participants took 850 mg of metformin twice a day and were provided standard advice about diet and physical activity.

- **Placebo group.** Group participants took a placebo twice a day instead of metformin and were provided standard advice about diet and physical activity.

DPP participants who developed diabetes remained in the study and received additional care from their own physicians if good blood glucose control could not be maintained.

After DPP ended all participants were provided a modified group version of the DPP's Lifestyle Change program.

Diabetes Prevention Program Outcomes Study (DPPOS)

DPPOS Goal

The DPPOS is following DPP participants to see if participants who took part in the DPP Lifestyle Change Program or who are continuing to take metformin have a delay in the development of type 2 diabetes over time and if they experience fewer health problems such as cancer, cardiovascular diseases, nerve damage, kidney disease, eye disease, and age-related health problems such as trouble with physical function and difficulties with thinking or memory.

DPPOS Results

Ten-Year Findings

At the 10-year follow-up:

- participants who took part in the DPP Lifestyle Change Program continued to have a delay in the development of diabetes by 34 percent—and developed diabetes about four years later—compared with participants who took a placebo. Participants from the DPP Lifestyle Change Program ages 60 and older had a delay in the development of diabetes by 49 percent.

- participants who continued to take metformin had a delay in the development of diabetes by 18 percent—and developed diabetes about two years later—compared with participants who took a placebo.

- participants from the DPP Lifestyle Change Program and participants who continued to take metformin or took a placebo all improved their risk factors for cardiovascular diseases, such as high blood pressure and cholesterol. However, the participants from the DPP Lifestyle Change Program achieved these results with fewer blood pressure and cholesterol-lowering medications.

- the DPP Lifestyle Change Program was shown to be cost-effective and metformin was shown to be cost-saving.

Fifteen-Year Findings

At the 15-year follow-up:

- participants from the DPP Lifestyle Change Program continued to have a delay in the development of diabetes by 27 percent compared with participants who took a placebo.

- participants who continued to take metformin had a delay in the development of diabetes by 18 percent compared with participants who took a placebo.

- about half (55 percent) of participants from the DPP Lifestyle Change Program and 56 percent of participants who continued to take metformin developed diabetes compared with 62 percent of participants who took a placebo.

- there were no overall differences in small blood vessel problems such as those found in eyes, nerves, and kidneys between participants from the DPP Lifestyle Change Program and participants who continued to take metformin or took a placebo. However, women from the DPP Lifestyle Change Program developed fewer small blood vessel problems than participants who continued to take metformin or took a placebo. Participants who did not develop diabetes had a 28 percent lower rate of small blood vessel problems compared with participants who developed diabetes.

Focus

In early 2016 the NIDDK, in partnership with the National Heart Lung and Blood Institute (NHLBI) and National Cancer Institute (NCI), began funding a third phase of DPPOS—proposed to last 10 years—to find out if people who are at high risk for type 2 diabetes and take metformin have lower rates of cardiovascular diseases and cancer, as suggested by several earlier small-scale studies.

DPPOS Study Design

The DPPOS follow-up study started in 2002. All 3,149 surviving participants of DPP groups were eligible for the DPPOS, including those with and without diabetes. Of the 3,149 surviving participants, 2,776 (88%) joined the DPPOS. Similar proportions of each DPP group joined the DPPOS and remained in their original groups. There were some changes to the treatments each group received:

- **Lifestyle change group.** Group participants received quarterly group lifestyle change classes throughout the study and two group classes yearly to reinforce self-management behaviors for weight loss.

- **Metformin group.** Group participants received quarterly group lifestyle change classes throughout the study. Participants continued to take metformin and were told that they were taking metformin.

- **Placebo group.** Group participants received quarterly group lifestyle change classes throughout the study. Participants did not take a placebo pill.

DPPOS participants who developed diabetes remained in the study and received additional care from their own physicians if good blood glucose control could not be maintained.

Chapter 60

Diabetes Drug May Prevent Recurring Strokes

Pioglitazone, a drug used for type 2 diabetes, may prevent recurrent stroke and heart attacks in people with insulin resistance but without diabetes. The results of the Insulin Resistance Intervention after Stroke (IRIS) trial, presented at the International Stroke Conference (ISC) 2016 in Los Angeles and published in the New England Journal of Medicine (NEJM), suggest a potential new method to prevent stroke and heart attack in high-risk patients who have already had one stroke or transient ischemic attack. This large, international study was supported by the National Institutes of Health's (NIH) National Institute of Neurological Disorders and Stroke (NINDS).

The IRIS trial is the first study to provide evidence that a drug targeting cell metabolism may prevent secondary strokes and heart attacks even before diabetes develops. Insulin regulates metabolism and keeps blood sugar levels from getting too high, along with many other processes, in the body. Insulin resistance is a condition in which the body produces insulin but does not use it effectively.

"This study represents a novel approach to prevent recurrent vascular events by reversing a specific metabolic abnormality thought to increase the risk for future heart attack or stroke," said Walter J. Koroshetz, M.D., director of the NINDS.

This chapter includes text excerpted from "Diabetes Drug May Prevent Recurring Strokes," National Institutes of Health (NIH), February 17, 2016.

"The IRIS trial supports the value of more research to test the vascular benefits of other interventions such as exercise, diet, and medications that have similar effects on metabolism as pioglitazone," said Walter N. Kernan, M.D., professor of general medicine at Yale University School of Medicine, New Haven, Connecticut, and lead author of the study.

More than 3000 patients from seven countries who had experienced an ischemic stroke or transient ischemic attack within the previous six months were randomized to receive pioglitazone or placebo for up to five years in addition to standard care. Ischemic stroke and transient ischemic attacks can occur when a cerebral blood vessel becomes blocked, cutting off the delivery of oxygen and nutrients to brain tissue.

In this study, stroke or heart attack occurred in nine percent of participants taking pioglitazone and 11.8 percent of patients on placebo, which was a relative decrease of 24 percent. The results suggest that 28 strokes or heart attacks may be prevented for every 1000 patients who take pioglitazone for up to five years.

Insulin resistance is a hallmark of type 2 diabetes but also occurs in more than 50 percent of people with ischemic stroke who do not have diabetes. People with diabetes are known to have increased risk of stroke. Previous research suggested that insulin resistance increases risk for stroke, but the IRIS trial was the first to treat it and suggested that the therapy reduced the risk of recurrent stroke and heart attacks. However, pioglitazone is not U.S. Food and Drug Administration (FDA)-approved for the uses studied in the IRIS trial.

In this study, pioglitazone also reduced the risk of diabetes by 52 percent in the study participants.

The study evidenced an additional known side effect of the drug, which is an increased risk of bone fractures. To help doctors and patients choose the best strategy for preventing recurring strokes, future studies will attempt to identify a person's risk of bone fractures due to pioglitazone. As approved for use in medical practice, the drug also carries additional side effects.

"More research is needed to determine the mechanisms by which pioglitazone decreases risk for stroke and heart attack and increases bone fracture risk, with the hope of developing strategies that maximize benefit and minimize serious side effects in our patients," said Dr. Kernan.

Chapter 61

Experimental Therapy Shows Promise for Type 1 Diabetes

Patients with difficult cases of type 1 diabetes were helped by transplants of insulin-producing islet cells. The experimental therapy helped to prevent dangerous drops in blood sugar levels.

People with diabetes have trouble managing and using blood glucose, a sugar that serves as fuel for the body. When blood glucose levels rise, islet cells in the pancreas normally make and secrete hormones such as insulin. Insulin triggers cells to take up sugar from the blood.

In type 1 diabetes, the immune system attacks and destroys these insulin-producing cells. People with type 1 diabetes must regularly measure their blood glucose and use insulin injections to maintain their blood sugar levels.

When blood sugar levels drop too low (hypoglycemia), symptoms like shaking or sweating usually warn people to eat or drink to raise their blood sugar levels. However, many people with type 1 diabetes can't tell when their blood sugar is too low. This raises their risk for severe hypoglycemia, which can cause seizures, loss of consciousness, and death.

One strategy to treat type 1 diabetes is to transplant pancreatic islets from deceased human donors. To test this experimental procedure, the National Institutes of Health (NIH)-funded researchers

This chapter includes text excerpted from "Experimental Therapy Shows Promise for Type 1 Diabetes," *NIH News in Health*, National Institutes of Health (NIH), June 2016.

studied 48 people with hard-to-treat type 1 diabetes. Participants received at least one transplant of pancreatic islets.

During the first year after treatment, 88 percent of participants were free of severe hypoglycemic events, had near-normal control of blood glucose levels, and were able to tell when their blood sugar was low. After two years, 71 percent still had these positive effects. Some people had side effects. Researchers are still monitoring the patients to assess the benefits and risks of this therapy.

"While still experimental, and with risks that must be weighed carefully, the promise of islet transplantation is undeniable and encouraging," says Dr. Griffin P. Rodgers, director of the NIH's National Institute of Diabetes and Digestive and Kidney Diseases (NIDDK).

Chapter 62

Pancreatic Islet Transplantation

Chapter Contents

Section 62.1

What Is Pancreatic Islet Transplantation?

This section includes text excerpted from "Pancreatic Islet Transplantation," National Institute of Diabetes and Digestive and Kidney Diseases (NIDDK), September 2013. Reviewed September 2018.

What Are Pancreatic Islets?

Pancreatic islets, also called islets of Langerhans, are tiny clusters of cells scattered throughout the pancreas. The pancreas is an organ about the size of a hand located behind the lower part of the stomach.

Pancreatic islets contain several types of cells, including beta cells, that produce the hormone insulin. The pancreas also makes enzymes that help the body digest and use food.

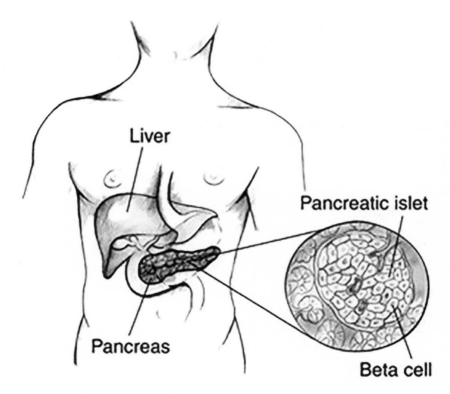

Figure 62.1. *Pancreatic Islets*

When the level of blood glucose, also called blood sugar, rises after a meal, the pancreas responds by releasing insulin into the bloodstream. Insulin helps cells throughout the body absorb glucose from the bloodstream and use it for energy.

Diabetes develops when the pancreas does not make enough insulin, the body's cells do not use insulin effectively, or both. As a result, glucose builds up in the blood instead of being absorbed by cells in the body.

In type 1 diabetes, the beta cells of the pancreas no longer make insulin because the body's immune system has attacked and destroyed them. The immune system protects people from infection by identifying and destroying bacteria, viruses, and other potentially harmful foreign substances. A person who has type 1 diabetes must take insulin daily to live. Type 2 diabetes usually begins with a condition called insulin resistance, in which the body has trouble using insulin effectively. Over time, insulin production declines as well, so many people with type 2 diabetes eventually need to take insulin.

What Is Pancreatic Islet Transplantation?

The two types of pancreatic islet transplantation are:

- Allotransplantation

- Autotransplantation

Pancreatic islet allotransplantation is a procedure in which islets from the pancreas of a deceased organ donor are purified, processed, and transferred into another person. Pancreatic islet allotransplantation is currently labeled an experimental procedure until the transplantation technology is considered successful enough to be labeled therapeutic.

For each pancreatic islet allotransplant infusion, researchers use specialized enzymes to remove islets from the pancreas of a single, deceased donor. The islets are purified and counted in a lab. Transplant patients typically receive two infusions with an average of 400,000 to 500,000 islets per infusion. Once implanted, the beta cells in these islets begin to make and release insulin.

Pancreatic islet allotransplantation is performed in certain patients with type 1 diabetes whose blood glucose levels are difficult to control. The goals of the transplant are to help these patients achieve normal blood glucose levels with or without daily injections of insulin and to reduce or eliminate hypoglycemia unawareness—a dangerous condition in which a person with diabetes cannot feel the symptoms of hypoglycemia, or low blood glucose. When a person feels the symptoms of hypoglycemia, steps can be taken to bring blood glucose levels back to normal.

Pancreatic islet allotransplants are only performed at hospitals that have received permission from the U.S. Food and Drug Administration (FDA) for clinical research on islet transplantation. The transplants are often performed by a radiologist—a doctor who specializes in medical imaging. The radiologist uses X-rays and ultrasound to guide the placement of a thin, flexible tube called a catheter through a small incision in the upper abdomen—the area between the chest and hips—and into the portal vein of the liver. The portal vein is the major vein that supplies blood to the liver. The islets are then infused, or pushed, slowly into the liver through the catheter. Usually, the patient receives a local anesthetic and a sedative. In some cases, a surgeon performs the transplant using general anesthesia.

Patients often need two or more transplants to get enough functioning islets to stop or reduce their need for insulin injections.

Pancreatic islet autotransplantation is performed following total pancreatectomy—the surgical removal of the whole pancreas—in patients with severe and chronic, or long lasting, pancreatitis that cannot be managed by other treatments. This procedure is not considered experimental. Patients with type 1 diabetes cannot receive pancreatic islet autotransplantation. The procedure is performed in a hospital, and the patient receives general anesthesia. The surgeon first removes the pancreas and then extracts and purifies islets from the pancreas. Within hours, the islets are infused through a catheter into the patient's liver. The goal is to give the body enough healthy islets to make insulin.

What Happens after Pancreatic Islet Transplantation?

Pancreatic islets begin to release insulin soon after transplantation. However, full islet function and new blood vessel growth from the new islets take time. Transplant recipients usually take insulin injections until the islets are fully functional. They may also receive various medications before and after transplantation to promote successful implantation and long-term functioning of the islets. However, the autoimmune response that destroyed transplant recipients' own islets in the first place can happen again and attack the transplanted islets. Although the liver has been the traditional site for infusing the donor islets, researchers are investigating alternative sites, such as muscle tissue or another organ.

What Are the Benefits and Risks of Pancreatic Islet Allotransplantation?

The benefits of pancreatic islet allotransplantation include improved blood glucose control, reducing or eliminating the need for insulin injections to control diabetes, and preventing hypoglycemia. An alternative to islet transplantation is whole organ pancreas transplantation that is performed most often with kidney transplantation. The advantages of whole organ pancreas transplantation are less dependence on insulin and longer duration of organ function. The main disadvantage is that a whole organ transplant is a major surgery that involves a greater risk of complications and even death.

Pancreatic islet allotransplantation can also help reverse hypoglycemia unawareness. Research has shown that even partial islet function after a transplant can eliminate hypoglycemia unawareness.

Improved blood glucose control from a successful allotransplant may also slow or prevent the progression of diabetes problems, such as heart disease, kidney disease, and nerve or eye damage. Research to evaluate this possibility is ongoing.

The risks of pancreatic islet allotransplantation include the risks associated with the transplant procedure—particularly bleeding and blood clots. The transplanted islets may not function well or may stop functioning entirely. Other risks are the side effects from the immunosuppressive medications that transplant recipients must take to stop the immune system from rejecting the transplanted islets. When a patient has received a kidney transplant and is already taking immunosuppressive medications, the only additional risks are the islet infusion and the side effects from the immunosuppressive medications given at the time of allotransplantation. Immunosuppressive medications are not needed in the case of an auto-transplant because the infused cells come from the patient's own body.

Collaborative Islet Transplant Registry Data

In its 2010 annual report, the Collaborative Islet Transplant Registry (CITR) presented data on 571 patients who received pancreatic islet allotransplants between 1999–2009. Although most procedures were pancreatic islet allotransplants alone, 90 procedures were done in conjunction with a kidney transplant. The majority of the islet transplant patients received one or two infusions of islets; at the end of the decade, the average number of islets received per infusion was 463,000.

According to the report, about 60 percent of transplant recipients achieved insulin independence—defined as being able to stop insulin injections for at least 14 days—during the year following transplantation.

By the end of the second year, 50 percent of recipients were able to stop taking insulin for at least 14 days. However, long-term insulin independence is difficult to maintain, and eventually, most recipients needed to start allotransplant.

The report identified factors linked to better outcomes for recipients, including:

• Age—35 years or older

• Lower pretransplant triglyceride, or blood fat, levels

• Lower pretransplant insulin use

The report noted that even partial function of the transplanted islets can improve blood glucose control and reduce the amount of insulin needed after loss of insulin independence.

What Is the Role of Immunosuppressive Medications?

Immunosuppressive medications are needed to prevent rejection—a common problem with any transplant.

Scientists have made many advances in islet transplantation in recent years. In 2000, islet transplantation researchers at the University of Alberta in Edmonton, Canada, reported their findings in the *New England Journal of Medicine*. Their transplant protocol, known as the Edmonton protocol, has since been adapted by transplant centers around the world and continues to be refined.

The Edmonton protocol introduced the use of a new combination of immunosuppressive medications, also called anti-rejection medications, including daclizumab (Zenapax), sirolimus (Rapamune), and tacrolimus (Prograf). Researchers continue to develop and study modifications to the Edmonton protocol, including improved medication regimens that promote successful transplants. Medication regimens vary from one transplant center to another. Examples of other immunosuppressive medications used in islet transplantation include antithymocyte globulin (Thymoglobulin), alemtuzumab (Campath), basiliximab (Simulect), belatacept (Nulojix), etanercept (Enbrel), everolimus (Zortress), and mycophenolate mofetil (CellCept, Myfortic). Researchers are also evaluating nonimmunosuppressive medications, such as exenatide (Byetta) and sitagliptin (Januvia).

Immunosuppressive medications have significant side effects, and their long-term effects are still not fully known. Immediate side effects may include mouth sores and gastrointestinal problems, such as upset stomach and diarrhea. Patients may also have:

- Increased blood cholesterol, or blood fat, levels

- High blood pressure

- Anemia, a condition in which red blood cells are fewer or smaller than normal, which prevents the body's cells from getting enough oxygen

- fatigue

- Decreased white blood cell counts

- Decreased kidney function

- Increased susceptibility to bacterial and viral infections

Taking immunosuppressive medications also increases the risk of developing certain tumors and cancers.

Scientists are seeking ways to achieve immune tolerance of the transplanted islets, in which the patient's immune system no longer recognizes the islets as foreign. Immune tolerance would allow patients to maintain transplanted islets without long-term use of immuno-suppressive medications. For example, one approach is to transplant islets encapsulated with a special coating, which may help to prevent rejection.

What Are the Obstacles to Pancreatic Islet Allotransplantation?

The shortage of islets from donors is a significant obstacle to wide-spread use of pancreatic islet allotransplantation. According to the Organ Procurement and Transplantation Network (OPTN), in 2011 there were about 8,000 deceased organ donors available in the United States. However, only 1,562 pancreases were recovered from donors in 2011. Also, many donated pancreases are not suitable for extracting islets for transplants because they do not meet the selection criteria, and islets are often damaged or destroyed during processing. Therefore, only a small number of islet transplants can be performed each year.

Researchers are pursuing various approaches to solve this shortage of islets, such as transplanting islets from a single, donated pancreas, using only a portion of the pancreas from a living donor, or using islets from pigs. Researchers have transplanted pig islets into other animals, including monkeys, by encapsulating the islets with a special coating or by using medications to prevent rejection. Another approach is creating islets from other types of cells, such as stem cells. New technologies could then be employed to grow islets in the lab.

Financial barriers also prevent the widespread use of islet allotransplantation. Until the transplantation technology is considered successful enough to be labeled therapeutic rather than experimental, the costs of islet allotransplants must be covered by research funds. Health insurance companies and Medicare generally do not cover experimental procedures. Federal law also does not allow healthcare providers or hospitals to charge patients or health insurance companies for research procedures. Some patient advocates and islet researchers feel that islet allotransplantation is close to having a therapeutic label. The National Institutes of Health (NIH) currently supports studies that are working toward obtaining FDA licensure to reclassify islet allotransplantation as therapeutic. In other countries, such as Canada, and Scandinavia, islet allotransplantation is no longer considered experimental and is an accepted therapy in certain patients.

Eating, Diet, and Nutrition

A person who receives a pancreatic islet transplant should follow a meal plan worked out with a healthcare provider and dietitian. Immunosuppressive medications taken after the transplant can cause changes in a person's body, such as weight gain. A healthy diet after the transplant is important to control weight gain, blood pressure, blood cholesterol, and blood glucose levels.

Section 62.2

Islet Transplantation Restores Blood Sugar Control in Type 1 Diabetes

This section includes text excerpted from "Islet Transplantation Restores Blood Sugar Control in Type 1 Diabetes," National Institutes of Health (NIH), April 26, 2016.

Diabetes is a disorder in the regulation and use of glucose in the blood. Glucose is a sugar that serves as fuel for the body. When blood glucose levels rise, beta cells in the islets of the pancreas normally make and secrete the hormone insulin. Insulin triggers cells to take up sugar from the blood.

In type 1 diabetes, the body's own immune system attacks and destroys pancreatic beta cells. People with type 1 diabetes require lifelong treatment that involves frequent (three or more times daily) measurement of blood glucose and administration of insulin to maintain blood sugar levels.

If blood sugar levels become very low (hypoglycemia), symptoms such as tremors and sweating typically prompt a person to eat or drink to raise their blood sugar levels. However, about one in three people with type 1 diabetes can't tell when their blood sugar is low. This impaired awareness puts them at risk for severe hypoglycemia, which can lead to seizures, loss of consciousness, and death.

One strategy to treat type 1 diabetes is to replace the destroyed beta cells with pancreatic islets transplanted from deceased human donors. An international team of researchers—the National Institutes of Health (NIH)-sponsored Clinical Islet Transplantation Consortium (CITC)—set out to evaluate the effectiveness and safety of this experimental procedure. The study was designed with guidance from the U.S. Food and Drug Administration (FDA) to potentially serve as the basis for future licensure for the manufacture of purified human pancreatic islet cells.

The scientists enrolled 48 people who had type 1 diabetes for more than five years, impaired awareness of hypoglycemia, and frequent hypoglycemic events despite expert care. The participants received at least one transplant of islets and were given immunosuppressive drugs to prevent their immune systems from rejecting the transplants. The research was supported by the NIH's National Institute of Allergy and Infectious Diseases (NIAID), National Institute of Diabetes and

Digestive and Kidney Diseases (NIDDK), and other NIH components. Results appeared online on April 18, 2016, in *Diabetes Care.*

During the first year after the initial transplant, 88 percent of participants were free of severe hypoglycemic events, had near-normal control of blood glucose levels, and had restored hypoglycemic awareness. After two years, 71 percent continued to meet these criteria for transplant success.

Adverse reactions included bleeding associated with the transplant procedure as well as infections and lowered kidney function associated with the immune-suppressing drugs. Although some of the side effects were serious, none led to death or disability.

"While still experimental, and with risks that must be weighed carefully, the promise of islet transplantation is undeniable and encouraging," says NIDDK Director Dr. Griffin P. Rodgers. The researchers are continuing to monitor the participants to assess the benefits and risks of the transplant therapy.

Section 62.3

Islet Transplantation Improves Quality of Life for People with Hard-to-Control Type 1 Diabetes

This section includes text excerpted from "Islet Transplantation Improves Quality of Life for People with Hard-to-Control Type 1 Diabetes," National Institutes of Health (NIH), March 21, 2018.

Quality of life (QOL) for people with type 1 diabetes who had frequent severe hypoglycemia—a potentially fatal low blood glucose (blood sugar) level—improved consistently and dramatically following transplantation of insulin-producing pancreatic islets, according to findings published online March 21 in Diabetes Care. The results come from a Phase three clinical trial funded by the National Institute of Allergy and Infectious Diseases (NIAID) and the National Institute of Diabetes and Digestive and Kidney Diseases (NIDDK), both part of the National Institutes of Health (NIH).

The greatest improvements were seen in diabetes-related quality of life. Islet recipients also reported better overall health status after transplant, despite the need for lifelong treatment with immune-suppressing drugs to prevent transplant rejection. Researchers observed these improvements even among transplant recipients who still required insulin therapy to manage their diabetes.

The trial enrolled 48 people with type 1 diabetes who had hypoglycemia unawareness—an impaired ability to sense drops in blood glucose levels—and experienced frequent episodes of severe hypoglycemia despite receiving expert care.

Previously reported clinical outcomes from the trial showed that islet transplantation prevents severe hypoglycemia and improves blood glucose awareness and control. The study was conducted by the NIH-funded Clinical Islet Transplantation Consortium (CITC).

"Although insulin therapy is life-saving, type 1 diabetes remains an extremely challenging condition to manage," said NIAID Director Anthony S. Fauci, M.D. "For people unable to safely control type 1 diabetes despite optimal medical management, islet transplantation offers hope for improving not only physical health but also overall quality of life."

Pancreatic islets release the hormone insulin, which helps control blood glucose levels. In type 1 diabetes, the body's immune system attacks and destroys the insulin-producing cells in islets. People with the disease must take insulin to live, but insulin injections or pumps cannot control blood glucose levels as precisely as insulin released naturally from the pancreas. Even with diligent monitoring, blood glucose can often reach levels that are higher or lower than normal.

A low blood glucose level, or hypoglycemia, typically is accompanied by tremors, sweating, nausea and/or heart palpitations. These symptoms prompt the person to eat or drink to raise their blood glucose. However, some people do not experience these early warning signs. This impaired awareness of hypoglycemia raises the risk of potentially life-threatening severe hypoglycemic events, during which the person is unable to treat himself or herself. These episodes can lead to accidents, injuries, coma, and death.

"People with type 1 diabetes who are at high risk for hypoglycemic events have to practice caution every moment, even while sleeping. It is an exhausting endeavor that—like the events themselves—can keep them from living full lives," said NIDDK Director Griffin P. Rodgers, M.D. "Although islet transplantation remains experimental, we are very encouraged by these findings, as we are by the rapid improvements in other treatments to help people with type 1 diabetes monitor and manage their blood glucose, including artificial pancreas technology."

All 48 study participants received at least one islet transplant. One year after their first transplant, 42 participants (88 percent) were free of severe hypoglycemic events, had established near-normal blood glucose control, and had restored awareness of hypoglycemia. Only a small number of functional insulin-producing cells are necessary to restore hypoglycemic awareness, but this amount may not be sufficient to fully regulate a person's blood glucose levels. Approximately half of the transplant recipients needed to continue taking insulin to control their blood glucose levels.

The study design incorporated four well-established, commercially available quality-of-life surveys that were given to participants repeatedly before and after islet transplantation. Two of the surveys were specific for diabetes, while two assessed health more generally.

"This study was very rigorous both in terms of the number of measures used to assess quality of life and the number of evaluations performed," said paper co-author Nancy D. Bridges, M.D., chief of the Transplantation Branch at NIAID. "Islet transplant recipients not only reported a decrease in concerns and fears related to their diabetes, but also felt better overall, despite the need to take daily immunosuppressive drugs to prevent transplant rejection."

Reported improvements in quality of life were similar among islet recipients who still needed to take insulin to manage their diabetes and those who did not. The researchers concluded that elimination of severe hypoglycemia and the associated fears accounted for these improvements, appearing to outweigh concerns about the need to continue insulin injections.

Islet transplantation is an investigational therapy in the United States. While promising for people whose type 1 diabetes cannot be controlled with standard treatments, the procedure is not appropriate for most people with type 1 diabetes, as there are risks associated with the transplant procedure, such as bleeding, as well as side effects of immunosuppressive medications, such as decreased kidney function and increased susceptibility to infections.

In the NIH-funded trial, investigators at eight study sites in North America used a standardized manufacturing protocol to prepare purified islets from the pancreases of deceased human donors. The study was designed, after discussions with the U.S. Food and Drug

Administration (FDA), to provide evidence to support licensure of the manufactured islet product. The NIAID, the regulatory sponsor of the study, has submitted final reports and clinical trial data to the FDA, laying the groundwork for individual universities and companies to submit biologics license applications for the manufacture of purified human pancreatic islets.

Chapter 63

Artificial Pancreas

Chapter Contents

Section 63.1

Introduction to Artificial Pancreas

This section includes text excerpted from "The Artificial
Pancreas Device System," U.S. Food and Drug
Administration (FDA), March 26, 2018.

The U.S. Food and Drug Administration (FDA) has been working together with diabetes patient groups, diabetes care providers, medical device manufacturers, and researchers to advance the development of an artificial pancreas.

There have been tremendous strides made in the research and development of an artificial pancreas device system. On September 28, 2016, the FDA approved the first hybrid closed-loop system, the Medtronic's MiniMed 670G System, intended to automatically monitor blood sugar and adjust basal insulin doses in people with type 1 diabetes. There are also many research projects underway looking at the feasibility of these device systems in hospital settings.

What Is Artificial Pancreas Device System?

The artificial pancreas device system (APDS) is a system of devices that closely mimics the glucose-regulating function of a healthy pancreas.

Most artificial pancreas device systems consists of three types of devices already familiar to many people with diabetes: a continuous glucose monitoring (CGM) system and an insulin infusion pump. A blood glucose device (such as a glucose meter) is used to calibrate the CGM.

A computer-controlled algorithm connects the CGM and insulin infusion pump to allow continuous communication between the two devices. Sometimes an artificial pancreas device system is referred to as a "closed-loop" system, an "automated insulin delivery" system, or an "autonomous system for glycemic control."

An artificial pancreas device system will not only monitors glucose levels in the body but also automatically adjusts the delivery of insulin to reduce high blood glucose levels (hyperglycemia) and minimize the incidence of low blood glucose (hypoglycemia) with little or no input from the patient.

The illustration below describes the parts of a type of artificial pancreas device system and shows how they work together.

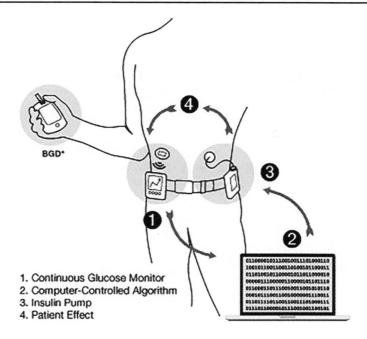

1. Continuous Glucose Monitor
2. Computer-Controlled Algorithm
3. Insulin Pump
4. Patient Effect

Figure 63.1. *Artificial Pancreas System*

1. **Continuous glucose monitor (CGM).** A CGM provides
   a steady stream of information that reflects the patient's
   blood glucose levels. A sensor placed under the patient's skin
   (subcutaneously) measures the glucose in the fluid around the
   cells (interstitial fluid) which is associated with blood glucose
   levels. A small transmitter sends information to a receiver.
   A CGM continuously displays both an estimate of blood
   glucose levels and their direction and rate of change of these
   estimates.

   - **Blood glucose device (BGD).** As of now, to get the most
     accurate estimates of blood glucose possible from a CGM, the
     patient needs to periodically calibrate the CGM using a blood
     glucose measurement from a BGD; therefore, the BGD still
     plays a critical role in the proper management of patients
     with an APDS. However, over time, it's anticipated that
     improved CGM performance may do away with the need for
     periodic blood glucose checks with a BGD.

2. **Control algorithm.** A control algorithm is software
   embedded in an external processor (controller) that receives

451

information from the CGM and performs a series of mathematical calculations. Based on these calculations, the controller sends dosing instructions to the infusion pump. The control algorithm can be run on any number of devices including an insulin pump, computer or cellular phone. The FDA does not require the control algorithm to reside on the insulin pump.

3. **Insulin pump.** Based on the instructions sent by the controller, an infusion pump adjusts the insulin delivery to the tissue under the skin

4. **The patient.** The patient is an important part of APDS. The concentration of glucose circulating in the patient's blood is constantly changing. It is affected by the patient's diet, activity level, and how his or her body metabolizes insulin and other substances.

Section 63.2

Research on Artificial Pancreas

This section includes text excerpted from "The Miracle of an Artificial Pancreas," MedlinePlus, National Institutes of Health (NIH), May 31, 2017.

Thanks to investments in research, improved methods for managing type 1 diabetes are on the horizon, including the artificial pancreas. The artificial pancreas is an integrated system that monitors blood glucose (sugar) levels automatically and provides insulin or a combination of insulin and a second hormone to people with type 1 diabetes.

A successful artificial pancreas would be a life-changing advance for many people with type 1 diabetes. This closed-loop system would replace reliance on testing by fingerstick or continuous monitoring systems and separate, nonintegrated delivery of insulin by shots or a pump.

The first of several major research efforts to test and refine artificial pancreas systems is now underway. Four separate projects, funded by the National Institute of Diabetes and Digestive and Kidney Diseases (NIDDK), are designed to be the potential last steps between testing the automated devices and requesting regulatory approval for permanent use.

"These studies aim to collect the data necessary to bring artificial pancreas technology to the people who need it," said Guillermo Arreaza-Rubín, M.D., director of the NIDDK's Diabetes Technology Program Opens a fresh window. "Results from these studies could change and save lives."

Previously, researchers and participants worked together to test artificial pancreas devices in short-term trials, with varying levels of patient supervision. In 2016, the U.S. Food and Drug Administration (FDA) approved a hybrid model of an artificial pancreas, an automated system that requires users to adjust insulin intake at mealtimes. A fully automated system will sense rising glucose levels, including at mealtimes, and adjust insulin automatically.

In addition to easing the burden of management for people with type 1 diabetes or their caregivers, in shorter studies, the devices brought glucose levels closer to normal than traditional management. The National Institutes of Health (NIH) research has found that early, tight control of blood glucose helps reduce diabetes complications including nerve, eye, and kidney diseases.

The four research projects began in 2017–18. They have been conducted in larger groups over longer periods of time than the earlier trials, and in largely glucose-regulating conditions. The participants will live at home and monitor themselves, going about their normal lives, with remote monitoring by study staff.

"Managing type 1 diabetes requires a constant juggling act between checking blood glucose levels frequently and delivering just the right amount of insulin while taking into account meals, physical activity, and other aspects of daily life, where a missed or wrong delivery could lead to potential complications," said Andrew Bremer, M.D., Ph.D., the NIDDK program official overseeing the studies. "Unifying the management of type 1 diabetes into a single, integrated system could lift so much of that burden."

Studies will look at factors including safety, efficacy, user-friendliness, physical and emotional health of the participants, and cost. The Jaeb Center for Health Research (JCHR) in Tampa, Florida, will serve as coordinating center for all of the trials.

"For many people with type 1 diabetes, the realization of a successful, fully automated artificial pancreas is a dearly held dream. It signifies a life freer from nightly wake-up calls to check blood glucose or deliver insulin, a life freer from dangerous swings of blood glucose," said NIDDK director Griffin P. Rodgers, M.D., M.A.C.P. "Nearly 100 years since the discovery of insulin, a successful artificial pancreas would mark another huge step toward better health for people with type 1 diabetes."

Chapter 64

Clinical Trials and Diabetes

What You Need to Know about Clinical Trials

Clinical trials are a part of clinical research and at the heart of all medical advances. Clinical trials look at new ways to prevent, detect, or treat disease. Treatments might be new drugs or new combinations of drugs, new surgical procedures or devices, or new ways to use existing treatments. The goal of clinical trials is to determine if a new test or treatment works and is safe. Clinical trials can also look at other aspects of care, such as improving the quality of life for people with chronic illnesses.

Where Can You Find Information about Current Clinical Trials?

Information about clinical trials conducted by the National Institutes of Health (NIH), the National Institute of Diabetes and Digestive and Kidney Diseases (NIDDK), and other federal and private organizations can be found at ClinicalTrials.gov (www.clinicaltrials.gov).

This chapter contains text excerpted from the following sources: Text under the heading "What You Need to Know about Clinical Trials" is excerpted from "Clinical Trials," National Institute of Diabetes and Digestive and Kidney Diseases (NIDDK), June 15, 2007. Reviewed September 2018; Text under the heading "Clinical Research in Diabetes" is excerpted from "Clinical Trials for Diabetes," National Institute of Diabetes and Digestive and Kidney Diseases (NIDDK), November 2016.

The ClinicalTrials site offers information about the location of clinical trials, their design and purpose, participation criteria, and additional information about the disease and treatment under study.

Who Participates in Clinical Trials?

Many different types of people participate in clinical trials. Some are healthy, while others may have illnesses. A healthy volunteer is a person with no known significant health problems. A patient volunteer has a known health problem. You can learn more about the types of people who participate in clinical trials and view personal stories from people who participated in the NIDDK clinical research.

How Can You Participate in a Clinical Trial?

Find a clinical trial that's right for you by searching ClinicalTrials. gov. If you are a healthy volunteer, contact the study coordinator listed for the clinical trial. If you are a patient volunteer talk with your doctor. You may need a referral to participate in a study.

Clinical Research in Diabetes

The National Institute of Diabetes and Digestive and Kidney Diseases (NIDDK) and other components of the National Institutes of Health (NIH) conduct and support research into many diseases and conditions. The NIDDK is the primary institute at the NIH that funds diabetes research, including clinical trials.

What Are Clinical Trials for Diabetes?

Clinical trials are part of clinical research and at the heart of all medical advances. Clinical trials look at new ways to prevent, detect, or treat disease. Scientists are conducting research to learn more about diabetes, including the following studies:

- **The Glycemia Reduction Approaches in Diabetes (GRADE):** A Comparative Effectiveness Study is following more than 5,000 people across the country who have type 2 diabetes to find out which combination of two diabetes medicines is best for blood glucose, also called blood sugar, management; has the fewest side effects; and is the most helpful for overall health in long-term diabetes treatment.

- **TrialNet** is conducting research studies around the world, including risk screening for relatives of people with type 1 diabetes, monitoring for people at risk, and innovative clinical trials aimed at slowing down or stopping the disease.

Researchers also use clinical trials to look at other aspects of care, such as improving the quality of life for people with chronic illnesses. What Clinical Trials for Diabetes Are Open?

Below is a list of selected clinical trials that are open and recruiting, but you can expand or narrow your search.

- Type 1 diabetes—includes studies funded by the NIH or other U.S. government agencies

- Type 2 diabetes—includes studies funded by the NIH or other U.S. government agencies

- Gestational diabetes—includes studies funded by the NIH; other U.S. government agencies; and individuals, universities, or other organizations

What Have We Learned about Diabetes from National Institute of Diabetes and Digestive and Kidney Diseases (NIDDK)-Funded Research?

The NIDDK has supported many research projects to learn more about diabetes. For example:

- **Look AHEAD:** Action for Health in Diabetes. The Look AHEAD study showed that people who were overweight or obese and had type 2 diabetes can lose weight and maintain that weight loss through a program of healthy eating and increased physical activity. The study also showed that weight loss provides added health benefits, such as better physical mobility and improved blood glucose, blood pressure, and cholesterol levels. The trial has been extended to study the long-term results of weight loss through healthy eating and physical activity programs in older adults with type 2 diabetes.

- **Diabetes Control and Complications Trial (DCCT) and Epidemiology of Diabetes Interventions and Complications (EDIC).** The DCCT showed that intensive treatment with insulin to maintain blood glucose levels as close to normal as safely possible greatly lowered participants' chances of developing eye, nerve, and kidney disease. The EDIC study has continued to follow DCCT participants for the past 20+ years. EDIC has shown that there are long-term benefits of early and intensive blood glucose control for the future development of diabetes-related complications such as heart, kidney, nerve, and eye disease; and that early and intensive control also lengthens life.

- **Diabetes Prevention Program (DPP) and Diabetes Prevention Program Outcomes Study (DPPOS).** The DPP showed that people who are at high risk for type 2 diabetes can prevent or delay the disease by making lifestyle changes that include weight loss through dietary changes and increased physical activity. Taking metformin, a safe and effective generic medicine used to treat diabetes, was also found to prevent the disease, although to a lesser degree. The DPPOS has continued to follow DPP participants to see if the lifestyle changes they made during the DPP or taking metformin continues to prevent or delay type 2 diabetes over time. To date, the DPPOS has shown that people can prevent or delay type 2 diabetes for at least 15 years with lifestyle changes or metformin.

Part Eight

Additional Help and Information

Chapter 65

Recipes for People with Diabetes and Their Families

What Is Diabetes?

Diabetes means that your blood glucose (blood sugar) is too high. Glucose comes from the food we eat. An organ called the pancreas makes insulin. Insulin helps glucose get from your blood into your cells. Cells take the glucose and turn it into energy.

When you have diabetes, your body has a problem making or properly using insulin. As a result, glucose builds up in your blood and cannot get into your cells. If the blood glucose stays too high, it can damage your body.

What Are the Symptoms of Diabetes?

Common symptoms of diabetes include the following:

- Having to urinate often
- Being very thirsty
- Feeling very hungry or tired
- Losing weight without trying

Text in this chapter is excerpted from "Recipes for People with Diabetes and Their Families," Centers for Disease Control and Prevention (CDC), July 22, 2015.

But many people with diabetes have no symptoms at all.

Why Should I Be Concerned about Diabetes?

Diabetes is a very serious disease. Do not be misled by phrases that suggest diabetes is not a serious disease, such as "a touch of sugar," "borderline diabetes," or "my blood glucose is a little bit high."

Diabetes can lead to other serious health problems. When high levels of glucose in the blood are not controlled, they can slowly damage your eyes, heart, kidneys, nerves, and feet.

What Are the Types of Diabetes?

There are three main types of diabetes:

- **Type 1 diabetes**: In this type of diabetes, the body does not make insulin. People with type 1 diabetes need to take insulin every day.

- **Type 2 diabetes**: In this type of diabetes, the body does not make enough insulin or use insulin well. Some people with type 2 diabetes have to take diabetes pills, insulin, or both. Type 2 diabetes is the most common form of diabetes.

- **Gestational diabetes**: This type of diabetes can occur when a woman is pregnant. It raises the risk that both she and her child might develop diabetes later in life.

Good News! You Can Control Diabetes

Diabetes can be managed. You can successfully manage diabetes and avoid the serious health problems it can cause if you follow these steps:

- Ask your doctor how you can learn more about your diabetes to help you feel better today and in the future.

- Know your diabetes "ABCs."

- Make healthy food choices and be physically active most days. Following this advice will help you keep off extra pounds and will also help keep your blood glucose under control.

- Check your blood glucose as your doctor tells you to.

- If you are taking diabetes medications, take them even if you feel well.

- To avoid problems with your diabetes, see your healthcare team at least twice a year. Finding and treating any problems early will prevent them from getting worse. Ask how diabetes can affect your eyes, heart, kidneys, nerves, legs, and feet.

- Be actively involved in your diabetes care. Work with your healthcare team to come up with a plan for making healthy food choices and being active—a plan that you can stick to.

Creating a Healthy Meal Plan

This chapter is a place to start creating healthy meals. Ask your doctor to refer you to a registered dietitian or a diabetes educator who can help you create a meal plan for you and your family. The dietitian will work with you to come up with a meal plan tailored to your needs.

Your meal plan will take into account things like:

- Your blood glucose levels

- Your weight

- Medicines you take

- Other health problems you have

- How physically active you are

Making Healthy Food Choices

- Eat smaller portions. Learn what a serving size is for different foods and how many servings you need in a meal.

- Eat less fat. Choose fewer high-fat foods and use less fat for cooking. You especially want to limit foods that are high in saturated fats or trans fat, such as:

  - Fatty cuts of meat

  - Whole milk and dairy products made from whole milk

  - Cakes, candy, cookies, crackers, and pies

  - Fried foods

  - Salad dressings

  - Lard, shortening, stick margarine, and nondairy creamers

- Eat more fiber by eating more whole-grain foods. Whole grains can be found in:

  - Breakfast cereals made with 100 percent whole grains

  - Oatmeal

  - Whole grain rice

  - Whole-wheat bread, bagels, pita bread, and tortillas

- Eat a variety of fruits and vegetables every day. Choose fresh, frozen, canned, or dried fruit and 100 percent fruit juices most of the time. Eat plenty of veggies like these:

  - Dark green veggies (e.g., broccoli, spinach, brussel sprouts)

  - Orange veggies (e.g., carrots, sweet potatoes, pumpkin, winter squash)

  - Beans and peas (e.g., black beans, garbanzo beans, kidney beans, pinto beans, split peas, lentils)

- Eat fewer foods that are high in sugar, such as:

  - Fruit-flavored drinks

  - Sodas

  - Tea or coffee sweetened with sugar

- Use less salt in cooking and at the table. Eat fewer foods that are high in salt, such as:

  - Canned and package soups

  - Canned vegetables

  - Pickles

  - Processed meats

- Never skip meals. Stick to your meal plan as best you can.

- Limit the amount of alcohol you drink.

- Make changes slowly. It takes time to achieve lasting goals.

Following a meal plan that is made for you will help you feel better, keep your blood glucose levels in your target range, take in the right amount of calories, and get enough nutrients.

Where Can You Learn More about Making a Diabetes Meal Plan?

- Contact a registered dietitian to make a meal plan just for you.

- Visit the American Dietetic Association (ADA) website to find a nutrition professional that can help you develop a healthy meal plan (www.eatright.org).

- Visit the American Association of Diabetes Educators (AADE) to find a diabetes educator (www.diabeteseducator.org).

- Visit the American Diabetes Association (ADA) website for more information on carbohydrate counting and the exchange method (www.diabetes.org).

- Visit www.diabetes.org/food-and-fitness/food/planningmeals/ carb-counting to get more information on carbohydrate counting.

Where Can You Learn How to Read Food Labels?

You can learn a lot about foods by reading food labels. Visit these websites to learn more about reading food labels:

- U.S. Food and Drug Administration (FDA) (www.cfsan.fda. gov/~dms/foodlab.html)

- U.S. Department of Agriculture (USDA) (www.fns.usda.gov/tn/ Resources/Nibbles/healthful_labels.pdf)

- American Diabetes Association (ADA) (www.diabetes.org/food- andfitness/food/what-can-i-eat/taking-a-closer-look-atlabels. html)

Recipes

Spanish Omelet / Tortilla Española

This tasty dish provides a healthy array of vegetables and can be used for breakfast, brunch, or any meal! Serve with fresh fruit salad and a whole grain dinner roll.

Ingredients

- 5 small potatoes, peeled and sliced vegetable cooking spray

- ½ medium onion, minced

- 1 small zucchini, sliced

- 1½ cups green/red peppers, sliced thin

- 5 medium mushrooms, sliced

- 3 whole eggs, beaten

- 5 egg whites, beaten Pepper and garlic salt with herbs, to taste

- 3 ounces shredded part-skim mozzarella cheese

- 1 tbsp. low-fat parmesan cheese

Directions

- Preheat oven to 375°F.

- Cook potatoes in boiling water until tender.

- In a nonstick pan, add vegetable spray and warm at medium heat.

- Add onion and sauté until brown. Add vegetables and sauté until tender but not brown.

- In a medium mixing bowl, slightly beat eggs and egg whites, pepper, garlic salt, and low-fat mozzarella cheese. Stir egg-cheese mixture into the cooked vegetables.

- In a 10-inch pie pan or ovenproof skillet, add vegetable spray and transfer potatoes and egg mixture to pan. Sprinkle with low-fat parmesan cheese and bake until firm and brown on top, about 20–30 minutes.

- Remove omelet from oven, cool for 10 minutes, and cut into five pieces.

Exchanges

Meat	2
Bread	2
Vegetable	2/3
Fat	2

Note: Diabetic exchanges are calculated based on the American Diabetes Association (ADA) Exchange System.

Beef or Turkey Stew

This dish goes nicely with a green leaf lettuce and cucumber salad and a dinner roll. Plantains or corn can be used in place of the potatoes.

Ingredients

- 1 pound lean beef or turkey breast, cut into cubes
- 2 tbsp. whole wheat flour
- ¼ tsp. salt (optional)
- ¼ tsp. pepper
- ¼ tsp. cumin
- 1½ tbsp. olive oil
- 2 cloves garlic, minced
- 2 medium onions, sliced
- 2 stalks celery, sliced
- 1 medium red/green bell pepper, sliced
- 1 medium tomato, finely minced
- 5 cups beef or turkey broth, fat removed
- 5 small potatoes, peeled and cubed
- 12 small carrots, cut into large chunks
- 1¼ cups green peas

Directions

- Preheat oven to 375°F.
- Mix the whole wheat flour with salt, pepper, and cumin. Roll the beef or turkey cubes in the mixture. Shake off excess flour.
- In a large skillet, heat olive oil over medium-high heat. Add beef or turkey cubes and sauté until nicely brown, about 7–10 minutes.
- Place beef or turkey in an ovenproof casserole dish.
- Add minced garlic, onions, celery, and peppers to skillet and cook until vegetables are tender, about 5 minutes.

- Stir in tomato and broth. Bring to a boil and pour over turkey or beef in casserole dish. Cover dish tightly and bake for 1 hour at 375°F.

- Remove from oven and stir in potatoes, carrots, and peas. Bake for another 20–25 minutes or until tender.

Exchanges

Lean Meat	3
Vegetable	2 1/3
Bread	2 2/3
Fat	1

Note: Diabetic exchanges are calculated based on the American Diabetes Association (ADA) Exchange System.

Caribbean Red Snapper

This fish can be served on top of vegetables along with whole grain rice and garnished with parsley. Salmon or chicken breast can be used in place of red snapper.

Ingredients

- 2 tbsp. olive oil
- 1 medium onion, chopped
- ½ cup red pepper, chopped
- ½ cup carrots, cut into strips
- 1 clove garlic, minced
- ½ cup dry white wine
- ¾ pound red snapper fillet
- 1 large tomato, chopped
- 2 tbsp. pitted ripe olives, chopped
- 2 tbsp. crumbled low-fat feta or low-fat ricotta cheese

Directions

- In a large skillet, heat olive oil over medium heat. Add onion, red pepper, carrots, and garlic. Sauté mixture for 10 minutes. Add wine and bring to boil. Push vegetables to one side of the pan.

- Arrange fillets in a single layer in center of skillet. Cover and cook for 5 minutes.

- Add tomato and olives. Top with cheese. Cover and cook for 3 minutes or until fish is firm but moist.

- Transfer fish to serving platter. Garnish with vegetables and pan juices.

Exchanges

Meat	2
Vegetable	1¼
Bread	½
Fat	2

Note: Diabetic exchanges are calculated based on the American Diabetes Association (ADA) Exchange System.

Two Cheese Pizza

Serve your pizza with fresh fruit and a mixed green salad garnished with red beans to balance your meal.

Ingredients

- 2 tbsp. whole wheat flour
- 1 can (10 ounces) refrigerated pizza crust
- Vegetable cooking spray
- 2 tbsp. olive oil
- ½ cup low-fat ricotta cheese
- ½ tsp. dried basil 1 small onion, minced
- 2 cloves garlic, minced
- ¼ tsp. salt (optional)
- 4 ounces shredded part-skim mozzarella cheese
- 2 cups mushrooms, chopped
- 1 large red pepper, cut into strips

Directions

- Preheat oven to 425°F.

- Spread whole wheat flour over working surface. Roll out dough with rolling pin to desired crust thickness.

- Coat cookie sheet with vegetable cooking spray. Transfer pizza crust to cookie sheet. Brush olive oil over crust.

- Mix low-fat ricotta cheese with dried basil, onion, garlic, and salt. Spread this mixture over crust.

- Sprinkle crust with part-skim mozzarella cheese. Top cheese with mushrooms and red pepper.

- Bake at 425°F for 13–15 minutes or until cheese melts and crust is deep golden brown.

- Cut into 8 slices.

Exchanges

Meat	2½
Bread	3
Vegetable	1
Fat	3¾

Note: Diabetic exchanges are calculated based on the American Diabetes Association (ADA) Exchange System.

Rice with Chicken, Spanish Style

This is a good way to get vegetables into the meal plan. Serve with a mixed green salad and some whole wheat bread.

Ingredients

- 2 tbsp. olive oil

- 2 medium onions, chopped

- 6 cloves garlic, minced

- 2 stalks celery, diced

- 2 medium red/green peppers, cut into strips

- 1 cup mushrooms, chopped

- 2 cups uncooked whole grain rice

- 3 pounds boneless chicken breast, cut into bite-sized pieces, skin removed
- 1½ tsp. salt (optional)
- 2½ cups low-fat chicken broth Saffron/Sazón™ for color
- 3 medium tomatoes, chopped
- 1 cup frozen peas
- 1 cup frozen corn
- 1 cup frozen green beans Olives or capers for garnish (optional)

Directions

- Heat olive oil over medium heat in a nonstick pot. Add onion, garlic, celery, red/green pepper, and mushrooms. Cook over medium heat, stirring often, for 3 minutes or until tender.
- Add whole grain rice and sauté for 2–3 minutes, stirring constantly to mix all ingredients.
- Add chicken, salt, chicken broth, water, Saffron/Sazón™, and tomatoes. Bring water to a boil.
- Reduce heat to medium-low, cover, and let the casserole simmer until water is absorbed and rice is tender, about 20 minutes.
- Stir in peas, corn, and beans and cook for 8–10 minutes. When everything is hot, the casserole is ready to serve. Garnish with olives or capers, if desired.

Exchanges

Meat	5
Bread	3
Vegetable	1
Fat	1

Note: Diabetic exchanges are calculated based on the American Diabetes Association (ADA) Exchange System.

Pozole

Only a small amount of oil is needed to sauté meat.

Ingredients

- 2 pounds lean beef, cubed
- 1 tbsp. olive oil
- 1 large onion, chopped
- 1 clove garlic, finely chopped
- ¼ tsp. salt tsp. pepper
- ¼ cup fresh cilantro, chopped
- 1 can (15 ounces) stewed tomatoes
- 2 ounces tomato paste
- 1 can (1 pound 13 ounces) hominy

Directions

- In a large pot, heat olive oil. Add beef and sauté.
- Add onion, garlic, salt, pepper, cilantro, and enough water to cover meat. Stir to mix ingredients evenly. Cover pot and cook over low heat until meat is tender.
- Add tomatoes and tomato paste. Continue cooking for about 20 minutes.
- Add hominy and continue cooking another 15 minutes, stirring occasionally. If too thick, add water for desired consistency. Option: Skinless, boneless chicken breasts can be used instead of beef cubes.

Exchanges

Meat	3
Bread	1
Vegetable	½
Fat	1

Note: Diabetic exchanges are calculated based on the American Diabetes Association (ADA) Exchange System.

Chapter 66

Financial Help for Diabetes Care

How Costly Is Diabetes Management and Treatment?

Diabetes management and treatment is expensive. According to the American Diabetes Association (ADA), the average cost of healthcare for a person with diabetes is $13,741 a year—more than twice the cost of healthcare for a person without diabetes.

Many people who have diabetes need help paying for their care. For those who qualify, a variety of government and nongovernment programs can help cover healthcare expenses. This chapter is meant to help people with diabetes and their family members find and access such resources.

What Is Health Insurance?

Health insurance helps pay for medical care, including the cost of diabetes care. Health insurance options include the following:

- Private health insurance, which includes group and individual health insurance

This chapter includes text excerpted from "Financial Help for Diabetes Care," National Institute of Diabetes and Digestive and Kidney Diseases (NIDDK), May 2014. Reviewed September 2018.

473

- Government health insurance, such as Medicare, Medicaid, the Children's Health Insurance Program (CHIP), TRICARE, and veterans' healthcare programs

Starting in 2014, the Affordable Care Act (ACA) prevents insurers from denying coverage or charging higher premiums to people with preexisting conditions, such as diabetes. The ACA also requires most people to have health insurance or pay a fee. Some people may be exempt from this fee.

Does Medicare Cover Diabetes Services and Supplies?

Medicare helps pay for the diabetes services, supplies, and equipment listed below and for some preventive services for people who are at risk for diabetes. However, coinsurance or deductibles may apply. A person must have Medicare Part B or Medicare Part D to receive these covered services and supplies.

Medicare Part B helps pay for:

- diabetes screening tests for people at risk of developing diabetes

- diabetes self-management training

- diabetes supplies such as glucose monitors, test strips, and lancets

- insulin pumps and insulin if used with an insulin pump

- counseling to help people who are obese lose weight

- flu and pneumonia shots

- foot exams and treatment for people with diabetes

- eye exams to check for glaucoma and diabetic retinopathy

- medical nutrition therapy services for people with diabetes or kidney disease, when referred by a healthcare provider

- therapeutic shoes or inserts, in some cases

Medicare Part D helps pay for:

- diabetes medications

- insulin, excluding insulin used with an insulin pump

- diabetes supplies such as needles and syringes for injecting insulin

People who are in a Medicare advantage plan or other Medicare health plan should check their plan's membership materials and call for details about how the plan provides the diabetes services, supplies, and medications covered by Medicare.

What Other Federal Programs Can Help?

The following federal programs can provide more resources for people with diabetes:

- U.S. Department of Veterans Affairs (VA)
- TRICARE
- The Indian Health Service (IHS)
- The Hill-Burton Free and Reduced-Cost Health Care Program
- Bureau of Primary Health Care (BPHC)
- U.S. Social Security Administration (SSA)
- Social Security Disability Insurance (SSDI)
- Supplemental Security Income (SSI)
- Women, Infants, and Children (WIC)

The VA runs hospitals and clinics that serve veterans who have service-related health problems or who simply need financial aid.

TRICARE—the healthcare program serving uniformed service members, retirees, and their families worldwide—is available to people who are:

- active duty service members
- military retirees
- family members of an active duty service member or a military retiree
- members of the National Guard/Reserves on active duty for 30 days
- family members of someone who is in the National Guard/Reserves on active duty for 30 days

TRICARE for Life is a specific TRICARE plan that offers secondary coverage for people who have Medicare Part A and Part B.

The Indian Health Service may help members of federally recognized American Indian or Alaska Native tribes. American Indians or Alaska Natives may also be eligible for help from public, private, and state programs.

The Hill-Burton Free and Reduced-Cost Health Care Program can help people who are uninsured and need help with the cost of hospital care. Although the program originally provided hospitals with federal grants for modernization, today it provides free or reduced-fee medical services to people with low incomes. The U.S. Department of Health and Human Services (HHS) administers the program.

The Bureau of Primary Health Care (BPHC), a service of the Health Resources and Services Administration (HRSA), offers primary and preventive healthcare to medically underserved populations through community health centers. For people with no insurance, the Bureau bases fees for care on family size and income. To find local health centers, call 888-ASK-HRSA (888-275-4772) and ask for a directory, or visit findahealthcenter.hrsa.gov.

The Social Security Administration (SSA) can provide information about eligibility for Medicare. People can contact the agency at 800-772-1213, visit the agency website at www.socialsecurity.gov, or check with their local Social Security office to learn if they are eligible for Medicare.

The Social Security Administration also provides the following programs:

- SSDI is a federal insurance plan that pays a monthly amount to people who cannot work. People earn SSDI work credits when they pay Social Security taxes. A person must have enough credits based on age to qualify. Then, if an illness or injury prohibits a person from working for at least a year, SSDI payments may be an option.

- SSI is a federal safety net program that pays a monthly amount to disabled children and adults who earn little and have few assets. A person who gets SSI may be able to get food stamps and Medicaid, too.

Women, Infants, and Children (WIC) provides the following services to low-income pregnant, breastfeeding, and postpartum women, as well as infants and children up to age 5 who are at nutritional risk:

- Supplemental foods
- Healthcare referrals
- Nutrition education
- Breastfeeding information

The U.S. Department of Agriculture (USDA) administers the program. Applicants must meet residential, financial need, and nutrition risk criteria to be eligible for assistance. Having gestational diabetes is considered a medically-based nutrition risk and would qualify a woman for assistance through the WIC program if she meets the financial need requirements and has lived in a particular state the required amount of time. The WIC website provides a page of contact information for each state and for American Indian and Alaska Native tribes.

What Other State Programs Can Help?

The following state programs can provide more resources for people with diabetes:

- Medicare Savings Programs (MSPs)
- State Health Insurance Assistance Programs (SHIPs)
- State Pharmaceutical Assistance Programs (SPAPs)

Medicare Savings Programs (MSPs). Some states may pay Medicare premiums, deductibles, and coinsurance if a person has low income and few assets. A city or county department of social services can determine whether a person is eligible.

State Health Insurance Assistance Program (SHIP). SHIPs get money from the federal government to give free health insurance advice to those with Medicare. SHIP counselors can help people choose a Medicare health plan or a Medicare Prescription Drug Plan. A person can find a SHIP counselor at www.shiptalk.org. A person who needs more health insurance should talk with a SHIP counselor or a social worker.

State Pharmaceutical Assistance Program (SPAP). Several states have SPAPs that help certain people pay for prescription drugs. Each SPAP makes its own rules about how to provide drug coverage to its members.

How Can a Person Save Money on Diabetes Medications and Medical Supplies?

People should talk with their healthcare providers if they have problems paying for diabetes medications. Some people do not fill prescriptions or take less medication than what a provider prescribes in order to save money; however, healthcare providers advise against taking less than the prescribed amount of medication. Less expensive generic medications for diabetes, blood pressure, and cholesterol are available. If a healthcare provider prescribes medications that a person cannot afford, the person should ask the healthcare provider about cheaper alternatives.

Healthcare providers may also be able to assist people who need help paying for their medications and diabetes testing supplies, such as glucose test strips, by providing free samples or referring them to local programs. Drug companies that sell insulin or diabetes medications often have patient assistance programs. Each patient assistance program has its own eligibility criteria.

The websites below provide links to programs that can help patients determine if they qualify for the different types of assistance and find free or low-cost healthcare. People can also search these websites for needed diabetes testing supplies by using keywords such as "glucose test strips" or the names of specific diabetes medications.

- The Partnership for Prescription Assistance (PPA) website at www.PPARx.org lists more than 475 programs that help pay for medications. The drug companies that produce medications provide many of these programs. People can find programs and apply for help by calling 888-477-2669.

- NeedyMeds is a nonprofit group that helps people find programs that help pay for medications. The NeedyMeds website at www. NeedyMeds.org allows the user to search a list of programs by medication or manufacturer name. Some of the forms to apply are online.

- RxAssist has a website at www.rxassist.org that provides information about drug company programs, state programs, discount drug cards, copay help, and more.

- Rx Outreach is a nonprofit pharmacy that provides affordable medications to people in need. The Rx Outreach website at www. rxoutreach.org provides information about the medications offered and how to apply.

- The National Council on Aging (NCOA) provides benefit information for seniors with limited income and resources at www.benefitscheckup.org.

HRSA offers a free nylon filament—similar to a bristle on a hairbrush—to check feet for nerve damage.

Also, some programs for the homeless may be able to provide help. A person can contact a local homeless shelter for more information about how to obtain free medications and medical supplies. People can access the number or location of the nearest homeless shelter online or in the phone book under "Human Service Organizations" or "Social Service Organizations."

Where Can a Person Find Help Paying for Prosthetic Care?

People who have had an amputation may need assistance in paying their rehabilitation expenses and the cost of a prosthesis. The following organizations provide financial assistance or information about finding resources for people who need prosthetic care:

Amputee Coalition
900 East Hill Ave., Ste. 290
Knoxville, TN 37915
Toll-Free: 888-AMP-KNOW (888-267-5669)
TTY: 865-525-4512
Website: www.amputee-coalition.org

Limbs for Life Foundation
218 East Main St.
Oklahoma City, OK 73104
Toll-Free: 888-235-5462
Phone: 405-605-5462
Fax: 405-843-5123
Website: www.limbsforlife.org
E-mail: admin@limbsforlife.org

Where Can a Person Find Help Paying for Kidney Dialysis and Transplantation?

Kidney failure, also called end-stage renal disease, is a complication of diabetes. People of any age with kidney failure can get Medicare if they meet certain criteria.

What Is Assistive Technology and What Organizations Might Provide Assistance?

Assistive technology is any device that assists, adapts, or helps to rehabilitate someone with a disability so he or she may function more safely, effectively, and independently at home, at work, and in the community. Assistive technology may include:

- computers with features that make them accessible to people with disabilities

- adaptive equipment, such as wheelchairs

- bathroom modifications, such as grab bars or shower seats

The following organizations may be able to provide information, awareness, and training in the use of technology to assist people with disabilities:

Alliance for Technology Access (ATA)
1119 Old Humboldt Rd.
Jackson, TN 38305
Toll-Free: 800-914-3017
Phone: 731-554-5ATA (731-554-5282)
TTY: 731-554-5284
Fax: 731-554-5283
E-mail: atainfo@ataccess.org
Website: www.ataccess.org

United Cerebral Palsy (UCP)
1825 K St. N.W., Ste. 600
Washington, DC 20006
Phone: 800-872-5827 or 202-776-0406
Website: www.ucp.org/resources/assistive-technology

Chapter 67

Glossary of Terms Related to Diabetes

A1C: A test that measures a person's average blood glucose level over the past two to three months.

acanthosis nigricans: A skin condition characterized by darkened skin patches; common in those with insulin resistance.

albumin: The main protein in blood. People who are developing diabetic kidney disease leak small amounts of albumin into the urine. As the amount of albumin in the urine increases, the kidneys' ability to filter the blood decreases.

alpha-glucosidase inhibitor: A class of oral medicine for type 2 diabetes that slows down the digestion of foods high in carbohydrate. The result is a slower and lower rise in blood glucose after meals.

angiotensin-converting enzyme (ACE) inhibitor: An oral medicine that lowers blood pressure. It also helps slow down kidney damage in diabetics.

autoimmune disease: A disorder of the body's immune system in which the immune system mistakenly attacks and destroys body tissue that it believes to be foreign.

This glossary contains terms excerpted from documents produced by several sources deemed reliable.

autonomic neuropathy: A type of neuropathy affecting the lungs, heart, stomach, intestines, bladder, or genitals.

beta cell: A cell that makes insulin. Beta cells are located in the islets of the pancreas.

biguanide: A class of oral medicine used to treat type 2 diabetes that lowers blood glucose by reducing the amount of glucose produced by the liver. Also used to treat insulin resistance.

blood glucose: The main sugar found in the blood and the body's main source of energy. Also called blood sugar.

blood glucose level: The amount of glucose in a given amount of blood. In the United States, blood glucose levels are noted in milligrams per deciliter, or mg/dL.

blood glucose meter: A small, portable machine used by people with diabetes to check their blood glucose levels.

body mass index (BMI): A measure used to evaluate body weight relative to a person's height. BMI is used to find out if a person is underweight, normal weight, overweight, or obese.

calorie: A unit of energy in food. Carbohydrates, fats, protein, and alcohol in the foods and drinks we eat provide food energy or "calories."

carbohydrate: One of the three main nutrients in food. Foods that provide carbohydrate are starches, vegetables, fruits, dairy products, and sugars.

carbohydrate counting: A method of meal planning for people with diabetes based on counting the number of grams of carbohydrate in food.

cholesterol: Cholesterol is a fat-like substance that is made by your body and found naturally in animal foods such as dairy products, eggs, meat, poultry, and seafood.

diabetic ketoacidosis: An emergency condition in which extremely high blood glucose levels, along with a severe lack of insulin, result in the breakdown of body fat for energy and an accumulation of ketones in the blood and urine.

diabetic retinopathy: Damage to the small blood vessels in the retina. Loss of vision may result. Also called diabetic eye disease.

dialysis: The process of cleaning wastes from the blood artificially. The two major forms of dialysis are hemodialysis and peritoneal dialysis.

gastroparesis: A form of neuropathy that affects the stomach. Digestion of food may be incomplete or delayed, resulting in nausea, vomiting, or bloating, making blood glucose control difficult.

glaucoma: An increase in fluid pressure inside the eye that may lead to vision loss.

glucagon: A hormone produced by the alpha cells in the pancreas that raises blood glucose.

glucose: One of the simplest forms of sugar.

glucose gel: Pure glucose in gel form used for treating hypoglycemia.

glucose tablets: Chewable tablets made of pure glucose used for treating hypoglycemia.

healthy weight: Healthy weight status is often based on having a body mass index (BMI) that falls in the normal (or healthy) range. A healthy body weight may lower the chances of developing health problems such as type 2 diabetes and heart disease.

high-density lipoprotein (HDL): A compound made up of fat and protein that carries cholesterol in the blood to the liver, where it is broken down and excreted. Commonly called "good" cholesterol, high levels of HDL cholesterol are linked to a lower risk of heart disease.

hyperglycemia: Higher than normal blood glucose.

hypertension: A condition present when blood flows through the blood vessels with a force greater than normal. Also called high blood pressure.

hypoglycemia: Also called low blood glucose, a condition that occurs when one's blood glucose is lower than normal, usually below 70 mg/dL. If left untreated, hypoglycemia may lead to unconsciousness.

hypoglycemia unawareness: A state in which a person does not feel or recognize the symptoms of hypoglycemia.

impaired glucose tolerance (IGT): A condition in which blood glucose levels are higher than normal but are not high enough for a diagnosis of diabetes. IGT, also called Prediabetes, is a level of 140–199 mg/dL two hours after the start of an oral glucose tolerance test.

incidence: The number of new cases of a given disease during a given period in a specified population. It also is used for the rate at which new events occur in a defined population.

inhaled insulin: A type of insulin under development taken with a special device that enables the user to breathe in insulin through the mouth.

insulin: A hormone that helps the body use glucose for energy. The beta cells of the pancreas make insulin. When the body cannot make enough insulin, insulin is taken by injection or other means.

insulin pen: A device for injecting insulin that looks like a fountain pen and holds replaceable cartridges of insulin.

insulin pump: An insulin-delivering device about the size of a deck of cards that can be worn on a belt or kept in a pocket.

insulin resistance: The body's inability to respond to and use the insulin it produces.

islet transplantation: Moving the islets from a donor pancreas into a person whose pancreas has stopped producing insulin.

islets: Groups of cells located in the pancreas that make hormones that help the body break down and use food.

jet injector: A device that uses high pressure instead of a needle to propel insulin through the skin and into the body.

ketone: A chemical produced when there is a shortage of insulin in the blood and the body breaks down body fat for energy.

ketosis: A ketone buildup in the body that may lead to diabetic ketoacidosis.

lactic acidosis: A serious condition in which there is a buildup of lactic acid in the body.

lancet: A spring-loaded device used to prick the skin with a small needle to obtain a drop of blood for blood glucose monitoring.

lipoprotein: A compound made up of fat and protein that carries fats and fat-like substances, such as cholesterol, in the blood.

low-density lipoprotein (LDL): A compound made up of fat and protein that carries cholesterol in the blood from the liver to other parts of the body.

maturity-onset diabetes of the young (MODY): A monogenic form of diabetes that usually first occurs during adolescence or early adulthood.

metabolic syndrome: A grouping of health conditions associated with an increased risk for heart disease and type 2 diabetes.

metabolism: The process that occurs in the body to turn the food you eat into energy your body can use.

nephropathy: Disease of the kidneys.

neuropathy: Disease of the nervous system. The three major forms in people with diabetes are peripheral neuropathy, autonomic neuropathy, and mononeuropathy.

oral glucose tolerance test (OGTT): A test to diagnose prediabetes and diabetes, given after an overnight fast. Test results show how the body uses glucose over time.

pancreas: An organ that makes insulin and enzymes for digestion. The pancreas is located behind the lower part of the stomach and is about the size of a hand.

pancreas transplantation: A surgical procedure to take a healthy whole or partial pancreas from a donor and place it into a person with diabetes.

peripheral neuropathy: Nerve damage that affects the feet, legs, or hands. Peripheral neuropathy causes pain, numbness, or a tingling feeling.

physical activity: Any form of exercise or movement.

portion size: The amount of a food served or eaten in one occasion. A portion is not a standard amount. The amount of food it includes may vary by person and occasion.

prediabetes: A condition in which blood glucose levels are higher than normal but are not high enough for a diagnosis of diabetes.

rapid-acting insulin: A type of insulin with an onset of fifteen minutes, a peak at thirty to ninety minutes, and a duration of three to five hours.

saturated fat: This type of fat is solid at room temperature. Saturated fat is found in full-fat dairy products (like butter, cheese, cream, regular ice cream, and whole milk), coconut oil, lard, palm oil, ready-to-eat meats, and the skin and fat of chicken and turkey, among other foods.

sulfonylurea: A class of oral medicine for type 2 diabetes that lowers blood glucose by helping the pancreas make more insulin and by helping the body better use the insulin it makes.

triglycerides: A type of fat in your blood, triglycerides can contribute to the hardening and narrowing of your arteries if levels are too high.

type 1 diabetes: A condition characterized by high blood glucose levels caused by a total lack of insulin. Occurs when the body's immune system attacks the insulin-producing beta cells in the pancreas and destroys them.

type 2 diabetes: A condition characterized by high blood glucose levels caused by either a lack of insulin or the body's inability to use insulin efficiently.

Chapter 68

Directory of Diabetes-Related Resources

American Association of Clinical Endocrinologists (AACE)
245 Riverside Ave.
Ste. 200
Jacksonville, FL 32202
Phone: 904-353-7878
Fax: 904-353-8185
Website: www.aace.com

American Association of Diabetes Educators (AADE)
200 W. Madison St.
Ste. 800
Chicago, IL 60606
Toll-Free: 800-338-3633
Website: www.diabeteseducator.org

American Diabetes Association (ADA)
National Service Center (NSC)
2451 Crystal Dr.
Ste. 900
Arlington, VA 22202
Toll-Free: 800-DIABETES
(800-342-2383)
Website: www.diabetes.org

Diabetes Canada (DC)
1400-522 University Ave.
Toronto, ON M5G 2R5
Toll-Free: 800-BANTING
(800-226-8464)
Website: www.diabetes.ca
E-mail: info@diabetes.ca

Resources in this chapter were compiled from several sources deemed reliable; all contact information was verified and updated in September 2018.

Centers for Disease Control and Prevention (CDC)
1600 Clifton Rd.
Atlanta, GA 30329-4027
Toll-Free: 800-CDC-INFO
(800-232-4636)
Toll-Free TTY: 888-232-6348
Website: www.cdc.gov

Diabetes Action Research and Education Foundation
6701 Democracy Blvd.
Ste. 300
Bethesda, MD 20817
Phone: 202-333-4520
Fax: 202-558-5240
Website: www.diabetesaction.org
E-mail: info@diabetesaction.org

Diabetes Insipidus Foundation
Website: www.diabetesinsipidus.org

Diabetes Teaching Center
University of California, San Francisco (UCSF)
400 Parnassus Ave.
Fifth Fl.
San Francisco, CA 94143
Phone: 415-353-2266
Fax: 415-353-2392
Website: www.diabetes.ucsf.edu
E-mail: diabetesteachingcenter@ucsfmedctr.org

Johns Hopkins Diabetes Center
601 N. Caroline St.
Ste. 2008
Baltimore, MD 21287
Phone: 410-955-5000
TTY: 410-955-6217
Website: www.hopkinsmedicine.org/diabetes/directions

Joslin Diabetes Center
One Joslin Pl.
Boston, MA 02215
Phone: 617-309-2400
Website: www.joslin.org

National Center for Complementary and Integrative Health (NCCIH)
National Institutes of Health (NIH)
9000 Rockville Pike
Bethesda, MD 20892
Toll-Free: 888-644-6226
Toll-Free TTY: 866-464-3615
Toll-Free Fax: 866-464-3616
Website: nccih.nih.gov
E-mail: info@nccih.nih.gov

National Institute of Diabetes and Digestive and Kidney Diseases (NIDDK)
9000 Rockville Pike
Bethesda, MD 20892
Toll-Free: 800-860-8747
Toll-Free TTY: 866-569-1162
Website: www.niddk.nih.gov
E-mail: healthinfo@niddk.nih.gov

National Institute on Aging (NIA)
31 Center Dr. MSC 2292
Bldg. 31, Rm. 5C27
Bethesda, MD 20892
Toll-Free: 800-222-2225
Phone: 301-496-1752
Toll-Free TTY: 800-222-4225
Website: www.nia.nih.gov
E-mail: niaic@nia.nih.gov

Office of Minority Health Resource Center (OMHRC)
Toll-Free: 800-444-6472
Phone: 240-453-2882
Fax: 301-251-2160
Website: www.minorityhealth.
hhs.gov/omh/browse.
aspx?lvl=1&lvlid=3
E-mail: info@minorityhealth.
hhs.gov

Diabetes-Related Bone Diseases

National Institutes of Health (NIH) Osteoporosis and Related Bone Diseases~National Resource Center (NIH ORBD~NRC)
2 AMS Cir.
Bethesda, MD 20892-3676
Toll-Free: 800-624-BONE
(800-624-2663)
Phone: 202-223-0344
TTY: 202-466-4315
Fax: 202-293-2356
Website: www.bones.nih.gov
E-mail: NIHBoneInfo@mail.nih.
gov

Diabetic Eye Disease

American Academy of Ophthalmology (AAO)
655 Beach St.
San Francisco, CA 94109
Phone: 415-561-8500
Fax: 415-561-8533
Website: www.aao.org

EyeCare America
Toll-Free: 877-887-6327
Fax: 415-561-8567
Website: www.aao.org/
eyecare-america
E-mail: eyecareamerica@aao.org

National Eye Institute (NEI)
31 Center Dr. MSC 2510
Bethesda, MD 20892-2510
Phone: 301-496-5248
Website: www.nei.nih.gov
E-mail: 2020@nei.nih.gov

Prevent Blindness America (PBA)
211 W. Wacker Dr.
Ste. 1700
Chicago, IL 60606
Toll-Free: 800-331-2020
Website: www.preventblindness.
org
E-mail: info@preventblindness.
org

Diabetes-Related Foot Problems

National Institute of Arthritis and Musculoskeletal and Skin Diseases (NIAMS)
1 AMS Cir.
Bethesda, MD 20892-3675
Toll-Free: 877-22-NIAMS
(877-22-64267)
Phone: 301-495-4484
TTY: 301-565-2966
Fax: 301-718-6366
Website: www.niams.nih.gov
E-mail: NIAMSinfo@mail.nih.gov

Diabetes-Related Heart Disease

American Heart Association (AHA)
7272 Greenville Ave.
Dallas, TX 75231
Toll-Free: 800-242-8721
Website: www.americanheart.org

National Heart, Lung, and Blood Institute (NHLBI)
31 Center Dr.
Bldg. 31
Bethesda, MD 20892
Website: www.nhlbi.nih.gov

Diabetic Kidney Disease

American Association of Kidney Patients (AAKP)
14440 Bruce B. Downs Blvd.
Tampa, FL 33613
Toll-Free: 800-749-AAKP
(800-749-2257)
Fax: 813-636-8122
Website: www.aakp.org
E-mail: info@aakp.org

National Kidney Disease Education Program (NKDEP)
3 Kidney Information Way
Bethesda, MD 20892
Toll-Free: 866-4-KIDNEY
(866-454-3639)
Toll-Free TTY: 866-569-1162
Fax: 301-402-8182
Website: www.nkdep.nih.gov
E-mail: nkdep@info.niddk.nih.gov

National Kidney Foundation (NKF)
30 E. 33rd St.
New York, NY 10016
Toll-Free: 855-NKF-CARES
(855-653-2273)
Website: www.kidney.org
E-mail: nkfcares@kidney.org

Diabetes-Related Mouth Problems

National Institute of Dental and Craniofacial Research (NIDCR)
31 Center Dr. MSC 2190
Bldg. 31, Rm. 5B55
Bethesda, MD 20892-2190
Toll-Free: 866-232-4528
Phone: 301-496-4261
Fax: 301-496-9988
Website: www.nidcr.nih.gov/
about-us/advisory-committees/
orientation-handbook/contacts
E-mail: nidcrinfo@mail.nih.gov

Juvenile Diabetes

Barbara Davis Center for Childhood Diabetes (BDC)
1775 Aurora Ct.
Aurora, CO 80045
Phone: 303-724-6779
Fax: 303-724-6839
Website: www.ucdenver.
edu/academics/colleges/
medicalschool/centers/
BarbaraDavis/Pages/contact.
aspx

Children with Diabetes (CWD)
Website: www.
childrenwithdiabetes.com

Juvenile Diabetes Research Foundation International (JDRF)
26 Bdwy.
14th Fl.
New York, NY 10004
Toll-Free: 800-533-CURE
(800-533-2873)
Website: www.jdrf.org
E-mail: info@jdrf.org

Nemours Foundation
10140 Centurion Pkwy N.
Jacksonville, FL 32256
Phone: 904-697-4100
Website: www.nemours.org

University of Chicago Diabetes Research and Training Center (DRTC)
5801 S. Ellis
Chicago, IL 60637
Website: drtc.bsd.uchicago.edu

Vanderbilt Diabetes Research and Training Center (DRTC)
2215 Garland Ave.
802 Light Hall
Nashville, TN 37232-0165
Phone: 615-343-1065
Fax: 615-322-0308
Website: diabetescenters.org/
centers/vanderbilt-university

Index

Index

Page numbers followed by 'n' indicate a footnote. Page numbers in *italics* indicate a table or illustration.

LONGWOOD PUBLIC LIBRARY
800 Middle Country Road
Middle Island, NY 11953
(631) 924-6400
longwoodlibrary.org

LIBRARY HOURS

Monday-Friday	9:30 a.m. - 9:00 p.m.
Saturday	9:30 a.m. - 5:00 p.m.
Sunday (Sept-June)	1:00 p.m. - 5:00 p.m.